Lecture Notes in Computer Science   9498

Commenced Publication in 1973
Founding and Former Series Editors:
Gerhard Goos, Juris Hartmanis, and Jan van Leeuwen

More information about this series at http://www.springer.com/series/7409

Naveen Kumar · Vasudha Bhatnagar (Eds.)

Big Data Analytics

4th International Conference, BDA 2015
Hyderabad, India, December 15–18, 2015
Proceedings

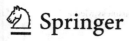 Springer

Editors
Naveen Kumar
Department of Computer Science
University of Delhi
Delhi
India

Vasudha Bhatnagar
Department of Computer Science
University of Delhi
Delhi
India

ISSN 0302-9743   ISSN 1611-3349 (electronic)
Lecture Notes in Computer Science
ISBN 978-3-319-27056-2   ISBN 978-3-319-27057-9 (eBook)
DOI 10.1007/978-3-319-27057-9

Library of Congress Control Number: 2015955359

LNCS Sublibrary: SL3 – Information Systems and Applications, incl. Internet/Web, and HCI

Printed on acid-free paper

Springer International Publishing AG Switzerland is part of Springer Science+Business Media
(www.springer.com)

Preface

Big data is no longer just a buzz word. It is a serious analytics area, requiring a rethinking of platforms, computing paradigms, and architectures. Big data analytics is now quintessential for a wide variety of traditional as well as modern applications, which has orchestrated intense research efforts in recent years.

This volume contains the papers presented at the 4th International Conference on Big Data Analytics (BDA 2015) held during December 15–18, 2015, in Hyderabad, India. The aim of the conference was to highlight recent advancements in the area while stimulating fresh research. There were 61 submissions in the research track. Each submission was reviewed by on average 2.5 Program Committee members. The committee decided to accept nine papers, which are included in this volume. The volume also includes nine invited papers. The volume is divided into four sections: *Security and Privacy, Commerce, Models and Algorithms, and Medicine.*

The section "Big Data: Security and Privacy" includes two papers. Barker describes the current state of the art and makes a call to open a dialog between the analytics and privacy communities. Agarwal et al. discuss online radicalization and civil unrest as two important applications of open source social media intelligence. The authors also discuss open research problems, important papers, publication venues, research results, and future directions.

The section "Big Data in Commerce" includes four papers. Singh discusses information exploration in e-commerce databases and identifies limitations in the query and result panel that deter exploratory search. Add-on extensions are proposed to address these limitations. Reddy proposes a framework to harvest the page views of the Web by forming clusters of similar websites. Anand et al. propose the utility-based fuzzy miner (UBFM) algorithm to efficiently mine a process model driven by a utility threshold. The utility can be measured in terms of profit, value, quantity, or other expressions of user's preference. The work incorporates statistical and semantic aspects while driving a process model. Bansal et al. integrate the notion of discount in state-of-the-art utility-mining algorithms and propose an algorithm for efficiently mining high-utility itemsets.

The section "Models and Algorithms" includes papers on a wide range of algorithms. Bhatnagar emphasizes that a completely new rethink of the solution from the perspective of the powers of the Map-Reduce paradigm can provide substantial gains. He presents an example of the design of a model-learning solution from high-volume monitoring data from a manufacturing environment. Toyoda addresses the requirement to increase the resilience and safety of transportation systems in view of the 2020 Olympic games in Tokyo, amidst predictions of big earthquakes. Based on large-scale smart card data from the Tokyo Metro subway system and vehicle recorder data, the author presents methods to estimate passenger flows, changes in the flows after accidents, and visualizes traffic with social media streams. Kiran and Kitsuregawa review issues involved in finding periodic patterns in the context of time series and transactional databases. They describe the basic model of finding periodic patterns, and its limitations, and suggest approaches to address them. Bhardwaj and Dash propose a novel density-based clustering algorithm for distributed environments using the MapReduce programming paradigm. Goel and Chaudhary present an incremental approach for mining formal concepts from a context that is assumed to be present in the form of object-attribute pairs. The approach utilizes the Apache Spark framework to discover and eliminate the redundant concepts in every iteration. Sachdev et al. present an implementation of the alpha-miner algorithm in MySQL and Cassandra using SQL and CQL with the aim of conducting a performance benchmarking and comparison of the alpha-miner algorithm on row-oriented and NoSQL column-oriented databases. Nagpal and Gaur propose a novel algorithm to filter out both irrelevant and redundant features from the data set using a greedy technique with gain ratio.

The last section, "Big Data in Medicine," addresses the applications of big data in the area of medicine. Talukder reviews the science and technology of big data translational genomics and precision medicine with respect to formal database systems. The paper presents two big-data platforms iOMICS (deployed at Google cloud) for translational genomics and DiscoverX (deployed at Amazon Web Services) for precision medicine. Adhil et al. present a clinical expert system (CES) that uses the clinical and genomic marker of the patient combined with a knowledge-base created from distributed, dissimilar, diverse big data. The system predicts the prognosis using a cancer registry compiled between 1997 and 2012 in the USA. Agarwal et al. present an integrative analytics approach for cancer genomics that takes the multiscale biological interactions as key considerations for model development. Sharma et al. propose a class-aware exemplar discovery algorithm, which assigns preference value to data points based on their ability to differentiate samples of one class from others. Goel et al. suggest a system for predicting the risk of cardiovascular disease based on electrocardiogram tests. The authors also discuss a recommendation system for suggesting nearby relevant hospitals based on the prediction.

In closing, we wish to thank the supporting institutes: NIT-Warangal, the University of Delhi, University of Aizu, and the Indian Institute of Technology Delhi. Thanks are also due to our sponsors: KDNuggets, NIT Warangal, Tata Consultancy Services, and Springer. We take this opportunity to thank Niladri Chatterjee (Student Symposium Chair), and Ramesh Agrawal (Tutorial Chair) for helping us in organizing the respective tracks. We gratefully acknowledge the Program Committee members and external reviewers for their time and diligent reviews. Thanks are due to Steering Committee members for their guidance and advisory role. The Organizing Committee and student volunteers of BDA 2015 deserve special mention for their support.

Last but not the least, we appreciate and acknowledge the EasyChair conference management system, which transformed the tedious task of managing submissions into an enjoyable one.

December 2015   Naveen Kumar
                                                                    Vasudha Bhatnagar

Organization

Steering Committee Chair

S.K. Gupta   IIT Delhi, India

Proceedings Chair

Subhash Bhalla   University of Aizu, Japan

General Chair

D.V.L.N. Somayajulu   NIT Warangal, India

Program Chairs

Naveen Kumar   University of Delhi, India
Vasudha Bhatnagar   University of Delhi, India

Tutorial Chair

R.K. Agrawal   JNU, New Delhi

Student Symposium Chair

Niladri Chatterjee   IIT Delhi, India

Organizing Chairs

P. Krishna Reddy   IIIT Hyderabad, India
R.B.V. Subramanyam   NIT Warangal, India

Finance Chairs

D.V.L.N. Somayajulu   NIT Warangal, India
Vikram Goyal   IIIT Delhi, India

Sponsorship Chair

T. Ramesh   NIT Warangal, India

Website Chair

R.B.V. Subramanyam   NIT Warangal, India

Publicity Chair

Vikram Goyal   IIIT Delhi, India

Steering Committee

Alexander Vazhenin   University of Aizu, Japan
D. Jankiram   IIT Madras, India
Jaijit Bhattacharyya   KPMG, India
Manish Gupta   Xerox Research Centre, India
Mukesh Mohania   IBM Research, India
N. Vijayaditya   Formerly at NIC, India
Nirmala Datla   HCL Technologies, India
R.K. Arora   Formerly at IIT Delhi, India
R.K. Datta   Formerly at IMD, India
S.K. Gupta (Chair)   IIT Delhi, India
Subhash Bhalla   University of Aizu, Japan
T. Srinivasa Rao   NIT Warangal, India

Program Committee

Muhammad Abulaish   Jamia Millia Islamia, India
Vijay Aggarwal   Jagan Institute of Management Studies, India
Ramesh Agrawal   Jawaharlal Nehru University, India
Avishek Anand   L3S Research Center, Germany
Rema Ananthanarayanan   IBM India Research Lab, New Delhi
Zeyar Aung   Masdar Institute of Science and Technology,
                             United Arab Emirates
Amitabha Bagchi   Indian Institute of Technology, Delhi, India
Amit Banerjee   South Asian University, New Delhi, India
Srikanta Bedathur   IBM India Research Lab, New Delhi, India
Subhash Bhalla   University of Aizu, Japan
Raj Bhatnagar   University of Cincinnati, USA
Vasudha Bhatnagar   University of Delhi, India
Arnab Bhattacharya   Indian Institute of Technology, Kanpur, India
Xin Cao   Queen's University Belfast, UK
Niladri Chatterjee   Indian Institute of Technology, Delhi, India
Debashish Dash   Institute of Genomics and Integrative Biology, India
Prasad Deshpande   IBM India Research Lab, India
Dejing Dou   University of Oregon, USA
Shady Elbassuoni   American University of Beirut, Lebanon

Anita Goel	Dyal Singh College, University of Delhi, India
Vikram Goyal	Indraprastha Institute of Information Technology, Delhi, India
Rajeev Gupta	IBM India Research Lab, New Delhi
S.C. Gupta	Indian Institute of Technology, Delhi, India
Renu Jain	CSJM University, India
Kalapriya Kannan	HP Research, India
Sharanjit Kaur	AND College, University of Delhi, India
Akhil Kumar	Penn State University, USA
Naveen Kumar	University of Delhi, India
Ulf Leser	Institut für Informatik, Humboldt-Universität zu Berlin, Germany
Aastha Madan	International Institute of Information Technology, Banglore, India
Ravi Madipadaga	Carl Zeiss
Sameep Mehta	IBM India Research Lab, Delhi, India
Yasuhiko Morimoto	Hiroshima University, Japan
Saikat Mukherjee	Siemens Medical Solutions, India
Mandar Mutalikdesai	Siemens Technology and Services Pvt. Ltd., India
S.K. Muttoo	University of Delhi, India
Ankur Narang	Data Science Mobileum Inc., India
Anjaneyulu Pasala	Infosys Limited, India
Dhaval Patel	IIT Roorkee, India
Nishith Pathak	Ninja Metrics, India
Lukas Pichl	International Christian University, Japan
Krishna Reddy Polepalli	IIIT, Hyderabad, India
Vikram Pudi	IIIT, Hyderabad, India
Mangsuli Purnaprajna	Honeywell Technology Solutions, India
Santhanagopalan R.	International Institute of Information Technology, Bangalore, India
Ramakrishnan Raman	Honeywell Technology Solutions, India
Maya Ramanath	Indian Institute of Technology, Delhi, India
Sreenivasan Sengamedu	Yahoo Labs, India
Mark Sifer	University of Wollongong, Australia
Alok Singh	University of Hyderabad, India
Manish Singh	Indian Institute of Technology, Hyderabad, India
Srinath Srinivasa	International Institute of Information Technology, Bangalore, India
Shamik Sural	Indian Institute of Technology, Kharagpur, India
Ashish Sureka	Software Analytics Research Lab, India
Asoke Talukedar	InterpretOmics, Bangalore, India
Durga Toshniwal	Indian Institute of Technology, Roorkee, India
Chenthamarakshan Vijil	IBM India Research Lab, India

Additional Reviewers

de Silva, N.H.N.D.
Gupta, Anamika
Gupta, Shikha
Kafle, Sabin

Kundu, Sonia
Puri, Charu
Saxena, Rakhi

Contents

Big Data in Medicine

Big Data: Security and Privacy

Privacy Protection or Data Value: Can We Have Both?

Ken Barker[(✉)]

University of Calgary, Calgary, AB, Canada
kbarker@ucalgary.ca

Abstract. Efforts to derive maximum value from data have led to an expectation that this is "just the cost of living in the modern world." Ultimately this form of data exploitation will not be sustainable either due to customer dissatisfaction or government intervention to ensure private information is treated with the same level of protection that we currently find in paper-based systems. Legal, technical, and moral boundaries need to be placed on how personal information is used and how it can be combined to create inferences that are often highly accurate but not guaranteed to be correct. Agrawal's initial call-to-arms in 2002 has generated a large volume of work but the analytics and privacy communities are not truly communicating with the goal of providing high utility from the data collected but in such a way that it does not violate the intended purpose for which it was initially collected [2]. This paper describes the current state of the art and makes a call to open a true dialog between these two communities. Ultimately, this may be the only way current analytics will be allowed to continue without severe government intervention and/or without severe actions on behalf of the people from whom the data is being collected and analyzed by either refusing to work with exploitative corporations or litigation to address the harms arising from the current practices.

1 Introduction

Users provide information about themselves to either receive a value of some kind or because they are compelled to do so for legal or moral reasons. For example, a patient needing health care due to an illness or injury must disclose to their physician personal information that is considered in almost all cultures to be highly private so they can receive the health care they need. The reason the information is being disclosed is to receive the medical care they need to maintain or regain their health. There is an expectation, and indeed a high ethical standard (Hippocratic Oath: Article 8) that compels this information be kept private and not used for any other purpose.[1] This example is often cited in the literature

---

[1] There are societally and individually acceptable deviations from this high standard such as informing an insurance company about the costs of the service so the physician can be paid. However, this is done with the explicit informed consent of the patient and there is an expectation that this information will be kept private and will not be used for any other purpose.

© Springer International Publishing Switzerland 2015
N. Kumar and V. Bhatnagar (Eds.): BDA 2015, LNCS 9498, pp. 3–20, 2015.
DOI: 10.1007/978-3-319-27057-9_1

to motivate the need for privacy and the expectations implied here are often applied to other interactions that occur. However, there are interactions that occur where there is no expectation of privacy or that a "private" communication will be kept confidential. For example, a person interviewed by a press reporter does not have the same expectation that the communication will be protected. In fact, the exact opposite is the expectation and both parties entering into such a communication understand that the reason for the conversation is to capture the discussion with the purpose of writing a very public story. Analytic advocates argue that data collection is often done with both parties understanding that the information collected will be used for many forms of analysis well beyond its apparent initial purpose. For example, search query data submitted to a search engine is not considered "private" by the search engine provider and in many cases, the collection of such data is the basis of their business model. However, police investigations now regularly include searches of suspects browser search histories for evidence that might link the suspect to the crime. It is a fairly obvious claim that this was not the intention of the suspect and as a result will likely feel privacy is being violated.

A commonly held myth is that privacy cannot be protected; that people no longer care about their privacy because any interactions in the modern world, by definition, requires that we forfeit our privacy; and that we should simply accept it and live without concern about it only because we gave up our right to privacy a long time ago. Clearly this myth is easily revealed as "false" by virtue of the large number of things each individual does in their daily lives to protect their privacy. Very few people would consider cameras in the bathroom a reasonable privacy of violation even if there might be substantial public good that might accrue from such cameras. The ubiquity of public survivance cameras does not imply the public accepts being monitored everywhere so there are societal limits that restrict the extent to which cameras can be used. Why should there these limits not also be placed on other forms of survivance?

Analytics, is effectively survivance. Click stream data describes how a user interacts on a website and some would argue it reveals their intent. Mining of such data allows an analyst to predict a particular users interests and to tailor the way information is presented to the user. This tailoring, it is argued, is a "user value" because it allows the webpage to provides "opportunities of *specific* interest" to the user. The argument continues that this is a "win-win-win" because the webpage vendor can provide a marketing opportunity to third-parties by promising to deliver advertising content to users with the maximum likelihood of purchasing their products. This, in effect, creates a "third" winner and this the third-party product provider who is able to more effectively sell their product or service.

Unfortunately there are serious issues associated with this particular three way "win". First, even if we accept that analytics for the purpose of "adding value to the customer's experience" is an acceptable tradeoff, the data collected may be used in any number of unanticipated ways. A person who is interested in understanding how a disease impacts a friend could be denied insurance coverage if there was a large number of searches undertaken about a particular disease, even if the person does not have such a disease. A teenage person searching for information about date rape drugs so they can better understand how a friend may have been subjected to such a criminal act may be brought under suspicion as a result of the police investigation into who might have committed the crime.

Second, the analytics will combine data in ways that will produce inferences that are inaccurate. Data mining will fail to produce useful inferences if accuracy is considered sacrosanct. The *accuracy paradox* [9] demonstrate that accuracy can even improve when known errors are introduced into the system. This has led researchers to develop terms and definitions that are more appropriate for analytical work such as *precision* and *recall* when evaluating the effectiveness of their algorithms. This is not problematic when data is considered in aggregate but introduces significant issues if the analytics purports to identify instances that may introduce inaccurate descriptions of individuals. The primary goal of classification systems is to place individuals within each class so they can be considered largely homogeneous. When an instance is misclassified the potential harm is substantial and it is unlikely that anyone would agree to a privacy policy statement that explicitly allowed for such errors.

Third, the analytics will lead to unintended consequences. The famous case of Target™ identifying a pregnant teenager and "helpfully" providing product information is often touted as how precise and successful data analytics is [5]. However, it does not address the harm that comes from such "helpful" marketing campaigns. Although the father in this particular situation was quite polite in his response when he says, "[I]t turns out there's been some activities in my house I haven't been complete aware of," is exceptionally muted, it is clear that not all parents would react quite so calmly. If the father's trust in such analytics was so great that he assumed Target™'s analysis was indeed correct but that daughter had chosen to seek an abortion without her parent's consent, the consequences could have been even more significant. Target argues that this is providing value for their customer and admits that the goal is to capture a high value market segment but acknowledges that not everyone receives such "helpful" information in the same way [5] so they have taken steps to disguise how specific this one-to-one marketing is for individuals.[2]

2   Big Data

Big Data is a term that has been used since the inception of modern computer systems and in particular since the development of database management systems (DBMS). Unfortunately, it is a term that can only be defined relative to something and even when care is taken in its definition, gaps readily form that lead to disagreements. Absolute size does not work as demonstrated by the date of the inaugural *Very Large Data Base* conference that occurred in 1975 to

---

[2] One-to-One marketing "... means being willing and able to change your behaviour toward an individual customer based on what the customer tells you and what else you know about that customer." [8].

help deal with "large" databases which would be consider miniscule by today's systems. Gudiveda *et al.* [6] define big data as "data too large and complex to capture, process and analyze using current computing infrastructure" and then point to the popular characterization using five "V"s, which may not be applicable in all big data environments. The "V"s are:

- Volume - currently defined as terabytes (2^{40}) or even as large as exabytes (2^{60}).
- Velocity - data is produced at extremely high rates so streaming processes are required to help limit the volume.
- Variety - often data captures are very heterogeneous and may include structured, unstructured or semi-structured elements.
- Veracity - provenance is often crucial in determining if the source is valid, trustworthy, and of high quality.
- Value - the data should be of value either in itself or via subsequent analytics.

Each of these characteristics has a different impact on how big data is managed but since our focus here is on privacy, we consider briefly how each impacts on analytics and the nature of the data that is privacy sensitive. Volume, in and of itself, is not necessarily a privacy sensitive characteristic. For example, large volumes of radio telescope data does not contain data that is private. The challenges here are found in stream processing through sparse data which is not relevant to this paper. The amount of data collected is largely orthogonal to privacy issues but as the volume increases relative to the available compute power, there is a risk that privacy (or for that matter security) considerations will be displaced by the need for efficiency. Thus, volume introduces a risk but is not in itself a privacy threat.

Similarly the velocity with which data is received is not inherently problematic for privacy. The challenge becomes one of ensuring that any privacy requirements for the quickly arriving data is managed in a timely way. Much like volume, the strong temptation would be to sacrifice proper meta-data management (including privacy annotations) in the interest of simply collecting the data. Later we argue that data must be appropriately annotated with privacy provenance and if the collection mechanisms are too slow, this critical foundational step could be compromised.

A key aspect of big data is variety. The analytics that can be undertaken when large volumes of heterogeneous data is collected provides both an opportunities for tremendous insight and to invade privacy. Research into how to integrate and validate heterogeneous data sources has been underway for at least three decades. The new issues introduced by privacy meta-data that will likely be in conflict because they come from different sources, in different formats, will provide a rich set of research opportunities.

One of the critical features of any big data project is ensuring the veracity of the data collected. This will be critical in privacy as one of the key privacy obligations is to ensure that data collected can be checked for correctness. In addition, any data found to be incorrect must be deleted and possibly replaced with correct values. Thus, the veracity characteristic will be challenging because the data must be validated upon collection, maintained correctly throughout its lifecyle and deleted (really deleted) at the end of its life [7].

Data analytics is fundamentally motivated by the desire to derive value from data. In privacy research, this is often expressed as the privacy-utility tradeoff. Privacy is trivially guaranteed by not providing any access to the data collected, but this sacrifices all utility. Conversely, utility is maximized by eliminating any data access but this provides no data privacy at all. Thus, the definition of "value" in big data needs to be tempered by the responsibility to facilitate appropriate privacy for the data provider.

3 Privacy

Data ownership is likely a central issue in how people think about data privacy. If you, as an individual, believe that information about yourself is ultimately your "property" and should be controlled and disseminated by you, your perspective about privacy will likely hold that the individual owns that data and should have the right to determine how, or even if, it is used by others. If you, possibly thinking as a corporation, believe that information about those with whom you interact belongs to the corporation, then you will view the artifacts arising from interactions with individuals as your property. Some would argue that these artifacts are "shared" property so both parties have the right to claim ownership but this position is difficult to realize pragmatically when considering privacy. In other words, once a piece of private data is released, it cannot be easily retracted and protected from further disclosure.[3] This suggests that there are at least three distinct schools of thought when it comes to data ownership and we consider each below.

3.1 Individuals Own Data About Themselves

Medical data, religious beliefs, sexual orientation and political viewpoints are often considered private by individuals and most jurisdictions have laws that prevent, for example, an employer asking questions about these beliefs or view-points. However, if a person seeks treatment for a particular disease, they must reveal detailed medical histories to ensure their physician will treat them appropriately. This highly personal data is often believed to be owned by the patient and they have the right to control how it is used and to who it might be disseminated. However, hospitals collect this data and often in the interest of the greater good argue that this data, appropriately anonymized, should be used for medical research. The Hippocratic Oath (Article 8) requires that this not be done without explicit permission so patients are often asked to sign documents

---

[3] This is often the argument made by those who believe that "nothing is private" any longer and we should just accept this as a reality. However, the argument is self-evidently specious since the argument's proponents are often quite protective of some aspects of themselves as discussed earlier.

that allow their data to be used for this purpose.[4] Thus, the hospital is acknowledging that ownership of the data resides with the patient and the research to be done is with explicit permission from the patient (i.e. data owner).

3.2   Corporations Own Data Collected

Users interact with websites for many reasons but their primary purpose is the acquisition of some knowledge or service. The way users interact is often a high value commodity that the corporation can use for analytics for its own operation or to resell this behavioural information to other interested parties. For example, a search engine may collect the queries posed by users to help identify what is trending or of interest to its user community. The value may be substantial for organizations that want to communicate with the public about things that may be of interest. A political party that makes a policy statement would likely want to see if their announcement is generating interest and if it is being received favourably. This kind of data is often considered the property of the website and as such can be used to derive benefits for themselves. The corporation will attempt to protect the individual users by anonymizing the data through aggregation or using some other technique but it strongly believes this data is owned by them and it is likely that most people would agree with their claim.

An online shopping site will also collect similar search queries and use it in the same way as a search engine. However, the shopping site may have an opportunity to collect additional data in the event that a user makes a purchase. The user must enter data relevant to the purchase itself including name, address, contact information, credit card information and other details directly applicable the purchase. The shopping site will use this information in the first instance for the purpose of selling and delivering the purchased product but is now able to link very specific identifying information to the individual doing the search. Often these website will also install, often with permission, an artifact on the users computer so future trips to the site will also be readily tracked. The shopping site would claim that this data is owned by them. Few people would likely agree that information such as name, address, and credit card data is now "owned" by the website but this is the current state of the art and there is not typically a need for the company to delete the information after its initial intended use.

3.3   Shared Ownership of Data

One sharing mechanism suggested is that the data remains the property of the data owner but because they have willing shared it with the corporation, they

---

[4] It is unclear if this permission is collected in a completely non-coercive way. A patient might feel that by failing to sign such a document they may not receive the best possible care. Clearly this would not be the case but the perception may be a critical factor in providing such permission and this would likely be considered coercive in some way by a reasonable person. However, and much more likely, the patient is simply overwhelmed with the amount of documents required as they seek treatment so they may simply sign the documents presented to them with due consideration as they seek care.

have become co-owners of this data. The argument is initially compelling because the corporation should have the right to know who their customers are and the user clearly does not want to pass exclusive ownership of their data to anyone else. To understand the implications it is important to note that the purpose the user provided the information was to complete a sale. If the corporation fully agreed with this as the sole purpose for the collection of the data, it would willingly delete the data once the sale was complete and not claim any ownership. Unfortunately, the value of the interaction is not just in the sale but also in the information derived from the consumers behaviour during the purchasing process and afterward as related items can be suggested to that individual in a highly targeted way.

Perhaps there is another way to "share" the ownership of this data without violating the purpose for which it was provided. Some aspects of the interaction could reasonably be seen as the property of the corporation in the same way the search engine from Sect. 3.2 owned the search data. Clearly this would have to be unlinked from the more specific information that was collected for the sale itself but if this is done the corporation would have a strong claim to owning the data collected. Conversely, the demographic information would be deleted (or at least fully unlinked from the search data) so the ownership of the search data could be held by the corporation. This would address the ownership issue because each party would retain the portion of the data that is uniquely theirs.

3.4   Summary – Ownership

The issue of ownership is ultimately an extremely divisive one and may need to be considered in light of the specific situation. However, the general principles that seem to apply are:

Personal Data, of any kind, remains the property of the original owner and cannot be transferred to another without explicit, easily understood, informed consent.

Behavioural Data, such as click streams and search queries, are owned by the corporation but must not be linked to the individual either explicitly (as in Sect. 3.2) or through analysis.

Our earlier work has argued that ownership is not the key issue but rather who should have control over an individual's private data, for what purpose, and who should have access to it. This immediately lead to the question of how this control can be enforced in an environment where organizations have a vested interest in maximizing the value of any data they are able to collect. "[F]or knowledge itself is a power"[5] [3] is only true if that knowledge can be used. This raises the question of what principles should be applied when determining how the data is to be used.

---

[5] This quote is often paraphrased as "knowledge is power" but Sir Francis Bacon is actually speaking of the limits of God and that "knowledge" is in fact only a part of God's power. It also suggests that it must be weighed against other aspects of power including, in this case, Godly judgement.

4   Privacy Principles

Building on the core principles of U.S. Privacy Act (1974) [1], which articulated six principles that (1) ensured an individual can determine what data is collected; (2) guarantees that data collected is only used for the purpose for which it is collect; (3) provides access to your own data; (4) and information is current, (5) correct and (6) only used for legal purposes, the OECD developed a list of eight principles including: limited collection, data quality assurance, purpose specification, limited use, security safeguards, openness, individual participation and accountability to guide all agents follow best practices [4]. Agrawal *et al.* [2] collected these into a set of ten principles in their development of the seminal work on Hippocratic databases. The ten principles mirror those indicated by the governmental definitions but are described so they can be operationalized as design principles for a privacy-aware database. The principles are: (1) a requirement to specify the purpose; (2) acquiring explicit consent; (3) limiting collection to only required data; (4) limiting use to only that specified; (5) limiting disclosure of data as much as possible; (6) retention of the data is limited and defined; (7) the data is accurate; (8) security safeguards are assured; (9) the data is open to the provider; and (10) the provider can verify compliance to these principles.

Although there have been serious challenges to the appropriateness of each of these principles, privacy proponent generally support them and argue that if they were implemented in full in modern systems, privacy protection would be well supported. If we assume that these principles are necessary and sufficient to provide privacy protection then the key question is: Who should be ultimately in control of ensuring that private data (or private data derived from inference tools) is protected? We will consider both extremes of a continuum before considering possible middle ground between them.

At the one extreme, data about an individual should be fully under the control of the principle. In other words, information about me and its use should only be permitted in complete conformance with my *preferences*.[6] This would require that privacy meta-data be tightly linked to all data so anyone that has access to the data can determine precisely how or if the data can be used for the proposed purpose. Systems would have to be built that could operate based on the privacy meta-data and only use it if the principle specifically allowed for its use for a particular purpose. If the meta-data does not explicit allow for its use for a purpose, the system would have to ignore the data's value as a normal part of its operations.

At the other extreme, any data collected by an organization must be protected by the organization. In some ways, this is implied by the other end point but there is an important difference. Organizations often consider anonymization as sufficient protection of individual data privacy. In other words, the organization, once it acquires a data item, even if private and containing personally identifiable information, can use it as a normal part of their analytical

---

[6] *Preferences* are used here when discussing the desires of an individual with respect to data about them.

operations as long as it is not possible to link the data back to the individual. The organization should, though very few do, then guarantee that any information derived from this analysis is not used for any purpose other than that specified by the individual. Even if we accepted that an organization might promise to behave in accordance with this very high standard, the temptation to derive increased value from the linkage would be difficult to ignore. Furthermore, the success of data anonymization is highly questionable. For example, *k-anonymity* was almost immediately usurped by *l-diversity*, which was quickly shown to be fragile with the advent of *t-closeness*. This anonymity arm's race has continued unabated since the first papers appeared in the area and with each incremental refinement the amount of utility derivable from the data is reduced. The literature continues to blossom with yet another anonymization technique that almost always begins by showing how its predecessor fails. *Differential privacy*, originally intended for use in a statistical database, argues that in a sufficiently large repository, the addition of an individual's record is protected provided a key parameter holds. Differential privacy works as described provided the parameters are respected and the repository is sufficiently large. Ideally the systems works in a *non-interactive* environment with a trusted curator to compute and publish the statistics. In the *interactive* environment, source data must be retained in the repository, to allow for responses to queries that are not immediately captured by the "statistics" calculated *a priori*. The trusted curator must also remain as a part of the system for the lifetime of the database. However, Dwork argues that both are equivalent although the latter requires ongoing monitoring.

Anonymity could be guaranteed if corporations were willing to follow the OECD's principles and users fully understood the implications of their privacy choices, it would be possible to have users opt out of participation in any corporate processes that could lead to their data being exposed. There are two key issues that prevent this from occurring. First, and probably the most challenging is the business model of the Internet. The highest principle, since its inception, appears to be that the user should not have to pay for it. Unfortunately, users do pay for it, if not with money, then with their privacy and possibly with their security. This philosophy of "free services" and "increased value delivery" is now prevalent in all aspects of our daily activities including loyalty cards that require we give up much demographic information for what is ultimately a fairly small reward. Unfortunately this first issue may not be resolved until users see sufficient harm in the behaviour to compel corporations to behave differently. The tradeoff will be that services that we now expect for "free" will likely require some other form of remuneration.

The second issue may well be more tractable and must be put in place before governments can move to legislate appropriate corporate behaviour. Currently, we do not have the systems necessary to support the OECD's principles in a way that allows a company to provide a requested service and capture the users' preferences about how their personal data should be handled after the service is delivered. For example, the easy solution to protecting privacy would suggest that after the transaction was completed, any related data should be deleted immediately.[7] Corporations currently try to keep every data item collected for an undetermined period of time because of its high residual value.[8] The reasons for this are a mix of partial truths and current computing system's inability to provide sufficient information about how an individual wants their data treated. Once data is curated (either from a public or private database, from a customer transaction, or from inferencing multiple data points) there is no way to explicitly link each data item back to the customer's privacy preferences. The reason is that those preferences are not collected and even if they are, once the data has been "mined" (possibly legitimately), the privacy preferences are lost. However, this is ultimately a technical as opposed to a human behavioural challenge so techniques can be developed to provide user privacy if we want to do so.

5   A Call for a New Approach

Where do we go from here? Scott McNealy argues "you have zero privacy anyway ... get over it" and this rather self-serving statement reflects what some believe to be an intractable problem in the modern era. Some even take it further to say that we do not care about our privacy any longer because we live in such an omnipresent surveillance society. However, the statement is patently wrong. A few examples are sufficient to demonstrate the point. Very few of us would argue that peeping into a window to take photographs of us in the bathroom should be considered appropriate or acceptable. We strongly support the home, or facilities such as bathrooms, as very private places and few people live in glass houses where the exterior walls are also transparent to the world. Some might argue that this is not the same thing but consider the second example.

Probably the group that "lives online" more than any other is teenage girls. The argument often put forward, even after much training about dangers online, is that this group still insist on putting information about themselves readily on social networks. Unfortunately this misses the point. Teenage girls do not consider the kind of information they are putting online as particularly private (the potential dangers notwithstanding) so a generalization has been made that they simply do not care about their privacy. Clearly the first example would be appropriate here, as teenage girls would consider a bathroom to be an extremely private space, but the argument is made strongly if a parent looks at the young girl's cell phone. This is considered by that group to be a highly sensitive form of private communication as text messages to friends (and other data kept on the phone)

---

[7] We set aside legal issues associated with maintaining records of sales transaction to meet requirements such as tax regulations or service agreements. It would be easy to argue that this falls within the scope of the user's purpose anyway but we are instead concerned with the "permanent" storage of this data for unspecified or other purposes that are common practice today.

[8] Many claim that credit card information is not maintained without specific permission but recent leaks have included credit card information in addition to all information required to identify an individual.

makes this a much more personal item than the diary that may have been kept by an older generation. Any parent that invades this private space of a young person is likely to find that they have breached a trust and invaded privacy not unlike the bathroom example. Similar examples could be drawn for everyone. There are things about us and about what we do or in what we are interested that simply do not belong in the public domain. Thus, we do not get away from this issue because "we cannot do anything about it" or "we do not care about it."

We need to develop systems that simply do not allow our data (or data about us)[9] to be used without our prior approval and consent. For the sake of brevity, the core aspect is we must tie together the data we provide with the privacy preferences we have about how it can be used. The data should not be used without this associated provenance. In short, any data item d_i must be linked to the providers privacy preferences p_i in an uncouplable way $< d_i, p_i >$. This privacy tuple will be the basis that provides the privacy protection necessary to enforce preferences. Although, at the highest level, this sounds simple, it will ultimately require a change in how we treat, manage, move, use and ensure compliance for data access. The approach will provide demonstrable conformance to the privacy policies and agreements that are in place, and will ultimately meet the demanding requirements of the OECD's principles.

We can now turn to the obligations that will be necessary to realize this vision and this will act as a call-to-arms on delivering a privacy conscious data management process. Although many different players will be involved in ensuring any privacy protection system is operational and the commitments made are honoured, we will focus on only a few initial pieces. The reader will likely think of many more but will also find that the modest list provided here represents many years of interesting research and implementation.

5.1 User and Corporate Obligations

Users clearly need to engage more meaningful in protecting their own privacy. This is not a case of "blame the victim" but rather a call to support users in making appropriate decisions about when, how and to whom data about themselves is being released. The current approach of informed consent by a protracted and often barely comprehensible legal agreement, presented just as the user is about to access a system or install a piece of software, is at best disingenuous. Most users are known to not read these documents and it is unlikely anyone could identify a person who reads all such agreements before ticking the appropriate box and gaining access. Excellent work has been done for many years to make our systems user friendly and accessible. The same effort needs to be undertaken so users have equally friendly, accessible and understandable presentations of a system's privacy policies and implications. This goes beyond the initial presentation of a legal agreement to allow access but to the continuous monitoring of user

---

[9] A much harder problem that we can turn to later.

interactions with the system so the users are continuously informed about the impact of their decisions on their privacy. Several groups are working on usable privacy and there is some interesting work beginning to emerge but this work has not yet been picked up in sufficient numbers by the corporate community. This will ultimately be a strategic advantage for corporations who are able to meaningfully protect and inform their clients.

Corporations ultimately need to commit to only using data they collect for its intended purpose.[10] This will require that systems be built capable of capturing the privacy agreements in place and that corporations be able to demonstrate that any data in its control is conformant with those commitments.

5.2 System Obligations

Systems must be developed that capture $< d_i, p_i >$ and bind them in such a way that data is only accessible when explicit permission is given and access is provided for the intended and agreed to purpose. We refer to this agreement as the *privacy commitment* and use this term when referring to the organizations commitment to the user (data provider) and the user's agreement that they understand the agreement. To develop systems that allow data to be bound to privacy commitments will ultimately involve many aspects of the data management system. The balance of this paper will describe some of the key elements that must work together to satisfy privacy commitments and ensure that both parties (the organization and the data providers) function appropriately and in an auditable way.

Database management systems receive queries from users/applications and seek to optimize the database's organization to maximize throughput. At the highest level, this is done through a user interface, a query processor, a transaction manager, and a file system that collectively optimizes queries, ensures consistency, and returns only correct/verifiable results. Ultimately all of these components may need to be privacy-aware to provide an end-to-end solution that addresses all principles required by OECD. However, we will focus on two key elements. First, the acquisition of any data requires that privacy commitments are included and stored in the system (Sect. 5.3). Secondly, the query processor must inspect those privacy commitments to ensure that the data accesses are legitimate (Sect. 5.4).

The final preliminary element is how privacy might be compromised? This is often called the *attack model* and can be quite complex if all possible attacks are to be considered. For our purposes, we use a simple attack model where the data analyst, wishing to maximize data value, seeks to pose queries that are as

---

[10] The intended purpose is not defined by the company's desire to acquire as much information as possible and leverage it for maximum utility. Intended purpose is defined by an agreement between a well-informed user and the clearly stated intentions of the corporation. If the corporation desires to change their intention, this is done by returning to the user to get an updated agreement.

complete as possible.[11] This means that the analyst wants to have included all data items in the database and seeks to pose queries that will include all relevant data. The attack could be an attempt to identify a particular value such as a user's private information (e.g. salary). Alternatively the attack could be of the form of an aggregation query where the goal is to include all data elements in the calculation of the aggregation.

5.3   Data Acquisition Process

Data acquisition should include the capture of any information necessary to enforce *privacy commitments*. Privacy commitments are defined by negotiation between the data provider (user) and the data collector (organization).[12] The results of these negotiations are captured in a set of *privacy policies* that collectively define the privacy commitments. The negotiations process is most easily seen as an *a priori* process whereby each user provides their privacy *preferences* to the collector, which provides for the provider a statement of their privacy *practices*. Traditionally this has been a largely unidirectional conversation in that the organization has, through a privacy statement, indicated their practices and the users has either accepted it (and gained access) or declined (and been refused access). This approach has worked to the corporations advantage in the past but for the reasons described earlier will ultimately not be a sustainable model.

The question becomes: How can negotiations be undertaken with multiple users so they provide the maximum amount of access for the corporation while having their privacy interests protected? There are no current complete solutions to this problem. However, several elements must be brought together to realize one:

- Clear interfaces must be provides so users understand privacy choices and their impacts. Users should be able to easily set their preferences in light of the organizations practices and understand what benefits they derive from the choices they make and the risks they accept as a result.
- Organizational practices must be constructed to be "negotiable" in a clear and transparent way. The current all-or-nothing approach is unacceptable and does not allow for individual sensitivities nor for individual flexibility within their own choices.
- Users must be able to audit how their data is accessed. A clear privacy requirement is that of transparency and that can only occur with access that is reasonable, timely, and accurate.

---

[11] The "attack" here is a bit of a misnomer in that the analyst is probably only doing their job and not intending to attack or unethically compromise the users privacy. However, from the user's perspective, if they have not consented to participating in a particular kind of analysis, they will see the analyst job as an attack on their privacy.

[12] In the following we will use the terms "provider" and "collector" to represent more abstractly the concept of a user and organization, respectively.

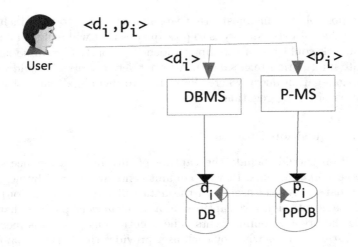

Fig. 1. Data acquisition requirements

– Users must be able to alter or withdraw their permission to access the data provided. This does not mean past access would be considered invalid but that future access is made in light of the changes made by the user. This also implies that the temporal aspects of privacy be included as a key part of the privacy commitments.

The reader will likely be able to identify many other open questions related to data acquisition and the user interface issues that must be in place to facilitate privacy commitments.

Although the interface challenge will be substantial, the output from the process should be a privacy policy that is linked to every collected data item. Figure 1 illustrates that any data item (d_i) acquired from the users is collected with its corresponding privacy policy (p_i) information. The data item itself will be stored in the database (DB) and the privacy information in the privacy-policy database (PPDB). Thus, both elements are retained in the system and used when queries are executed against the provided data. Figure 1 suggests that d_i is separated from p_i so the data can be managed using a traditional non-privacy-aware DBMS, while the privacy policy elements are maintained in a separate *privacy management system (P-MS)*. This architectural model depicts a compromise in that existing (or legacy) DBMSs will likely exist into the foreseeable future so managing privacy is likely to require a separate but tightly linked subsystem that only allows access when the privacy commitment can be honoured. Future, more secure, privacy-ware data management systems could more tightly link d_i with p_i so access is only possible to the data if the commitments are honoured. Unfortunately, current legacy systems would allow access to the DB without forcing privacy checking of the data with the PPDB. However, we do not consider this "super user" form of attack because we assume that the database administrator (DBA) is trustworthy. Recall that our attacker is an analyst who would not be given direct access to the DBMS because they are simply a system user.

5.4 Managing Private Queries

Fully supporting a privacy-aware data management system will involve many interacting architectural components. Our goal here is modest in that we consider only the processing of a high level query and introduce the key architectural components necessary to facilitate the production of appropriate results. We will begin by describing the components and then discuss how they provide privacy under the attack model presented earlier.

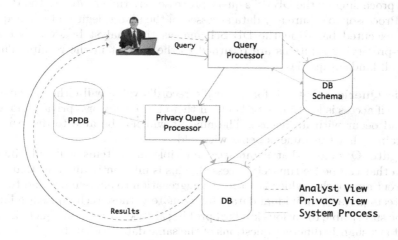

Fig. 2. Privacy preserving query processor architecture (Color figure online)

The analyst submits queries unaware of any underlying data flow and receives results back from the system in an opaque, privacy preserving way. Figure 2 depicts the analyst sending queries to the *query processor* based on view or database schema provided by the DBA. The database schema (DB Schema) is a euphemism for the schema, data directory and catalog necessary to pose queries (i.e. transactions) on the database (DB) itself. The relevant system level interactions are depicted by green arrows in Fig. 2 and all such interactions are opaque to the analyst. The query processor produces the data access plan in the normal way and passes its output onto the *Privacy Query Processor* (P-QP), which is responsible for modifying the query based on the privacy policy database (PPDB) that captures the privacy commitments for each data item. The P-QP modifies the access plan so the only data accessed are those conformant with the privacy commitments made between the organization and its users. Data that does exists outside of the commitments is never accessed.[13]

---

[13] The normal database operations, such as paging algorithms, may actually access some of the private data but since it is not seen at this level as a part of the modified query, it is not returned. There are associated exposures from paging in data that is not a part of the query *per se* because it is exposed in memory but this is not relevant to our simplified attack model.

Figure 2 also depicts the privacy protection afforded as a result of the architecture. The analyst will pose queries and the perceived flow is depicted by the dashed red arrows. The query is submitted to the query processor, which has provided the analyst with a view based on the DB Schema. The DB Schema facilitates access to the data itself that is stored in the database. The analyst sees *all* of the data legitimately afforded by that view so the result returned is seen as a complete answer to the query posed.

Privacy is provided by the **blue** arrows. Queries posed by the analyst, after normal processing by the DBMS's query processor are then routed to the Privacy Query Processor to ensure any data accessed in the plan is legitimate. The query that is executed based on the DB Schema, as the analyst believes, but only privacy-preserving solutions are returned to the analyst in the results. This is true of all kinds of queries:

Specific Queries: that ask for a specific record's value will either receive the value if access is legitimate or "null" if there is no value or a privacy violation would occur with its release. The analyst will not be able to discern with certainty that the value is being withheld.

Aggregate Queries: that summarize multiple data items will only include data that can be legitimately accessed. This is inherently different than most current approaches which trust in the aggregation to anonymize, and thereby protects privacy, individual data. Unfortunately, these techniques are known to be susceptible to various kinds of probing attacks or by multi-query attacks that ask slightly different questions of the same data to identify unique values in the database. The proposed architecture does not allow any data to be accessed unless it is permitted by the privacy commitments.

6   Summary

The primary purpose for this paper is to address the growing need to account for individual privacy in big data analytics. The first challenge is to understand that this issue is not restricted to "big data" but is certainly exacerbated by it. Governments, data provides, and the general public are becoming increasingly aware of the risks associated with the unrestrained use of data about us and will ultimately move to enforce limits on how it is used. Users do not currently fully understand privacy and how the data collected about them impacts on their daily lives; and this has been taken advantage of by many modern organizations. However, this unrestrained use of our personal data is fast approaching its limits.

Modern analytics will shortly be challenged in its fundamental assumptions. Current beliefs around ownership assume that data "generated" by analytics about an individual "belongs" to the analyst and can be used or resold without restraint (legal or ethical). This assumption will be challenged. An organization that is able to infer information about me with a high degree of accuracy should not be able to claim that they can use it even if it was not provided by me directly. Current mobile tracking systems and their associated analytics should not be used to make (possibly incorrect) assumptions about the person. For example, a police organization may request travel records from an insurance company to determine who might be frequently in "attendance" at a geolocation where a racist group has its offices. The insurance company collected the geolocation information for a completely different purpose such as reduced auto insurance rates because of the customer's claim to be a "good driver." It is entirely possible that those offices are geographically indistinguishable from an HIV clinic that the person is attending with a friend who has AIDS, but the police analytics cannot make such a semantic distinction so inappropriately flags the person as a member of a racist organization (in the interest of public safety). The insurance company's analytics reveals that the individual may be good driver but attends an HIV clinic so is denied coverage when attempting to renew their life insurance policy with this organization. The model described here would disallow both kinds of queries since they would violate the privacy commitments in place.

This paper has address societal and technical motivation for the creation of a privacy aware data management system. It has provided a very high level architecture and called for the development of one of the key enabling technologies that must be developed so users can make informed decisions about their privacy preferences. However, it has only scratched the surface. Fortunately, there is much activity underway.

The ultimate future challenge is that this requires not just technological solutions but also societal, governmental, legal, and corporate engagement. However, the technologists, should not start by saying that any solution we produce is doomed to failure without the committed involvement of all of these other players. In fact, these other players can abdicate responsibility for privacy solutions because there are no technological solutions available, which would lead to the vicious cycle where all stakeholders blame the lack of action of others for our collective inability to protect privacy.

Privacy protection or data value: can we have both? Although these two goals need to be held in tension and care must be made to ensure that systems are created that honour privacy commitments made in exchange for providing data, there is no reason we cannot have both. The motivation behind extracting maximum value from data to facilitate maximal dollar value is a powerful motivator for many modern data collectors. However, as with any technology, reasonable constraints must be placed on its use to ensure that it is used appropriately. Although governments might ultimately intervene to impose those constraints if industry cannot find a way to manage itself, there are only surmountable technical challenges that will ultimately prevent us from achieving utility while protecting privacy. This paper calls for two technical developments. First, data is only collected when the privacy information describing its use is collected with it. Secondly, that systems be developed that interrogates that privacy information before allowing access to the data. The idea itself is a simply one ... its implementation will be more challenging.

References

1. The privacy act of 1974 (September 26, 2003 1974). http://www.archives.gov/about/laws/privacy-act-1974.html
2. Agrawal, R., Kiernan, J., Srikant, R., Xu, Y.: Hippocratic databases. In: VLDB 2002: Proceedings of the 28th International Conference on Very Large Databases, vol. 28, pp. 143–154. VLDB Endowment, Hong Kong (2002)
3. Bacon, F.: Religious Meditations, Of Heresies (1597)
4. Bennett, C.: Regulating Privacy: Data Protection and Public Policy in Europe and the United States. Cornell University Press, Ithaca (1992)
5. Duhigg, C.: How companies learn your secrets. New York Times Mag. (2012)
6. Gudivada, V., Baeza-Yates, R., Raghavan, V.: Big data: promises and problems. Computer **48**(3), 20–23 (2015)
7. Mayer-Schonberger, V.: Delete: The Virtue of Forgetting in the Digital Age. Princeton University Press, Princeton (2011)
8. Peppers, D., Rogers, M., Dorf, B.: Is your company ready for one-to-one marketing? Harvard Bus. Rev. **77**, 151–160 (1999)
9. Zhu, X., Davidson, I.: Knowledge Discovery and Data Mining: Challenges and Realities. Information Science Reference. IGI Global, Hershey (2007)

Open Source Social Media Analytics for Intelligence and Security Informatics Applications

Swati Agarwal[1], Ashish Sureka[2(✉)], and Vikram Goyal[1]

[1] Indraprastha Institute of Information Technology, Delhi (IIITD), New Delhi, India
{swatia,vikram}@iiitd.ac.in
http://www.swati-agarwal.in, http://www.iiitd.edu.in/~vikram/
[2] Software Analytics Research Lab (SARL), New Delhi, India
ashish@iiitd.ac.in
http://www.software-analytics.in/

Abstract. Open-Source Intelligence (OSINT) is intelligence collected and inferred from publicly available and overt sources of information. Open-Source social media intelligence is a sub-field within OSINT with a focus on extracting insights from publicly available data in Web 2.0 platforms like Twitter (micro-blogging website), YouTube (video-sharing website) and Facebook (social-networking website). In this paper, we present an overview of Intelligence and Security Informatics (ISI) applications in the domain of open-source social media intelligence. We present technical challenges and introduce basic Machine Learning based framework, tools and techniques within the context of open-source social media intelligence using two case-studies. The focus of the paper is on mining free-form textual content present in social media websites. In particular we describe two important application: online radicalization and civil unrest. In addition to covering basic concepts and applications, we discuss open research problem, important papers, publication venues, research results and future directions.

Keywords: Information retrieval · Intelligence and Security Informatics · Machine learning · Mining user generated content · Open-Source Intelligence · Social media analytics

1 Introduction

Terrorism is not only a national problem specific to few countries experiencing terrorist incidents but an international and a global problem. Countering terrorism and building advanced technology based solutions to combat terrorism is a major concern and challenge to the government, law enforcement agencies and society [11,16]. Recent research and evidences demonstrate that Internet and social media platforms are increasing used by extremists and terrorists for planning and mobilization, recruitment, propagating hate and disseminating extreme political and religious beliefs. Social media platforms (such as YouTube

N. Kumar and V. Bhatnagar (Eds.): BDA 2015, LNCS 9498, pp. 21–37, 2015.
DOI: 10.1007/978-3-319-27057-9_2

video-sharing website and Twitter micro-blogging platform) are exploited for conducting extremist and terrorist activities due to low content publication barrier, wide reachability to a large number of people across countries and anonymity. Online radicalization has a major impact on society that contributes to the crime against humanity and main stream morality. Presence of such content in large amount on social media is a concern for website moderators (to uphold the reputation of the website), government and law enforcement agencies (locating such users and communities to stop hate promotion and maintaining peace in country). Hence, automatic detection and analysis of radicalizing content and protest planning on social media are two of the important research problems in the domain of ISI [4,10]. Monitoring the presence of such content on social media and keeping a track of this information in real time is important for security analysts working for law enforcement agencies. Mining publicly available open-source social media data for analysing, detecting, forecasting and conducting a root-cause analysis is an area that has attracted several researchers' attention [2,15] as shown in Fig. 1, the focus and scope of this paper is an intersection of three fields: (1) Online Social Media Platforms, (2) Intelligence and Security Informatics, and (3) Text Mining and Analytics. Online radicalization detection and civil unrest forecasting from social media data are subtopics (focus of this paper) within the broad area of Intelligence and Security Informatics. In this paper, we introduce the topic of online radicalization detection and civil unrest prediction, present technical challenges, problems and solution framework, literature survey, reference to case-studies and future research challenges.

Basic Definitions and Background Concepts

1.1   Online Social Media

Online Social Media Online Social Media and Web 2.0 (also referred to as the current generation of Web) consists of websites such as YouTube (video-sharing), Twitter and Tumblr (micro-blogging), Facebook (social networking), StackOverflow (community based question and answering), Delicious (social bookmarking), online wikis, message boards and discussion forums. Social media platforms are highly participatory and collaborative in nature in which users can easily share content and post messages and comments. According to information on Twitter website[1], there are about 500 million Tweets posted every day and the micro-blogging platform has 316 million monthly active users. According to information on YouTube website[2], YouTube has more than 1 billion users and 300 hours of video to the video-sharing platform every minute. According to SocialMedia-Today August 2015 statistics, 1.925 Billion users utilise their mobiles for Social Media platforms[3].

---

[1] https://about.twitter.com/company.

[2] https://www.youtube.com/yt/press/statistics.html.

[3] http://www.socialmediatoday.com/social-networks/kadie-regan/2015-08-10/
    10-amazing-social-media-growth-stats-2015.

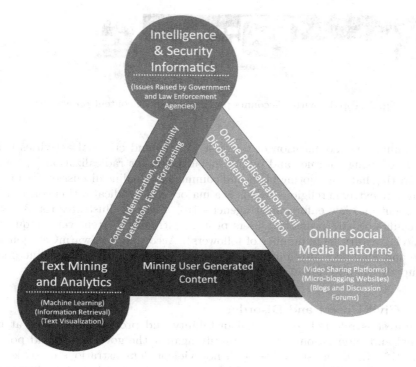

Fig. 1. Scope and focus of research area: an intersection of 3 topics and sub-topics (Online social media, text mining & analytics and Intelligence & Security Informatics)

1.2 Intelligence and Security Informatics

Intelligence and Security Informatics (ISI) is a field of study concerning investigation and development of counter terrorism, national and international security support systems and applications. ISI is a fast growing interdisciplinary area which has attracted several researchers and practitioners (form academia, government and industry) attention spanning across multiple disciplines like computer science, social sciences, political science, law and even medical sciences [16]. An example of ISI application is mining open-source (publicly available) social media data for terrorism forecasting or terrorism root cause analysis [13].

1.2.1 Online Radicalization

Online radicalization consists of using Internet as a medium by extremists and terrorists for conducting malicious activities such as promoting extreme social, religious and political beliefs, recruitment of youth, propagating hatred, forming communities, planning and mobilizing attacks [5–7,13]. Creating channels and video clips on how to make a bomb or a speech on racist propaganda and posting it on a popular video sharing website like YouTube falls under online radicalization [2,4,11]. Using a widely used micro-blogging platform such as Twitter

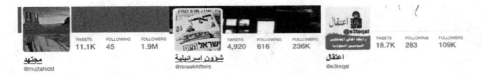

Fig. 2. Top 3 Twitter accounts posting extremist content on website

for planning and mobilization of terrorist attacks and criminal activities is an example of using Internet and online social media for radicalization [3]. Similarly, posting hate-promoting blogs and comments on online discussion forums to disseminate extreme religious beliefs is a major online radicalization concern for government and law enforcement agencies [16]. Figure 2 illustrates top 3 Twitter accounts of hate promoting users posting extremist content very frequently and having a very large number of followers[4]. According to SwarmCast journal article and Shumukh-al-islam posts, these are the three most important jihadi and support sites for Jihad and Mujahideen Twitter[5].

1.2.2   Civil Unrest and Disorder

Civil unrest is referred to as social instability and protest movements at the National and International level primarily against the government and policy-makers [12]. Civil unrest can be both non-violent demonstrations or strikes as well violent riots. The reason behind large scale civil unrest is mainly discontent in the society due to poor social and economic conditions [15]. The Arab Spring democratic uprising which originated in Tunisia in December 2010[6] and then propagated across various countries in the Arab world in the year 2011 is an example of intense civil unrest and disorder[7].

2   Technical and Computational Challenges

1. **Massive Size and Rich User Interaction.** The volume and variety of data in-terms of the modality such as free-form text, images, audio and video generated every day is so huge (refer to some statistics given in Sect. 1.1) that it poses hard computational challenges such as data processing and storage for researchers or application developers interested in analyzing the data [3,12]. In addition to the massive data size, the rich user interaction (such as friend, follower, subscriber, favorite and like relationship between various users) possible in social media increases data complexity, dimensions and variability which needs to be addressed.

---

[4] http://www.terrorismanalysts.com/pt/index.php/pot/article/view/426/html.

[5] http://jihadintel.meforum.org/identifier/149/shumukh-al-islam-forum.

[6] http://middleeast.about.com/od/humanrightsdemocracy/tp/
Arab-Spring-Uprisings.htm.

[7] http://www.npr.org/2011/12/17/143897126/the-arab-spring-a-year-of-revolution.

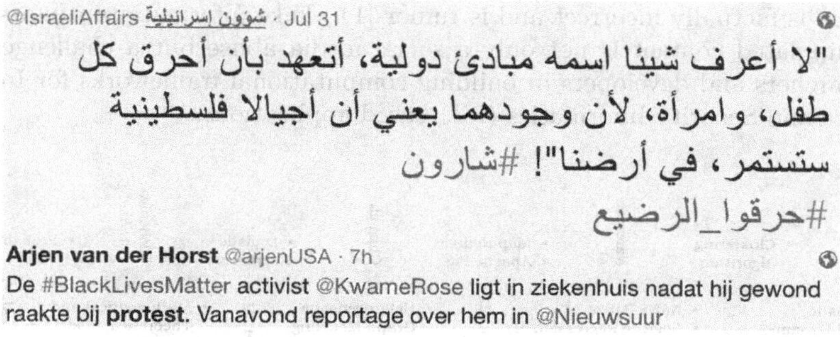

@IsraeliAffairs شؤون إسرائيلية · Jul 31

"لا أعرف شيئا اسمه مبادئ دولية، أتعهد بأن أحرق كل
طفل، وامرأة، لأن وجودهما يعني أن أجيالا فلسطينية
ستستمر، في أرضنا"! #شارون
#حرقوا_الرضيع

Arjen van der Horst @arjenUSA · 7h

De #BlackLivesMatter activist @KwameRose ligt in ziekenhuis nadat hij gewond
raakte bij **protest**. Vanavond reportage over hem in @Nieuwsuur

Fig. 3. Examples of multi-lingual posts on extremism and civil unrest

2. **High Velocity.** In addition to the overall quantity, the speed (for example few megabytes per second or minute or millions of rows per hour) at which data is generated poses data analytics challenges [1]. Real-time processing and storing of such high-velocity and massive flow of data is computationally challenging from the perspective of data ingestion [2].

3. **Multilingualism.** The web and social media is inherently multilingual. Content is posted in several different languages and processing them through automated algorithms requires linguistic resources for each language. Mining multilingual information is important and even essential for several Intelligence and Security Informatics (ISI) based application due the global diversity, user demographics and reach of the social media platforms and its users. Figure 3 shows examples of extremism and unrest related tweets posted in Arabic and Dutch language respectively.

4. **Noisy Content.** A huge amount of content on social media is of low quality (such as spam) and in general of low relevance (such as posting a message on what one had for breakfast or lunch) due to low barrier to publication [1,5,8]. Moreover, there are several issues such as grammatical mistakes, spelling errors, usage of non-standard acronyms and abbreviations, emoticons and incorrect capitalization of terms due to the informal nature of the content.

5. **Spam and Fake Accounts.** Spam, irrelevant and unsolicited messages as well as fake accounts is common in social media platforms [8]. Such content not only decreases the value of the website and the user experience but also poses technical challenges for social computing researchers in terms of data cleaning and pre-processing before building accurate data mining models.

6. **Data Annotation and Ground Truth.** Data annotation and ground-truth creation is a basis for several machine learning tasks such as predictive modeling and classification. Creating and annotating high quality ground-truth data at a large scale is effort intensive if done manually and a non-trivial technical challenge if done (semi)-automatically [3].

7. **Manipulation, Fabrication and Adversarial Behavior.** Deception, manipulation, misinformation, adversarial behaviors and credibility is a major issue in social media. Research shows that lot of content posted on social

media is factually incorrect and is rumor [14]. Fake information, rumors and manipulated content is not only a social media abuse but a challenges for researchers and developers in building computational frameworks for Intelligence and Security Informatics (ISI) based applications.

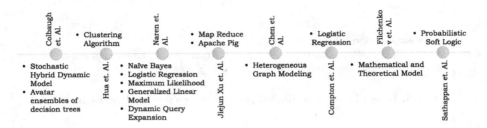

Fig. 4. Machine learning techniques used by researchers in existing literature of event forecasting in the domain of civil disobedience

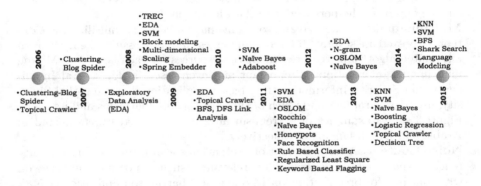

Fig. 5. Machine learning techniques used by researchers in existing literature of online radicalization and hate promotion detection

3   Machine Learning and Data Mining Techniques

In this Section, we discuss the most popular and common data mining techniques used by previous researchers in the area of detecting online radicalization and predicting civil unrest related events. Figure 4 illustrates a preview of these techniques used in existing literature in the domain of civil unrest event detection. Similarly, Fig. 5 shows a timeline of online radicalization techniques proposed over the past decade.

Based on our literature survey and analysis of previous work, we observe that ensemble learning on various machine learning techniques is a common approach to achieve better accuracy in the results. However, Ramakrishnan et al. [15]

proposed a different technique for different type of dataset/activities. They propose 5 different techniques for predicting events from 5 different models: volume based, opinion based, tracking of activities, distribution of events and cause of protest. In ensemble learning approach, Clustering, Logistic Regression and Dynamic Query Expansion (DQE) are the most commonly used techniques. We also observe that Named Entity Recognition (NER) is the most widely used phase in all techniques illustrated in Fig. 4. In named entity recognition, they extract various named entities present in the contextual metadata (tweets, Facebook comment, News article). For example, spatiotemporal expressions (locations and time related enetities), topic being discussed in the tweets or articles. They further use Dynamic Query Expansion and semi-automatic approaches to expand the list of extracted entities and keywords. They use various lexical sources (for example- WordNet[8], VerbOcean[9]) to extract similar and relevant keywords for their case study. Dynamic Query Expansion is an iterative process and converges once same keywords starts repeating. They further perform various clustering, regression (Logistic Regression) and classification (Naive Bayes) algorithm on these entities for event prediction.

We conducted a literature survey in the domain of online radicalization (extremist content, users and communities) detection on social media websites (video sharing websites, micro-blogging websites, blogs and forums) and we collected 37 articles (journal and conference proceedings). Therefore, we create a timeline of various deradicalization approaches that has been used by researchers over the past decade (refer to Fig. 5). Nowadays, social networking websites (Twitter, YouTube, Tumblr etc.) are some of the largest repositories of user generated content (contextual data) on web. Therefore, Text Classification KNN, Naive Bayes, SVM, Rule Based Classifier, Decision Tree, Clustering (Blog Spider), Exploratory Data Analysis (EDA) and Keyword Based Flagging (KBF) are the most commonly used techniques to identify hate promoting content on Internet. However, Topical Crawler and Link Analysis (Breadth First Search, Depth First Search, Best First Search) are common techniques to navigate through links and locate users with similar interest. Language modeling, n-gram and Boosting are other techniques used for mining textual data and classifying hate promoting content on web (social media, blogs, forums) [2]. Figure 5 also reveals that with the emergence of social media websites, Social Networking Analysis (SNA) became a popular techniques among researchers to locate hidden communities and groups. As we looked into the literature, we find that OSLOM (Order Statistics Local Optimization Method) is another common technique that has been used to locate hidden communities of extremist users. It is an open source visualization tool using a clustering algorithm designed to compute the similarity between two nodes (users) and locate their groups (network) sharing a common agenda. OSLOM uses an iterative process to identify internal structure of clusters and overlapping clusters (if possible). In order to detect hidden communities, it locally optimize the clusters by taking edge directions, edge weight, overlapping clusters and hierarchies of clusters into account.

---

[8] https://wordnet.princeton.edu.
[9] http://demo.patrickpantel.com/demos/verbocean/.

4   Case Studies

In this Section, we present two case studies in the area of Intelligence and Security Informatics. We describe our proposed solution approaches and algorithms for detecting online radicalization on YouTube and predicting civil unrest related events using an open source Twitter data.

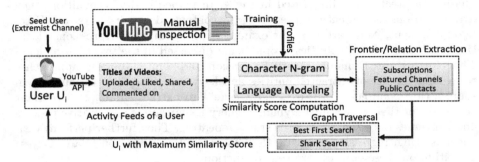

Fig. 6. A focused Crawler based framework for detecting hate promoting videos, users and communities on YouTube

4.1   Identification of Extremist Content, Users and Communities

Research shows that YouTube has become a convenient platform for many extremist groups to post negative videos disseminating hatred against a particular religion, country or person. These groups put forth hateful speech, offensive comments and promote certain ideology and beliefs among their viewers [2]. Social networking allows these extremist users to connect with other hate promoting users and groups, spreading extremist content, facilitating recruitment and forming their virtual communities [4]. Due to the dynamic nature of website, it is technically challenging and overwhelmingly impractical to detect such hate promoting videos and users by keyword based search. In this case study, we formulate our problem of identifying extremist content as a classification problem and use topical crawler based approach to locate such users and their hidden communities sharing a common agenda.

Figure 6 presents a general research framework for the proposed solution approach. The proposed method is a multi-step process primarily consisting of three phases, collection of training profiles, learning the statistical model and topical crawler. We perform a manual inspection on various YouTube channels and collect 35 hate promoting user profiles based upon their activity feeds such as titles and content of videos uploaded, commented, liked and favorited by the user. We build our training dataset by extracting contextual metadata of all activity feeds and profile summary of these 35 channels using YouTube API[10]. We also perform a characterization study on the contextual metadata and observe some

---

[10] https://developers.google.com/youtube/getting_started.

domain specific key-terms. We divide these terms into following 9 categories: important dates, religion, region, people name, negative emotions, communities, politics terms, war related terms and others. We apply character n-gram and language modeling on our training dataset and build our learning model. We use this learning model to compute the extent of similarity between contextual metadata of input channel and training data. We classify a YouTube channel as relevant (hate promoting) or irrelevant if the similarity score is above or below a threshold value. Further, To mine the relations among these hate promoting users, we build a focused crawler that follows the classifier and extract external links (connected users) to that profile. This focused crawler takes one YouTube channel (annotated as hate promoting channel) as a seed and classifies it using the learning model. We further extract the frontiers (featured channels, public contacts and subscribers) of this channel by parsing channel's YouTube home-page using jsoup HTML parser library[11]. We compute a similarity score for each frontier against training data and prioritize them in the descending order of their score. We execute our focused crawler for each frontier that results into a directed connected graph. In this graph, nodes represents the YouTube channel and edges represents the link between two channels (e.g. features channel). We further perform social network analysis on this graph to locate hidden communities and influential users playing major role in the community. As shown in the Fig. 6, in graph traversal phase, we use two different algorithms: Best First Search (BFS) and Shark Search (SS) traversal. In BFS algorithm, we extract the frontiers of a user channel only if it is classified as a relevant (hate promoting) channel. While in Shark Search algorithm, we explore the frontiers of both relevant and irrelevant users. Given a graph G, if B is a frontier of A and A is classified as irrelevant then in SS Algorithm, the similarity score of the B is reduced by a decay factor d that directly impacts on the priority of user. Therefore a frontier node of an irrelevant node has an inherited score of $score_{frontier} * d$. However, this inherited score is dynamic because as we traverse in the network, a node might have more than one parent (frontier of multiple channels). If a node has multiple parent nodes then we chose the $max(S_{P1}, S_{P2}.....S_{Pn},)$ where S_{Pi} is the inherited score of frontier for i_{th} parent.

Figure 7 (generated using ORA[12]) shows the cluster representation of network graph using Best First Search and Shark Search focused crawlers. Colors of nodes represents the variation in number of frontiers per user and the width of the edge represents the number of links between two users. Based on the network measurements, we find that the average clustering coefficient of graph for shark search focused crawler is very large in comparison to the graph for BFS focused crawler. Similarly, Fig. 7 also reveals that in BFS approach, network has 13 different clusters (represented as 13 different colors) for a total of 23 nodes. Among these 13 clusters, 6 clusters consists of only one user node which shows the difference in user channels. However, the cluster representation of network for shark search focused crawler contains only 7 clusters for 24 nodes. Unlike

---

[11] http://jsoup.org/apidocs/.

[12] http://www.casos.cs.cmu.edu/projects/ora/.

BFS focused crawler, in Shark search approach, only 2 clusters are formed with one node and we are able to find 3 existing strongly connected communities: C, D, E, H, I and B, C, D, E, G, H, I, J and A, D, E, G, where G has the maximum closeness centrality and connected to maximum number of users.

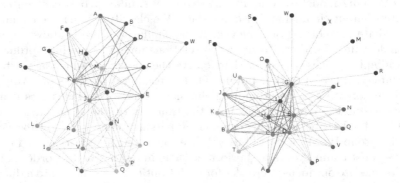

Fig. 7. Cluster graph representation for best first search (Left) Shark search Crawler (Right). Source: Agarwal et al. [4] (Color figure online)

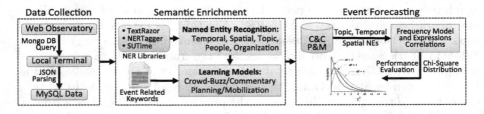

Fig. 8. A general research framework for mining Tweets and predicting civil unrest related events

4.2   Event Forecasting for Civil Unrest Related Events

We define the problem of civil unrest event prediction as the identification of several named entities expressions: spatial- location l where the protest is going to happen, temporal- time ti (can be date and time) of the protest and topic to- root cause of the protest. In this case study, we divide our problem into two sub-problems: (1) to perform a characterization study on open source Twitter dataset to investigate the feasibility of building event forecasting model. and (2) to evaluate the performance of machine learning and statistical based forecasting model by conducting experiments on real word Twitter data. Figure 8 presents the general research framework of our proposed approach for civil unrest event forecasting on micro-blogs. Figure 8 shows a high level architecture and design of proposed methodology that primarily consists of three phases: data collection, semantic enrichment and event forecasting. We conduct experiments on open

source Twitter dataset ('Immigration Tweets') downloaded from Southampton
Web Observatory[13]. This dataset consists of approximately $2M$ tweets where
each tweet contains at least of these 4 words: 'immigration', 'immigrant', 'migra-
tion' and 'migrant'. These tweets are collected in a time span of 5 months collected from October 1, 2013 to February 28, 2014. We use mongoDB queries to
access this data on our local terminal and further use JSON parsing to convert
it into mySQL. Since this dataset contains all tweets related to 'immigration',
we search popular media and news articles posted during this time span and
look for immigration related events happened worldwide. We find 5 such civil
unrest related events. However, in this paper we present a case study for only one
event i.e. 'Christmas Island Hunger Strike'. This event happened in Australia on
January 16, 2014 where nine asylum seekers stitch up their mouth with dental
floss and protested against new immigration law proposed by the country.

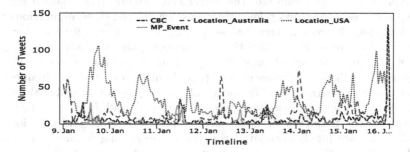

Fig. 9. Trend of crowd-buzz, mobilization and location based Tweets

As shown in the Fig. 8, we perform pre-processing on dataset and semantically enrich these tweets to achieve better accuracy in prediction. For semantic
enrichment of tweets, we use a trend based sliding window frame of 7 days
and extract only those tweets from the dataset that were published during that
time frame. For example, for 'Christmas Island Hunger Strike', we use tweets
posted from January 9 to 15. We make a hypothesis that before an event happens there are two types of tweets that are posted: people spreading the word
and discussing about the event (crowd-buzz and commentary) and organization
posting tweets for planning and mobilizing that event. Based on this hypothesis,
we train a multi-class classifier that classifies tweets into 3 categories: Crowd-
buzz and Commentary (C&C), Planning and Mobilization (P&M), Irrelevant
(not about the event). We use C&C and P&M tweets as two lead indicators that
helps in early detection of an event. These indicators filters relevant tweets to our
problem of civil unrest event forecasting from all other tweets and hence reduces
the traffic and extra computation of irrelevant tweets. Figure 9 shows the trend
of number of tweets being posted in every hour for 7 days sliding window time
frame. Figure 9 also reveals that relatively a very small fraction of these tweets
are C&C and P&M that increase the significance of filtering these tweets. In C&C

---

[13] https://web-001.ecs.soton.ac.uk/wo/dataset.

tweets, we use a lexicon based approach and look for the occurrence of various predefined key-terms particularly hashtags (collected by manual inspection and bootstrapping of tweets, related news and articles) relevant to the event. To classify P&M tweets, we train a machine learning classifiers that uses named entities (temporal, spatial, people, organization) of annotated P&M tweets as training dataset. Another input to the classifier is a lexicon of some key-terms related to planning and mobilization. For example- 'join us', 'spread the word', future tense related words. We use these P&M and C&C tweets to build our event prediction model. Research shows that spatio-temporal expressions are discriminatory features for predicting an event. We further include 'topic' as one more discriminatory feature and named entity. There can be multiple named entities in one tweet therefore we define 3 pairs of location-topic (l_i, to_i), topic-time (to_i, ti_i) and location-time (l_i, ti_i) for all expressions. We develop an adaptive version of Budak et al. [9] and compute the correlations among these named entities. To keep only significant and relevant entities, we discard those expressions that occur less than θ times in the dataset (C&C, M&P) where θ varies for all 3 categories of expressions. To find these significant pairs, we extract all expressions of x entity that are at least θ frequent in the dataset $F(x) > \theta N$ and further extract all those expressions of paired entity y that are ψ frequent for at least one x and vice versa. We select only those pairs of named entities that satisfy the following conditions: $F(x, y) > \lceil \psi F(x) \rceil$ and $F(y, x) > \lceil \varphi F(y) \rceil$. We compute the frequency of each pair in bipartite manner and only look for the pairs that are highly correlated and has no decreasing frequency in 7 days of sliding window. Since, these named entities are categorical attributes, we use Chi-Squared distribution to find correlation between two expressions. We define a pair of expressions to be significantly correlated if their $p\text{-}value$ <0.05 for their respective χ^2 and degree of freedom.

5   Characterization and Classification of Related Work

In this Section, we present a characterization based study on existing literature in the area of civil unrest related event forecasting (refer to Table 1) and hate & extremism detection (refer to Table 2). We analyze all relevant articles and create a list of facets to understand the current state-pf-the-art. Each facet is further classified into sub-categories and have their properties associated with them. Table 1 shows a list of all dimensions (Language, Features and Genre) and their sub-classes for the existing articles in the domain of civil disobedience prediction. Popular social media website allow users to post their content in various languages. The problem of civil unrest event detection can be a region specific as well as on across the globe. Therefore, translating multi-lingual text into English and extracting information (demographic, named entities- temporal, location, topic, people, organization) from translated text is useful for predicting a country or region specific events. Our analysis reveals that in 90 % of the papers researchers have been using English language text and among those in 60 % the articles, the proposed techniques are capable to address multi-lingual

text (English, Dutch, French, Portuguese and Spanish). We also observe that
75 % of the articles on civil unrest event forecasting focuses on events specific to
a region or country (e.g. Latin America).

Table 1. Various facets for classifying articles on civil unrest prediction

Facets	Categories	Description
Language	English	Mining only English language content
	Non-English	Text consisting Non-English language content
	Others	Testbed consisting of multi-lingual text
Features	Time	Presence of temporal expressions
	Location	Presence of spatial expressions
	Topic	Targeted or central topic of discussion
	Content	Mining text to extract event related information
	Demographic	Demographic and statistical based information
Genre	Regional	Predicting protests happened in one or specific region or country [Latin America]
	Global	Predicting any civil unrest related event happened worldwide

Table 2 shows a list of various dimensions for annotating and existing schol-
arly articles in the domain of online radicalization detection. Our investigation of
the literature reveals that among 37 articles, in 35 papers the proposed method
uses contextual metadata as a discriminatory feature to detect hate promoting content[14]. Similarly, in 16 articles, they use demographic information and
external links to find relation between two profiles and locate their communities. Similar to civil unrest event prediction related articles, we classify these
articles based on the language being addressed. Based on the meta-analysis we
find that among 37 articles, 14 articles are capable to mine the content written in Arabic language and script. Among these 14 articles, methods proposed
in 7 articles are capable to analyze other non-English language texts as well
(German, French). Based on the research aim of articles, we classify previous
researches into five genre of online radicalization: Anti-black communities are
a form of racism that promotes white supremacy. Jihad communities promote
their belief towards Islamic extremism (Sharia Law), also a part of religion based
communities where users post hate speech against some religion and promote
their ideologies. Hate and Extremism includes the others categories that are
undefined and covers political radicalization.

6   ISI Leading Conferences and Journals

The IEEE Intelligence and Security Informatics (ISI) series of conferences[15] is
the flagship conference on ISI which started in the year 2003 and has happened

---

[14] http://bit.ly/1L3x4zV.
[15] http://ieee-isi.org/.

Table 2. Various facets for annotating articles on extremism detection

Dimension	Categories	Description
Features	Text	contextual metadata (Title of Video, Tweet)
	Link	Links between two users (Friend, Follower)
	Demographic	Other demographic and statistical based metadata
Analysis	Content	Detecting the presence of extremist content on web
	User Profile	Identifying hate promoting users
	Community	Locating hidden communities of extremist users
Language	English	Text containing only English language content
	Arabic	content written in Arabic language including scripts
	Others	Posts consisting of any other Non-English language (excluding L2)
Genre	Anti-black	White communities targeting black people
	Jihad	Promotion of Jihad among followers on network
	Terrorism	Social media activities performed by terrorist groups
	Extremism	Promote hatred among various targeted audience
	Religion	Anti-religious content (example- Anti-Islamic Tweets)

in various countries such as USA, Taiwan, Canada, China and Netherlands. ISI is an annual conference and happens normally in the month of May or June. The European Intelligence and Security Informatics Conference (EISIC)[16] is also a leading international scientific conference bringing together researchers and practitioners working in the area of ISI. EISIC has established itself as a premier European conference on counter-terrorism and criminology. It was started in the year 2011 and has happened in various countries such as Greece, Denmark, Sweden, Netherlands and United Kingdom. The Pacific Asia Workshop on Intelligence and Security Informatics (PAISI)[17] is another prestigious forum on ISI which was started in the year 2006 is normally co-located to the Pacific-Asia Conference on Knowledge Discovery and Data Mining (PAKDD) every year. Security Informatics[18] is a high quality and high impact open-access Journal from Springer which publishes peer-reviewed articles on ISI. Studies in Conflict & Terrorism formerly known as Terrorism is a peer reviewed based open-accessed journal started in 1992. SICT is ranked in the International Relations category and in the Political Science category of the 2015 Thomson Reuters, 2015 Journal Citations Report.

7   Conclusions

Open source social media analytics for Intelligence and Security Informatics applications is an area that has attracted the attention of several researchers over

---

[16] http://www.eisic.eu/.

[17] http://www.business.hku.hk/paisi/.

[18] http://www.security-informatics.com/.

the past decade. In this paper, we discuss two important and major application of open source social media intelligence: online radicalization and civil unrest. We perform a comprehensive analysis of literature survey and we observe that even though there has been a lot of work in the domain of event prediction on social media websites, civil unrest event prediction by mining textual content in social media has recently gained the attention of researchers. We also find that the number of research papers on social media analytics for online radicalization detection are much more (about 7 times) than on civil disobedience detection[19]. Our analysis also reveals that Twitter plays a major role in facilitating mobilization and planning of civil unrest events in comparison to other social media platforms. It is interesting to observe that despite being the most popular video sharing website, YouTube has not been used in any of the existing research for protest planning or prediction. On the contrary, research shows that YouTube is the most widely used platform for online radicalization, hate and extremism promotion. We conduct a meta-analysis of exiting literature in the domain of online radicalization detection and civil unrest even prediction on social media platforms. Our analysis reveals a variety of machine learning, information retrieval and data mining approaches that has been used in past to investigate solution for these problems. Based on our analysis, we find that Clustering, Logistic Regression and Dynamic Query Expansion are the most commonly used techniques to predict upcoming events related to civil unrest or protest. Named Entity Recognition (NER) is a most common and widely used component in all above event prediction models. Graph modeling and Ensemble Learning are also some techniques adopted by researchers for the problem of event forecasting. Text Classification KNN, Naive Bayes, SVM, Rule Based Classifier, Decision Tree, Clustering (Blog Spider), Exploratory Data Analysis (EDA) and Keyword Based Flagging (KBF) are the most commonly used techniques to identify extremism and hate promoting content on Internet. However, for navigating through links and locating users with similar interest, Topical Crawler and Link Analysis (Breadth First Search, Depth First Search, Best First Search) are common graph traversal algorithms in use. Language modeling, character level n-gram and Boosting are other techniques used for mining textual data and classifying hate promoting content on web (social media, blogs and forums).

In this paper, we also present two case studies as two applications of open source social media analytics for Intelligence and Security Informatics. We present a classification framework for the problem of identifying hate promoting content on YouTube and a topical crawler based approach to locate such extremist users and their hidden communities sharing a common agenda. We conduct a series of experiments on YouTube videos and channels by varying various algorithmic parameters such as the similarity threshold for the language modelling based text classifier and n-grams. We conclude that by performing social network analysis on network graphs, we are able to locate hidden communities. We also identify the users who play major roles in the communities and

---

[19] http://bit.ly/1L3x4zV.

have highest centrality among all. We reveal the communities by dividing the network graph into clusters formed by similar users (refer to our previous work [2,4] for more details). For civil disobedience forecasting, we propose an approach for early detection of these events. In our approach we present a case study on immigration related event- Christmas Island Hunger Strike. To investigate the effectiveness of our approach, we conduct experiments on real world dataset downloaded from Southampton WebObservatory. We train a multi-class classifier to filter event related tweets (crowd-buzz and mobilization) which certainly improves the accuracy the accuracy of prediction and reduces the computational cost. We develop a frequency based model on these event related tweets (semantically rich) and find those pairs of named entities (spatial location, topics and temporal) expressions that are significantly correlated. We perform the χ^2 and p-value distribution on these pairs of named entities expressions and conclude that by detecting trend analysis of spatial, temporal and topic based entities in sliding window (7 days), we can predict civil unrest related events with high confidence score. We further perform an in-depth meta-analysis of existing literature and perform a characterization based classification of articles. Based on our analysis we find that contextual based metadata (title, description, comments) is most commonly used feature for identifying hate promoting content. However, to find the relation between user channels and to locate their hidden communities, demographic information and activity feeds of user profile are common discriminatory features. We observe that many of the existing techniques are capable to mine multi-lingual text such as Arabic and capture relevant information.

References

1. Agrawal, S., Sureka, A.: Copyright infringement detection of music videos on YouTube by mining video and uploader meta-data. In: Bhatnagar, V., Srinivasa, S. (eds.) BDA 2013. LNCS, vol. 8302, pp. 48–67. Springer, Heidelberg (2013)
2. Agarwal, S., Sureka, A.: A focused crawler for mining hate and extremism promoting videos on YouTube. In: 25th ACM Conference on Hypertext and Social Media (HT), pp. 294–296 (2014)
3. Agarwal, S., Sureka, A.: Learning to classify hate and extremism promoting tweets. In: Intelligence and Security Informatics Conference (JISIC), pp. 320–320 (2014)
4. Agarwal, S., Sureka, A.: Topic-specific YouTube crawling to detect online radicalization. In: Chu, W., Kikuchi, S., Bhalla, S. (eds.) DNIS 2015. LNCS, vol. 8999, pp. 133–151. Springer, Heidelberg (2015)
5. Agarwal, S., Sureka, A.: A topical crawler for uncovering hidden communities of extremist micro-bloggers on tumblr. In: 5th Workshop on Making Sense of Microposts (MICROPOSTS) (2015)
6. Agarwal, S., Sureka, A.: Using common-sense knowledge-base for detecting word obfuscation in adversarial communication. In: Workshop on Future Information Security (FIS) (2015)
7. Agarwal, S., Sureka, A.: Using KNN and SVM based one-class classifier for detecting online radicalization on Twitter. In: Natarajan, R., Barua, G., Patra, M.R. (eds.) ICDCIT 2015. LNCS, vol. 8956, pp. 431–442. Springer, Heidelberg (2015)

8. Aggarwal, N., Agarwal, S., Sureka, A.: Mining YouTube metadata for detecting privacy invading harassment and misdemeanor videos. In: Privacy, Security and Trust (PST), pp. 84–93 (2014)
9. Budak, C., Georgiou, T., Agrawal, D., El Abbadi, A.: Geoscope: online detection of geo-correlated information trends in social networks. Proc. VLDB Endow. **7**, 229–240 (2013)
10. Compton, R., Lee, C.: Detecting future social unrest in unprocessed Twitter data: emerging phenomena and big data. In: Intelligence and Security Informatics (ISI), pp. 56–60 (2013)
11. Fu, T., Huang, C.N., Chen, H.: Identification of extremist videos in online video sharing sites. In: 2009 IEEE International Conference on Intelligence and Security Informatics, ISI 2009, pp. 179–181, June 2009
12. Hua, T., Lu, C.T., Ramakrishnan, N.: Analyzing civil unrest through social media. Computer **46**(12), 80–84 (2013)
13. Kwok, I., Wang, Y.: Locate the hate: detecting Tweets against blacks. In: AAAI (2013)
14. Qazvinian, V., Rosengren, E., Radev, D.R., Mei, Q.: Rumor has it: identifying misinformation in microblogs. In: Proceedings of the Conference on Empirical Methods in Natural Language Processing, Stroudsburg, PA, USA, pp. 1589–1599 (2011)
15. Ramakrishnan, N., Butler, P., Muthiah, S.: 'Beating the news' with embers: forecasting civil unrest using open source indicators. In: Proceedings of the 20th ACM SIGKDD International Conference on Knowledge Discovery and Data Mining, KDD 2014, pp. 1799–1808. ACM, New York (2014)
16. Wang, M., Alan, C.G.: Intelligence and security informatics. In: Pacific Asia Workshop (PAISI) (2011)

Big Data in Commerce

Information Exploration in E-Commerce Databases

Manish Singh (✉)

Indian Institute of Technology, Hyderabad, India
msingh@iith.ac.in

Abstract. Many e-commerce sites struggle to present their data to users in an easily accessible manner, especially when the users have limited knowledge of what is contained in their database or lack technical expertise to form proper queries. Faceted navigation is a central tool that these e-commerce sites use to address this challenge. A typical faceted interface has two main component panels: a query panel and a result panel. Faceted browsing is primarily designed to help users quickly get to a specific item if they know the characteristics they are looking for. However, limitations in the query and the result panel deter effective faceted browsing, especially for users unfamiliar with the data. In this paper, we study why users are not able to explore e-commerce databases. We identify five limitations in the query and result panel that deter exploratory search using faceted browsing. We propose nine add-on extensions—four in the query panel and five in the result panel—to address these limitations.

1 Introduction

Users today have access to many large databases, yet find it difficult to access the records they want. In some cases, the challenge is to write correct SQL. But databases today often come with easy-to-use query interfaces. Users still find it difficult to specify the precise query conditions, due to limited familiarity with the data. Consider, for example, a user on a travel web site looking to book a hotel in a big city. If she knows her preferences for price, location, star rating, and other such relevant attributes, she can easily specify a query that will pull out a few good choices for her to consider from among the hundreds of hotels in the city. But, if she is unfamiliar with the city, she may not understand what typical prices are in the city or how all the 5-star hotels are clustered in the financial district or how there is a tradeoff between location and price. Without this knowledge of the data in the database, she is forced to depend on other data sources, such as advice from friends and relatives, social media, web documents, etc., to gain data familiarity and pose the right queries. In consequence, even after hours of effort she may be left with various doubts: "Did I make a good choice?" "Did I explore all my options?" "Did I spend more than I needed to?"

There are two types of search: *lookup* and *exploratory* [27,32,38]. In lookup search users have a specific well-defined search goal. Lookup search can be

© Springer International Publishing Switzerland 2015
N. Kumar and V. Bhatnagar (Eds.): BDA 2015, LNCS 9498, pp. 41–56, 2015.
DOI: 10.1007/978-3-319-27057-9_3

expressed as precise queries using structured query languages, such as SQL, XQuery and SPARQL, which are bit difficult for normal end-users. The more user-friendly solutions are forms, keyword search [13], faceted navigation [15,40], and so on. In contrast, in exploratory search users' goal is to learn about an unfamiliar information landscape through diverse, ill-defined and open-ended search queries. Through exploratory search users' aim is to gain a comprehensive understanding of data that will enable them to make more informed lookup queries. Users often have to go through an exploratory search phase before they can form informed lookup queries.

The existing search interfaces, such as forms, faceted navigation, keyword search with auto-completion, etc., are quite effective for lookup search. However, there are various limitations in relation to exploratory search. Supporting data exploration is difficult because: (a) Datasets are complex and heterogeneous, and (b) Users have diverse needs. It is easy, for example, to provide the user with some simple summary statistics, such as average price for a hotel room. However, this number is of only limited value to the user, perhaps because there is huge variance between different parts of the city or perhaps because the user is a backpacker looking for youth hostels whose price is poorly correlated with those at fancy hotels. What the user needs is a characterization of a portion of the data (which she has identified to the system) along dimensions that are of interest to her.

In this paper, we focus exclusively on e-commerce databases. We present the pains that users face in exploring e-commerce databases; the existing solutions that are used by e-commerce sites to provide easy access to users and their limitations. We also present techniques that can further enhance users' data exploration [36].

2   Search Interface in E-Commerce

Faceted navigation is a central tool that most e-commerce sites use to allow users browse through products. It is a type of categorization technique that is used to access a collection of items by their multiple classifications, or facets. It can be used to access both documents and structured databases, though we will primarily focus on its application to structured data.

Figure 1 is a screenshot of a typical faceted interface for browsing a database of cars. A basic faceted interface has two main component panels: a *query panel* and a *result panel*. The latter typically occupies the majority of the screen real estate and shows the set of currently selected items. The former is usually on the left (or top) side, and offers both user interface controls as well as a summary digest of the current query and the result set.

Due to the many benefits of faceted interface, many researchers in IR and Databases have worked on improving the usability of basic faceted interface by providing numerous add-on extensions to improve both the query and the result panel. The faceted interface shown in Fig. 1 is from `cars.com`, which is a major online car shopping company for buying and selling cars. Unlike

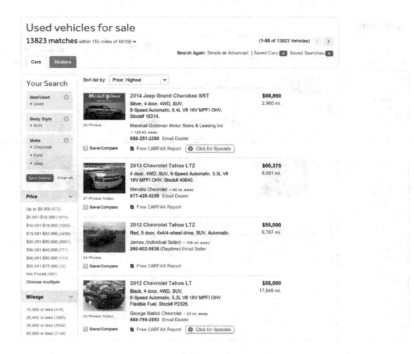

Fig. 1. This screen capture from `cars.com` represents a typical example of a faceted navigation interface. Like most such interfaces, it is divided between a small *query panel* on the left and a *results panel* on the right. The left-hand side also includes a small *summary digest* describing the overall result set.

`cars.com` that only deals with cars, problems become more acute at sites, such as `amazon.com`, `ebay.com`, etc., where they manage huge collection of highly heterogeneous items. Although `amazon.com` uses the basic faceted interface, but it is integrated with many useful add-on extensions, such as keyword search, ranking, etc., as shown in Fig. 2. Although the basic faceted interface is quite usable for exploring small databases having homogeneous (same set of attributes) collections of items, it is not very effective for exploring large databases having heterogeneous collection of items.

Following are some of the important components and add-on extensions that are found in typical faceted interfaces:

1. Facet: Facets refer to categories used to characterize information items in a collection. Each facet has a name, such as `Departments`, `Optical Zoom`, `Brand`, `Price`, etc. A facet can be *flat* or *hierarchical*. For hierarchical categories, such as `Department`, `Location`, etc., one can use hierarchical facets so that users can roll-up or drill-down in a hierarchy of categories. Since our primary focus is on relational databases with flat columns, we treat each relational attribute as a flat facet. In this paper, we use the terms facet, dimension, feature and attribute interchangeably.

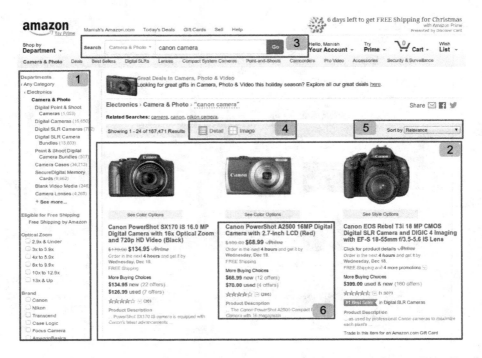

Fig. 2. This screen capture from `amazon.com` shows a typical search interface often seen in large e-commerce sites with heterogeneous data. Here faceted navigation is integrated with other search techniques, such as keyword search, ranking, etc.

Based on whether a facet can be queried, one can divide the facets into two groups: queriable and non-queriable facets. Since the queriable facets are typically shown in the main query panel, we can call them as *shown* facets. In a traditional faceted interface, the non-queriable facets are like additional features that users can possibly see for individual tuples, but they cannot query or get summary digest for such facets. We call these non-queriable facets as *hidden* facets or additional features.

2. Facet Value: For each facet, we enumerate a discrete set of facet values, with a preference to keep this set small. For facets with categorical domains, or with a small discrete numerical domain, the facet values are obtained directly from the domain. Where the number of values is very large, such as for most numerical domains, ranges of values are binned together to create a small number of discrete facet values. For example, an `Optical Zoom` facet might be shown with a few different discrete zoom ranges (e.g., 2.9x & under, 3x to 3.9x, 4x to 5.9x) as facet values. In a faceted interface, users select facet values using links or check boxes. Links usually indicate straightforward equals condition (single selection). For example, "I want to narrow down my search result to `Department` equals `Digital Camera`". Check boxes typically indicate an additive "or" condition (multiple selection). For example, "I want to narrow down my search result to Brand equals Canon, Nikon or Sony"

3. The Query Panel: The query panel is usually on the left (or top) side, and offers both user interface controls as well as a summary digest of the current query and the result set. In Fig. 1, the query panel has two separate parts: the users' current query at the top and summary digest at the bottom. The summary digest typically comprises all the facet values that appear in the current query result, grouped by their corresponding facet. The summary digest may also include a tuple count for each facet value. As users select facet values from the summary digest, the facet values become part of the users' current query. Users can select single or multiple facet values from any subset of the displayed facets.

In Fig. 1, the top part of the query panel shows the user's current query, where the user has selected single value for New/Used and Body Style, and several values for Make. The bottom part of query panel shows the summary digest of current query result in the form of all facet values that appear in the query result grouped by their facets. The summary digest has some amount of statistical information in the form of tuple counts next to each unchosen facet value (e.g., there are 87 cars with Price of Up to 5000). In many faceted interfaces, such as Fig. 2, the user's current query and the summary digest is shown in interleaved manner.

4. The Keyword Search Bar: The keyword search bar, labeled as box 3 in Fig. 2, is one of the most important extensions of the query panel. It is crucial in applications that require search over heterogeneous collection of items. Based on the keywords that users enter in the keyword search bar, the system determines the appropriate facets that should be shown on the left-side query panel. In this dissertation, we do not deal with the keyword search bar.

5. Result Panel: The result panel, labeled as box 2 in Fig. 2, typically occupies the majority of the screen real estate and shows the set of currently selected items. The results panel is scrollable, so the user can examine more results than can be displayed on the screen at once.

The basic faceted interface shows the query result in the result panel in some random order, and thus is not very usable for browsing large result sets. There are various existing add-on extensions to improve the usability of the result panel. For example, the designer can provide an appropriate ranking function to rank the result tuples. Even users can reorder their result set using provided sorting options, such as sort by Relevance, Price, etc., as shown in box 5 of Fig. 2. Users can also see the result in zoomed-in or zoomed-out view by using options—Detail, Image view—as shown in box 4.

6. Result Snippet: Since most datasets are high-dimensional, it is not possible to show all the attributes of each result tuple in the main result panel. Rather each result tuple is shown in the form of a snippet, where each snippet is a small subset of attribute values, as shown in box 6 of Fig. 2.

For a database with homogeneous data, one can show the same subset of attributes for all the tuples as snippet. This is the easiest form of snippet. However, most e-commerce applications have to handle heterogeneous data and they show different subset of attributes for each result tuple as snippet, as can be seen in both Figs. 1 and 2. To create such a variable format snippet, they create an additional attribute where they manually enter the snippet that should be shown whenever the particular tuple appears in the query result. Both the above types of snippets are static in the sense that they are not dependent on the users' query.

3   Obstacles in Exploratory Search

There are three factors that thwart exploratory search: (a) Limited feedback in the query panel, (b) Low adaptivity of the result panel, and (c) Information loss from hidden attributes. In this section, we explain each of these three obstacles.

3.1   Limited Feedback in the Query Panel

As discussed in Sect. 2, faceted navigation combined with keyword search is currently the most popular frontend for accessing e-commerce databases. Unlike traditional data navigation techniques, such as forms, hierarchical browsing, etc., that forced users to follow a predetermined navigation order, both faceted navigation and keyword search are designed to be *self-explorable*. In other words, they do not restrict users to follow a predetermined navigation order. Users can browse a faceted interface through independent facets based on their specific preference, or domain knowledge. However, giving too much independence, without suitable feedback, also leads to users feeling lost, especially when they are unfamiliar with the data.

Many e-commerce sites now provide feedback to users for keyword search through the autocompletion (word completion) feature, which predicts the rest of words as the user types in few words. This feature helps the e-commerce sites to more precisely select the facets that should be shown in the query panel and the items that should be shown in the result panel; when the user selects one of the standard options shown in the form of autocompletion choices. These e-commerce sites maintain mapping of which data to show based on the user's typed keywords. If the users are allowed to type in keywords without feedback, then there might be spelling errors or the keywords may not be the same keywords as used in the product description, and thus leading to search with no results or wrong results. Keyword search combined with autocompletion has greatly improved the exploration of e-commerce sites that deal with heterogeneous data.

While creating a faceted interface, designers want to choose a subset of attributes as facets that are important for most of the underlying data and are also independent. However, this independence assumption rarely holds true in real-life applications. When users make certain choices, it narrows their search space by automatically eliminating many other choices. For example, cars with eight-cylinder engines tend to be large and expensive; someone who chooses the eight-cylinder facet value will not select facet values inexpensive and compact.

Instead of providing users useful feedback information, such as information about their exploration direction, or relationship across facets and conditional distributions on facet values, the faceted interface leaves it to the users to manually figure out such information beyond a minimal summary digest that provides some counts.

A faceted interface devotes the bulk of its display space to show the result panel. Since it is not possible for users to manually look at thousands of result tuples that are shown in the result panel, most users do not really care about the result panel until they near the end of their exploration. Users spend most of their time exploring the summary digest, which is shown within the small left-hand query panel, because that is their only means to understand the space of available options and get to their desired result set.

The tuple counts given by the summary digest can be helpful guidance for the users, but are not nearly enough — they only provide information on the number of matches without characterizing them in any meaningful way.

3.2   Low Adaptivity of the Result Panel

The traditional faceted interface has a very simple presentation for the query and the result panel. Typically, the query panel shows a subset of attributes from the dataset as facets, which are shown in some fixed order, with each facet showing a list of facet values that are ordered by count or alphabetical order. Similarly, the result panel shows an unorganized list of result tuples, which users can often reorder by sorting along some provided sorting attribute, such as Price, Year, etc.

Some recent research work has addressed this low adaptivity aspect. For example, [4, 26] have looked at improving the adaptivity of query panel by ranking facets and facet values to minimize users' navigation cost. Similarly, the result panel can be made more user-adaptive by clustering the results [31, 39] and then allowing users to more easily find similar result tuples by using features such as more-like-this [3].

Limitation 2. Variable Speed Browsing — The result panel is not adaptive to allow the users to browse through large result sets at different browsing speeds and still be able to absorb the displayed information. The result panel that is normally used for presenting relational tuples, including faceted interface, cannot support variable-speed browsing. Faceted search often yields a large set of tuples as query result. If the result comprises tuples of alphanumeric values with few visual markers, it is hard to quickly browse such data, even if the result is sorted. When users try to scroll fast through such alphanumeric data, then everything seems like a fast-changing blur. The result panel can be more effective if it can become aware of users' browsing pattern, and dynamically adjust itself to the users' need. For example, instead of showing users a large number of tuples that they cannot assimilate during fast scrolling, it would be useful to show users fewer tuples that they can assimilate even while fast scrolling. The trick is to choose carefully the tuples to show so as to minimize information loss.

Limitation 2. Dynamic Result Snippet — Since most datasets are high-dimensional, it is not feasible to show all the attributes of each result tuple in the main result panel. Rather each result tuple is shown in the form of a snippet, where each snippet shows a subset of attribute values, as shown in Fig. 1. The easiest way to form such snippets is to show some fixed subset of attributes for all the result tuples. However, many e-commerce site show variable format snippet for each result tuple. To create such variable format snippet, they create an additional attribute where they store the snippet that should be shown whenever the particular tuple appears in the query result. Clearly, both the above snippets are static in nature, and they do not directly address users' search need. On the contrary, when we do web search, then many search engines return a dynamic snippet for each search result, where the snippet highlights why a particular document is relevant to the user's given query. The result panel of faceted interface will be more informative if it can show a snippet that is relevant to the user's given query or some known user preference.

3.3   Information Loss from Hidden Attributes

Even though faceted interfaces are designed to permit self-exploration by users, limited screen real estate (and user fatigue) often force interface designers to restrict the number of queriable facets that are shown to users in the query panel. For example, cars.com does not offer the number of cylinders in the engine as a queriable facet, even though this information is available as a hidden facet (additional feature) for each result tuple.

Designers often choose attributes that are globally important for all the tuples as queriable facets. The remaining attributes (hidden facets) may also be very important, but they may not be applicable for all the tuples or used frequently by all the users.

Following are some important limitations due to the existence of hidden facets:

Limitation 1. Expressing Selection — If users want to perform selection using hidden facets, then existing faceted interface do not provide any support to assist such selection. However, if users are shown the relationship between hidden facets and queriable (shown) facets, then users can easily express their selection in hidden facet(s) in terms of the queriable facets. We need to help users learn such insightful mappings between facets by providing appropriate feedback in the query panel.

Limitation 2. No Summary Feedback — Faceted interfaces almost ignores all the information present in the hidden facets. The only way users can see the information in hidden facets is by looking at the additional features for each individual tuple. Since many datasets are high-dimensional with number of attributes between 25 to a hundred or more [14] and the faceted interface shows only a few (typically less than 10) of those attributes as queriable facets, it means that users lose almost all the important information that is present in such high-dimensional data. Instead of ignoring all the hidden facets, it would be more useful if the appropriate information from hidden facets can be automatically combined with the queriable facets to provide better insight to users.

4   Extensions to Facilitate Exploratory Search

In this section, we give an overview of different techniques that can used to address the exploratory search obstacles presented in Sect. 3. We present the techniques that can be integrated with query panel in Sect. 4.1 and the techniques that can be integrated with the result panel in Sect. 4.2. We consider the following example:

Example 1. Consider a used car database, which contains a single table $\mathcal{D}$ with n attributes where each tuple represents a car for sale. The table has numerous attributes that describe details of the car, such as Price, Make, Model, BodyType, Drivetrain, Mileage, EngineSize, NumCylinders, Color, FuelEconomy, Power, Year, etc. Consider a user Mary, who is unfamiliar to car domain, trying to buy a used SUV car, using an interface similar to Fig. 1.

4.1   Exploratory Search in Query Panel

Faceted interface allows users to select facet values independently from any of the available queriable facets. As a result, users have exponential number of ways to explore faceted data. However, the existing query panel provides very limited feedback about these available exploration paths or the query result.

Following are some of features that one can provide in the query panel to facilitate exploratory search:

Extension 1. Compare Facet Values — In the Body Style facet Mary can see all the available body styles, such as SUV, Sedan, Hatchback, etc., along with their tuple counts in the current query result. But a faceted interface does not provide any means to see the detailed difference or similarity between these body styles. The problem becomes more acute when facets have many values. For example, Make and Model have more than 50 and 200 facet values respectively.

Although faceted interface by itself is not designed for supporting comparison, a user can use single selection to compare options. For example, Mary can have five separate windows where in each window she selects a particular body style with other query conditions being same. She can then compare the five body styles based on their summary digest. This kind of comparison is painful, particularly if one would like to compare many options. It is also limited to the counts available in the summary digest. One cannot use multi-selection option because it would commingle the list of facet values that are shown in other facets.

To allow comparison, some e-commerce sites provide users an additional interface to perform side-by-side comparison. In cars.com there is an option to compare different car models. A user can select a list of car models, and the system shows comparison across some fixed set of other attributes by showing simple statistical summaries, such as min-max range, mean etc. Since there are an exponential number of choices to compare and users are not even aware of what are the best options they should compare, even these additional interfaces provide very limited help to users.

One can use data analysis algorithms to automatically compute the relationship between the attribute values that the user wants to compare with values other attributes. For example, if the user wants to compare different Body Styles, we can show to the user how other attributes such as Price, Doors, Ground Clearance, etc., are related to different body styles.

Extension 2. Finding Themes — Each facet value often represents a very large set of diverse items. For example, body style SUV has sub-categories Compact, Mid-size, Full-size etc. Even a single sub-category can have very diverse cars due to difference in car manufacturers and the specific car model. If Mary wants to compare the five body styles using the single selection option (as described above), she will not be able to see all these different sub-categories or themes within each body style. If we show simple one column type of statistical summary (such as mean or median) for different body styles, it will seem that SUVs are quite costly compared to Sedans and Hatchbacks. Although there might be a small class of SUVs with price and other features similar to Sedans and Hatchbacks. This misleading summary may discourage Mary to explore SUVs further even though there are SUVs that meet her price criteria.

We can automatically compute these sub-categories by clustering cars of different body styles. We can label the clusters using values from different facets, and thereby helping users to understand sub-categories within each facet value.

Extension 3. Expressing Selections — In high-dimensional dataset, most of the dimensions are non-queriable or hidden facets. Users cannot express selection over such facets. For example, cars.com does not offer the number of cylinders in the engine as a queriable facet. If Mary wants to focus on V4 engines, she has no easy way to express that selection. Even worse, suppose Mary wants to choose a certain car body style, but this field is not encoded anywhere in the database, whether as a queriable or a hidden facet. There may be a way to express her preference as a selection on queriable facets (perhaps by indicating a certain combination of fuel efficiency and number of doors), but any such mapping from available queriable facets to her preferred dimension is entirely opaque. In the query panel if we can show to users how the values in queriable facets are related to the values in other facets, including hidden facets, then users can understand the relationship between hidden facet and queriable facets. This will enable them to query the hidden facets in terms of queriable facets.

Extension 4. Understanding Implicit Selections — Users often have an unspecified, complicated preference function that spans across multiple attributes. When they try to select optimal choice(s) along one attribute, it often leads to non-optimal choices in other attributes. In most real datasets, each attribute is dependent on many other attributes. When one selects a value from one attribute, it leads to implicit selection of values in other attributes. One cannot understand these implicit selections by observing one or few tuples. However, by looking at many tuples, one can statistically understand these implicit selections. For example, most SUVs in Mary's chosen year range will be costly compared to cheaper body types such as Hatchbacks, Wagons and Sedans. When users are about to select an attribute value, if we can show all the important implicit selections in other attributes, then users will not have to take this approach of trying to take an exploration path, and then later on retract because it does not satisfy the preference in some other attribute. If users see that the implicit selection in even one attribute is not according to their preference, they can save the effort of exploring further in that direction.

Given two result set $\mathcal{R}_1$ and $\mathcal{R}_2$, such that $\mathcal{R}_2 \subseteq \mathcal{R}_1$, we can determine the implicit selections by computing the statistical difference between $\mathcal{R}_1$ and $\mathcal{R}_2$ in terms of distribution of values in all the facets. The result set $\mathcal{R}_2$ is obtained from the result set $\mathcal{R}_1$ using a more constrained query.

4.2 Exploratory Search in Result Panel

The add-on extensions we presented in Sect. 4.1 can facilitate query formulation by providing better feedback to users through the query panel. However, there are phases during data exploration where users like to look at the query result to understand how they can alter, narrow down or expand their search condition. Not surprisingly, many user interface studies [5–7,17] have shown that users tend to browse quite often while searching for information, in addition to querying. These studies show that browsing is a rich and fundamental part of human information seeking behavior, and that querying is not the only mode of interaction with data. Users often formulate a more precise query after they have attained an understanding of the underlying data through quick exploratory browsing.

During faceted navigation users often start their exploration with a large result set (30K–40K tuples) and then gradually reduce it to a final result set of few tuples. Even during the interim stages of faceted navigation, users often look at sample results in the result panel to figure out the next facet value that they would like to select.

Following are some of features that one can provide in the result panel to facilitate exploratory search by providing users means to get quick sense of large result sets:

Extension 1. Information Visualization — There are many popular information visualization techniques, such as tag clouds [28,29], histograms, scatter plots, tree maps [25,35], parallel coordinate plots [21,22], etc., that can convey abstract information to users in intuitive ways. These techniques use visual representations and interaction techniques to help users see, explore and understand large amount of information at once. Some of these techniques convey important information through distinct text properties, such as font, color, etc. One can use these visualization techniques to help users quickly understand the data presented in the result panel.

Extension 2. Data Summarization — Large relational data is often summarized using data warehousing and OLAP technology [11,18,34]. There are also many data mining techniques, such as clustering [8,19,24,30,42] and decision trees [9,12], which can group data into meaningful groups according to some user given notion of similarity. For relational data some clustering based fast browsing interfaces are [31,37,39]. Many interesting data summarization techniques are presented in [20]. Web search result can be summarized and combined with some information visualization techniques to support fast browsing [28,29].

Extension 3. Ranked Results — Evaluating top-k query has been an important research in information retrieval and databases. Many results may satisfy a user's query. But by ranking the result set, these ranking algorithms enable the user to quickly locate the desired information by just browsing the top few results. For relational data, top-k ranking algorithms have been proposed in [2,10].

It is hard to design a top-k ranking algorithm that can simultaneously satisfy the information need of all users, because rankings change with change in users' preference. To satisfy most users, algorithms for computing top-k diverse set has been proposed, for example web queries [1,16] and SQL queries [12,33,41].

Extension 4. Skim through Results — Where user preferences are well understood, results may be scored and ranked. Information retrieval systems routinely present large result sets in this fashion. Users can then focus on the few top-ranked results and skim, or even ignore, the rest. However, in the database context there is usually insufficient information to rank with confidence. A common solution in the case of databases is to sort the result set on some attribute of importance: say `Price`, in our `cars.com` or `amazon.com` example. The user then has to scroll through this large result, reading through each tuple. While the data is sorted on the `Price` column, the user still has to focus on reading the other columns, which may not correlate with `Price`. Clearly, reading through each non-sort-key attribute of each tuple in a entire large result set is a slow and arduous task. Therefore, our task becomes that of supporting fast browsing (and more specifically, scrolling) over such a sorted relational result set.

Humans browse all the time, for example with newspapers and magazines. Visual cues in the layout assist users in browsing data quickly. Relational data tuples tend to comprise dense alphanumeric data, with few visual markers. Thus, there is a rather low maximum rate at which a human can skim tuples from a database. The only way to browse a database faster than this rate is to have the human eye see less than all the information.

To improve the usability of scrolling interfaces, we need variable-speed scrolling interface [37] that can automatically adjust the amount of information displayed based on the user's scrolling rate. The interface should display only a few selected tuples from each page, where the number of tuples is determined by the user's current scrolling speed. If some results seem interesting to the user while scrolling fast, the user can reduce the speed of scrolling, making the system show more tuples from the currently-viewed section of the data. In contrast to a typical sampling problem, the goal should be to identify tuples that provide the most information with respect to the entire scrolling session, and not just the page at hand.

Extension 5. Query Biased Snippet — When data is high-dimensional, we cannot show all the attributes of all the result tuples in the result panel because it will overwhelm users with information overload. Moreover, it will drastically increase the number of result pages that users have to browse because each page can fit only a few such high-dimensional tuples. To address these browsing issues, the existing faceted interface shows a query independent snippet for each result tuple, which sometimes has low relevance to the user's specific query. To make the result panel more informative we develop techniques to create a more informative snippet having both query independent and query dependent information that is relevant to the user's query and/or known user preference.

5   Evaluation

Addressing the limitations described above requires overcoming multiple challenges:

Challenge 1. Retaining Basic Faceted Interface — One common major challenge in designing any new add-on extension for faceted interface is to not alter the basic fundamental structure of faceted interface. A faceted interface provides one of the best means to query a database, and a concise and an easily understandable summary of the query result. Extensions that address specific limitations should be designed as add-ons that do not destroy the fundamental structure of faceted interface. For example, there are many limitations of the existing query panel due to limited feedback, hidden facets, etc. Ideally, one would like to address these limitations without introducing much change in the basic query panel structure. Similarly, the result panel should be improved in such a way that it looks very similar to the existing result panel, but it provides better quality information to users.

Challenge 2. Quality Evaluation — Most of the limitations that needs to be addressed are related to users' difficulty in understanding the information that is presented in the traditional faceted interface. For example, we highlight the difficulties that users face in understanding: the query panel, the result panel and the hidden facets. We claim that although users somehow manage to do things in the existing faceted interface, without even properly understanding what they are doing; they can do their navigation more effectively if we can provide them more informative query and result panel. In all the user studies we need to objectively measure users' better understanding through the use of our proposed add-on extensions.

Challenge 3. Performance Constraint — Faceted interface is a user-facing application. All user interface applications have strict computational constraint that requires small computation time ($< 500\,\text{ms}$) for providing real-time performance. Although the data mining algorithms needed to address the limitations are often computationally intensive, we need to design systems in such a way that we can provide real-time performance to users.

6 Conclusion

During the last few decades, database researchers have greatly improved the capability of databases both in terms of performance and functionality. But users' limited knowledge of what is contained in various databases and lack of technical expertise makes it very hard for them to directly interact with databases in a meaningful way. Managing a database system thus usually requires an army of database administrators, consultants, and other technical experts all busily helping users get data in and out of the database. To make databases more accessible to users, researchers in the past few years have started to look at the usability aspect of databases [23], such as usability in data storage, data access, data presentation, etc. In this paper we have focused on improving the usability in data presentation in e-commerce databases. We showed how one can combine machine learning, data mining, statistics, and information visualization to help users effectively explore through huge volumes of relational data. There are many popular data navigation techniques, such as clustering, ranking, faceted navigation, etc., with each one having its own strengths and weaknesses. Instead of focusing on a single navigation technique, we need to intelligently combine multiple such techniques in a way that enhances their strengths and cancels their weaknesses.

References

1. Agrawal, R., Gollapudi, S., Halverson, A., Ieong, S.: Diversifying search results. In: WSDM (2009)
2. Agrawal, S., Chaudhuri, S.: Automated ranking of database query results. In: CIDR (2003)
3. Apache solr (2014). http://lucene.apache.org/solr/
4. Basu Roy, S., Wang, H., Das, G., Nambiar, U., Mohania, M.: Minimum-effort driven dynamic faceted search in structured databases. In: CIKM (2008)
5. Bates, M.: Subject access in online catalogs: a design model. ASIS J 37(6), 357–376 (1986)
6. Bates, M.: The design of browsing and berrypicking techniques for the online search interface. Online Information Review (1989)
7. Belkin, N., Oddy, R., Brooks, H.: Ask for information retrieval. J. Documentation 38(2), 61–71 (1982)
8. Berkhin, P.: A survey of clustering data mining techniques. In: Kogan, J., Nicholas, C., Teboulle, M. (eds.) Grouping Multidimensional Data, pp. 25–71. Springer, Heidelberg (2006)
9. Chakrabarti, K., Chaudhuri, S., Hwang, S.: Automatic categorization of query results. In: SIGMOD, pp. 755–766. ACM (2004)
10. Chaudhuri, S., Das, G., Hristidis, V., Weikum, G.: Probabilistic ranking of database query results. In: VLDB (2004)
11. Chaudhuri, S., Dayal, U.: An overview of data warehousing and OLAP technology. ACM Sigmod Rec. 26(1), 65–74 (1997)
12. Chen, Z., Li, T.: Addressing diverse user preferences in SQL-query-result navigation. In: SIGMOD, pp. 641–652. ACM (2007)

13. Chu, E., Baid, A., Chai, X., Doan, A., Naughton, J.: Combining keyword search and forms for Ad Hoc querying of databases. In: SIGMOD, pp. 349–360. ACM (2009)
14. Das, G., Hristidis, V., Kapoor, N., Sudarshan, S.: Ordering the attributes of query results. In: SIGMOD, pp. 395–406. ACM (2006)
15. English, J., Hearst, M., Sinha, K. Swearingen, and K. Yee. Hierarchical faceted metadata in site search interfaces. In: CHI (2002)
16. Gollapudi, S., Sharma, A.: An axiomatic approach for result diversification. In: WWW (2009)
17. Goodchild, A.: An evaluation scheme for trader user interfaces. In: IFIP (1995)
18. Gray, J., Chaudhuri, S., Bosworth, A., Layman, A., Reichart, D., Venkatrao, M., Pellow, F., Pirahesh, H.: Data cube: a relational aggregation operator generalizing group-by, cross-tab, and sub-totals. Data Min. Knowl. Disc. 1(1), 29–53 (1997)
19. Guha, S., Rastogi, R., Shim, K.: Cure: an efficient clustering algorithm for large databases. In: ACM SIGMOD Record, vol. 27, pp. 73–84. ACM (1998)
20. Han, J., Kamber, M.: Data Mining: Concepts and Techniques. Morgan Kaufmann (2006)
21. Inselberg, A.: The plane with parallel coordinates. Vis. Comput. 1(2), 69–91 (1985)
22. Inselberg, A., Dimsdale, B.: Parallel coordinates. Human-Machine Interactive Systems, pp. 199–233. Springer, US (1991)
23. Jagadish, H., Chapman, A., Elkiss, A., Jayapandian, M., Li, Y., Nandi, A., Yu, C.: Making database systems usable. In: SIGMOD (2007)
24. Jain, A.K., Murty, M.N., Flynn, P.J.: Data clustering: a review. ACM Comput. Surv. (CSUR) 31(3), 264–323 (1999)
25. Johnson, B., Shneiderman, B.: Tree-maps: a space-filling approach to the visualization of hierarchical information structures. In: IEEE Conference on Visualization 1991, Proceedings, pp. 284–291. IEEE (1991)
26. Kashyap, A., Hristidis, V., Petropoulos, M.: Facetor: cost-driven exploration of faceted query results. In: CIKM, pp. 719–728. ACM (2010)
27. Koutrika, G., Lakshmanan, L.V., Riedewald, M., Stefanidis, K.: Exploratory search in databases and the web. In: EDBT/ICDT Workshops, pp. 158–159 (2014)
28. Koutrika, G., Zadeh, Z., Garcia-Molina, H.: Data clouds: summarizing keyword search results over structured data. In: EDBT (2009)
29. Kuo, B., Hentrich, T., Good, B. et al.: Tag clouds for summarizing web search results. In: WWW (2007)
30. Li, C., Wang, M., Lim, L., Wang, H., Chang, K.: Supporting ranking and clustering as generalized order-by and group-by. In: SIGMOD (2007)
31. Liu, B., Jagadish, H.: Using trees to depict a forest. In: VLDB (2009)
32. Marchionini, G.: Exploratory search: from finding to understanding. Commun. ACM 49(4), 41–46 (2006)
33. Qin, L., Yu, J.X., Chang, L.: Diversifying top-k results. VLDB Endowment 5(11), 1124–1135 (2012)
34. Sarawagi, S., Agrawal, R., Megiddo, N.: Discovery-driven exploration of OLAP data cubes. In: Schek, H.-J., Saltor, F., Ramos, I., Alonso, G. (eds.) EDBT 1998. LNCS, vol. 1377, pp. 168–182. Springer, Heidelberg (1998)
35. Shneiderman, B.: Tree visualization with tree-maps: 2-D space-filling approach. ACM Trans. Graph. (TOG) 11(1), 92–99 (1992)
36. Singh, M.: Effective Faceted Browsing. PhD thesis, The University of Michigan (2014)
37. Singh, M., Nandi, A., Jagadish, H.: Skimmer: rapid scrolling of relational query results. In: SIGMOD, pp. 181–192. ACM (2012)

38. White, R.W., Roth, R.A.: Exploratory search: beyond the query-response paradigm. Synth. Lect. Inf. Concepts Retrieval Serv. **1**(1), 1–98 (2009)
39. Wu, T., Li, X., Xin, D., Han, J., Lee, J., Redder, R.: DataScope: viewing database contents in Google Maps' way. In: VLDB (2007)
40. Yee, K.-P., Swearingen, K., Li, K., Hearst, M. Faceted metadata for image search and browsing. In: SIGCHI, pp. 401–408. ACM (2003)
41. Yu, C., Lakshmanan, L., Amer-Yahia, S.: It takes variety to make a world: diversification in recommender systems. In: EDBT (2009)
42. Zhang, T., Ramakrishnan, R., Livny, M.: Birch: an efficient data clustering method for very large databases. In: ACM SIGMOD Record, vol. 25, pp. 103–114. ACM (1996)

A Framework to Harvest Page Views of Web for Banner Advertising

P. Krishna Reddy[(✉)]

Center for Data Engineering, IIIT Hyderabad (IIIT-H),
Hyderabad, Telangana, India
pkreddy@iiit.ac.in

Abstract. Online advertising provides an opportunity for product sellers and service providers to reach customers and has become a key factor in the growth of economy. It is a major source of revenue for the major search engine and social networking sites. Search engine, context-specific and banner advertising are the major modes of online advertising. The banner advertisement mode has certain advantages over other modes of advertising. Currently, the number of websites registered comes to a billion. Each day, a typical website receives the number of visitors ranging from hundreds to millions. In a few years, the entire population of the globe is going to be connected to Internet and browse websites. It is possible for a product seller or service provider to reach every potential customer through banner advertising. In this paper, a framework is proposed to harvest the pages views of web by forming the clusters of similar websites. Rather than managing a single website, the publisher manages the aggregated advertising space of a collection of websites. As a result, the advertisement space could be expanded significantly and it will provide the opportunity for increased number of publishers to market the aggregated advertisement space of millions of websites to advertisers for reaching potential customers. It will also help in balancing the management of banner advertising market.

Keywords: Internet monetization · Computational advertising · Banner advertising · Internet marketing · Online advertising

1 Introduction

During the last decade, one could observe the rapid growth in the number of Internet users. In near future, one can expect that almost all population will be connected to Internet due to the reduction of connectivity and equipment costs. Due to the rapid expansion of the Internet, all the commercial activities are being shifted to online, and goods/service exchange through e-commerce is becoming the key driver of the economy. It is important to note that the cyber space allows constant visibility and accessibility to the products and services of business enterprises (seller) to the customer (buyer). In addition, the websites are available to the website visitors 24 hours a day.

© Springer International Publishing Switzerland 2015
N. Kumar and V. Bhatnagar (Eds.): BDA 2015, LNCS 9498, pp. 57–68, 2015.
DOI: 10.1007/978-3-319-27057-9_4

The evolution of the Internet had a profound impact on the advertising domain. The Internet provides an untapped opportunity for the advertisers and has become an attractive medium for advertising. Online advertising, also called online marketing or Internet advertising, is as popular as other advertising domains like television and news papers. It is a form of marketing and advertising which uses the Internet to deliver promotional marketing messages to consumers. It includes email marketing, search engine marketing, social media marketing, many types of display advertising (including web banner advertising), and mobile advertising [3]. In online advertising scenario, the ever increasing website visitors are the potential customers for the advertiser. The interactive nature of the medium can be used by the advertisers to hold the attention of the customer. These take the form of advertisement placements either in response to users web search queries, or at predetermined ad slots on publishers web pages [11]. Over traditional advertising, online advertising has the advantages of faster diffusion of information and the absence of geographical constraints. It has become a key factor in the growth of economy in the Internet age. It is a major source of revenue for the major search engine and social network sites.

Currently, banner advertisement mode is the major form of web advertising in addition to the contextual and sponsored search advertising [20]. It is approximately a US \$ 24 billion business [15]. A banner advertisement is described as a hypertext link that is associated with a box containing graphics which is redirected to a particular web page when a user clicks on the banner [6]. The Interactive Advertising Bureau developed standardized sizes and formats for banner ad placement [1]. A banner ad has become defined as a small graphical area on a web page, which include logos or messages to persuade the viewer to either click it or remember the brand advertised in a positive way. The banner advertisements can be in any form such as graphic images, animation, audio and video.

The following three entities are involved in banner advertising: advertiser, publisher and visitor. An advertiser is interested in endorsing products through banner advertisements. A publisher manages a website or an advertisement network that sells banner advertisement space. Finally, a visitor visits the web pages of a website which contains banners. Given budget constraints, an advertiser wants to advertise the products to the wider target audience segment which will result in enhanced sales. Given the ad slots, the objective of the publisher is to maximize the revenue by meeting the advertising demands of the maximum number of advertisers. A visitor is annoyed by the repeated display of banner advertisements. An advertisement should not infringe individual privacy. The publisher manages the advertisements.

The multiple issues concerning online banner advertising domain are as follows.

Auction mechanisms and charging schemes: The main challenge in auction mechanism design is the optimal allocation of advertising space for the multiple bids based on multiple factors. In addition, there is a complex problem of dealing with real time bids and dynamic advertising space for auction. Also, attracting advertisers with a pricing scheme which results in the higher return on investment for the advertiser is the key challenge. There are multiple pricing schemes offered by the publisher to charge fees for displaying the banner advertisement. For instance, cost-per-thousand impressions (CPM) model, cost-perclick (CPC), cost-per-event (CPE) model are the dominant models.

Scheduling and allocation of banner advertisements: Generally a website displays advertisements in consecutive time intervals and sells ad space to different advertisers. Since the maximum space to be used by advertisements on a given screen is always limited, the website owner may not be able to place all the advertisements that are competing for space in a given planning horizon. In order to maximize revenue, advertisements at a website should be scheduled optimally. Also, many advertisements compete for space on a given web page in any given scheduling horizon. Advertisements are updated at regular intervals of time and a rectangular slot with advertisements is displayed in each interval. As a result, each of these time intervals represents decisions to be made regarding which advertisements to present to the viewer. Users should not be annoyed by multiple display of the same advertisement. Also, the visitors to a website access the site based on their information needs and individual interests. The key challenge is to place the banner advertisement in an optimal manner to cover more target visitors by matching the similarity of advertisement and user interests.

Privacy issues: Most of the targeted advertising systems are based on the premise that the online behavior captures the user's interests. Tracking individual actions based on the online behavior is clearly infringement of individual privacy. The challenge is to develop approaches without infringing the privacy of the website visitors.

In addition to preceding research issues, we can also consider the building of banner advertising frameworks to increase the availability of page views or ad slots related to millions of websites as a research issue. In this paper, we have made an effort to provide a framework to harvest page views of millions of popular and unpopular websites. Currently, the number of websites hit a billion. Seventy five percent of websites are not active. A new website is registered every second [2]. Normally each of 25 million websites receives a certain number of visitors ranging from hundreds to millions. Currently, publishers manage the banner advertisement space of popular websites which receive a huge traffic. Millions of websites receive number of visitors ranging from hundreds to tens of thousands. The frameworks to manage the advertisement space of websites which receive relatively less number of visitors have to be developed. In the proposed framework, rather than managing the advertisement space of one single large site, a publisher manages the aggregated advertisement space of several sites of the similar category. So, the potential websites can be divided into clusters based on the topic and the interested publishers can manage the aggregated advertisement space of the cluster. As a result, there is an opportunity for the increased number of publishers to play role in connecting the sellers with buyers. Due to expanded advertising space, the products (or services) reach to large number of potential buyers. It will balance the management of advertisement space and result into the growth of the economy.

In the next section, we explain the related work. In Sect. 3, we explain the proposed framework. In Sect. 4, we discuss the design issues concerning to proposed framework. The last section contains summary and conclusions.

2 Related Work

We discuss the related work on the issues of banner advertising and website clustering.

In [23], a strategy was presented to model and predict the arrival and departure of users with Bluetooth enabled devices within an advertising system. It has been shown the performance of the bidding strategy proposed in that paper is better than the simple and randomized bidding strategies even in an uncertain environment. In [22], a mechanism was proposed under Cost Per Action (CPA) pricing model where the utility function of the advertisers is independent in an online advertising scenario. The proposed mechanism estimates the utility using sampling based learning algorithms and determines the pay based on the estimation. Florin Constatin et al. [11] proposed a model for auctioning ad slots in advance. In that work, the authors report the theoretical and practical problems pertaining to display advertising and study online pricing schemes where allocation decisions can be revoked with some cost. The solution proposed in [15] addresses the problem of trade-off in deciding which impressions to allocate to the guaranteed contract and which ones to the spot market for auction. Banner advertising has traditionally been sold via guaranteed contracts. A guaranteed contract is a deal between a publisher and an advertiser to allocate a certain number of impressions over a certain period, for a prespecified price per impression. However, as spot markets for banner advertisements, such as the Right Media Inc. [4] have grown in prominence, the selection of advertisements to show on a given page is increasingly being chosen based on price, using an auction [15].

Efforts are being made by Adler et al. [5] to solve scheduling problem by formulating as a standard bin packing problem. A greedy heuristic and random permutation technique was proposed to select and display subset of ads that fit an ad slot respectively to maximize the revenue. A Lagrangian decomposition method based approach has been proposed by Ali Amiri et al. [6] for scheduling of banner advertisements. Kumar et al. [20] proposed a genetic algorithm inspired from the standard multifit algorithm for the classic bin packing problem. In [19], a heuristic of Knapsack like problem is solved for every ad slot with an aim of maximizing expected revenue from K exposures of an ad with the specified constraints. The problem has also been studied by Nakamura et al. [21] as a linear programming problem. A variant of greedy algorithmic techniques to select the subset of advertisers that maximize the revenue is introduced in [13].

An approach to extract Coverage Patterns (CPs) from transactional dataset is proposed in [24]. Given a website clickstream transaction data over a period of time, the statistics of visitors behavior can be analyzed by processing the transactions. Set of web pages that can cover a certain percentage of transactions is called Coverage Pattern (CP). It was stated that the knowledge of CPs can be used for the placement of the banner advertisements on the web pages. Improved approaches for extracting CPs is presented in [25,26]. In [29], a model of content specific CPs and a methodology to extract content-specific CPs from clickstream data is proposed to capture the aspect of relevancy between the web pages and the banner ads to be displayed on the web pages. The notion of coverage and concept taxonomy has been employed by authors in [8] to group search keywords in the context of search engine advertising. The authors proposed an approach to advertise on the tail query keywords. A concept taxonomy was employed while creating the coverage patterns to ensure semantic relationships among the grouped keywords. Their results show considerable improvement with respect to utilization of advertisement space and achieved more diversity in capturing the eye balls for a particular advertisement.

To address the issue of targeted online banner advertising, a framework has been proposed in [14]. The approach is based on the idea of precisely targeting advertisements based on characteristics and behavior of individual users of information services. For example, visitors of a Travel page on an information service may be good targets for an advertisement for discount airfares, as would readers of the Travel section of a newspaper. Caruso et al. [9] proposed an approach for behavioral targeting using naive Bayesian model to maximize the profit by estimating the click frequency of banner advertisements. In [30], through experimental study on different strategies adopted by different advertising networks, the strategies adopted by different advertising networks such as *Taobao* and *AdSense* were discussed by considering the dataset from leading advertising network platforms and compare the strategies experimentally. It was shown that optimality of allocation depends primarily on platform targeting technology and demographical and categorical match of advertisements. In personalized systems, users long term activity is monitored. Many existing approaches to banner advertisement are based on demographic targeting or on information gained directly from the user. An approach for personalized web advertising has been proposed in [16]. It is based on knowledge extraction from the web pages content and historical user sessions as well as the current behavior of the online user, using data mining techniques.

In [10], the authors consider architecture of existing ad networks and present an online target advertising technique with a defined set of rules that ensure consumers privacy to avoid click frauds. Continuous monitoring of a users online habits, capturing and storing the data and linking with other databases is a privacy infringement. One of the aspects of privacy preserving advertising is not storing any data related to the web user on a long term basis. Kazienko et al. [16] propose an approach to address the issue of privacy preserving in banner advertising. The approach helps to capture immediate short-term user interests and select a suitable advertisement from the pool of available banners. An *AD ROSA* system has been proposed for an automatic web banner personalization, which integrates web usage and content mining techniques to minimize the user input and to respect the users privacy [17]. An experimental study has been conducted by Bleier et al. [7] on the effectiveness of retargeting technique for personalized banner advertising. The role of various factors like information and intrusive aspects in the effectiveness of the click through rates of the banner ads depending on the web browsing behavior of the customers was discussed.

Some of the research efforts related to website clustering are as follows. In [12], attempts are made to identify websites as a group to extract interesting information which can be used in various applications. In that paper, they introduce a new approach of website mining with an idea of considering each website as a super page and applied several classification techniques to classify the super pages like normal web pages classification. In [28], computer implemented methods are introduced to automatically associate resources like websites with a group user at given point of time. They define an approach to group by considering frequently accessed group of websites within a time bound by a user and thus provide valuable information about a particular group of users accessing a particular group of websites. In [18], they attempt to use unsupervised machine learning techniques to cluster website group home pages to identify similarity aspects of home pages of different website groups. In that paper, the authors use self organizing maps and principal component analysis based clustering techniques and validate the reliability of the clusters obtained.

3 Proposed Approach

We first explain the related terms and discuss the existing framework. Next, we present the proposed framework.

3.1 Existing Framework

We explain the notions website, ad slot, adslot pattern and advertisement space.

- **Website:** The number of web pages in the website can range from one to millions. The website is a collection of pages owned by individual or organization. We consider a group of web page as the website, if the advertisement space of a collection of web pages and corresponding click stream data is owned by one entity.
- **Ad slot:** Regarding banner advertising, the unit of advertising space to place a banner on the web page is called banner advertising slot or more commonly referred as an ad slot. A web page may have several ad slots.
- **Ad slot Pattern (AP):** A set of ad slots is called ad slot pattern. Each Ap has certain number of expected page views.
- **Advertising space (AS):** Consider n web pages. The ad slots of n pages is called the advertising space of n pages. Similarly, the ad slots of all pages of website (or a set of websites) are called as AS of a website (or a collection of websites).

The advertiser, publisher and visitor are the main entities in banner advertising. An advertiser wants that the advertisement should be reached to the large number of visitors. The publisher who manages the advertisement space makes efforts to maximize the revenue by covering the advertising requirements of as many advertisers as possible.

Normally, in the existing banner advertisement framework, a publisher manages the ad space for a single popular website or a collection of popular websites. The banner advertisement can be managed in a static manner in which the APs with certain number of page views are extracted and allocated to the advertiser and corresponding ads are placed in the ad slots. Also, the ads can be dynamically placed in the corresponding ad slot as and when a user clicks the corresponding web page. In this paper, we consider static framework to explain the existing and proposed framework.

The framework to manage AS of a website consists of two steps: Extraction of APs and Scheduling and allocation of APs. The framework is depicted in Fig. 1.

1. **Extraction of APs:** The input to this process is web pages and click stream data of the website. From the web pages, we know the web page id and available Ad slots. From click stream data, it is possible to extract the knowledge of APs concerning to the website. The output of this step is the sets of APs with the expected number of page views for each AP.
2. **Scheduling and allocation of APs:** Very large number of APs could be extracted from the AS of the website. Several advertisers put demand for advertisement space, such as number of page views with budget. The publisher follows appropriate scheduling and allocation strategy to maximize the revenue by allocating APs to advertisers.

The area of banner advertising is an active research area. Several approaches have been proposed in the literature (refer Related Work section) about the issues concerning auction mechanisms and charging schemes, scheduling and allocation of banner advertisements, methods to target customers, and privacy protection.

3.2   Proposed Framework

Currently about one billion websites are registered and 25 million websites are active [2]. Each website receives a certain number of visitors ranging from thousand to millions. For managing AS, normally, the publisher considers the popular

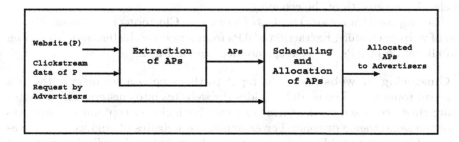

Fig. 1. Framework for managing the advertising space of a single website.

websites which contain a large number of web pages and receive huge traffic. It can be noted that millions of websites receive the number of visitors ranging from hundreds to tens of thousands. The frameworks to manage the advertisement space of websites who receive relatively less visitors have to be developed.

In near future, almost all the population is going to be connected to the Internet and spend time in browsing. We consider that every user who is connected to the Internet visits a certain number of websites, is the potential target for banner advertising. The main issue is to evolve an advertisement management framework which allows to exploit the page views of every user who is browsing the Web.

The basic idea is as follows. We can divide the websites into two groups: the websites which receive huge traffic and the websites which receive relatively less traffic. For example, a newspaper site is might be more popular and receive huge traffic as compared to the traffic received by the website of an educational institute. For banner advertising, the combined advertising space of several unpopular websites that receive relatively less traffic could be used to create potential AS similar to AS of the popular website. The main issue is to group the websites into meaningful clusters such that each cluster of websites receive certain type of traffic and provide AS which is marketable by a publisher. For example, a cluster of websites concerning medical educational institutions receive traffic consists of students, parents and teachers who are concerned to medical education and could become AS for promoting products related to pharmaceutical and medical domain.

We propose that it is possible to connect sellers with more potential buyers by providing a broad framework to harvest AS of Web by creating appropriate groups of websites. If we develop and operate frameworks to group the websites based on interests and enable thousands of publishers by assigning one or a few groups of websites to each publisher, it is possible to harvest page views of web to display ads. In the proposed framework, the publishers manage the AS of a cluster of websites of similar category. So, the potential websites can be divided into clusters based on the topic and the interested publishers can manage the advertisement space of a cluster of websites. As a result, there is an opportunity for increased number of publishers to play a role in connecting the sellers with buyers. As a result, the products or services reach to large number of potential buyers. It will also balance the management of banner advertisement space and accelerate the growth of the economy.

The proposed framework consists of four steps: Clustering of websites, Allocation of website clusters, Extraction of APs from a website cluster, and Scheduling and allocation of APs. These steps are depicted in Fig. 2.

1. **Clustering of websites:** The input to this step is a set of websites in a broad topic area. The module divides the websites into clusters. The websites are clustered based on the theme or topic. Each cluster contains the websites of the same theme or topic. For example, the websites of engineering educational institutes could be one cluster and the websites of medical educational institutes could be another cluster.

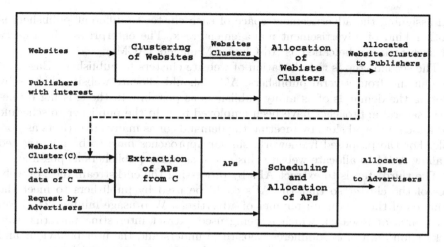

Fig. 2. Proposed framework for managing the advertising space of clusters of websites.

2. **Allocation of website clusters:** The input to this step is website clusters and publishers with interests. A publisher is willing to manage the advertisement space of a website cluster having specific interests. Based on the publishers' interests, the website clusters are allocated to publishers. For example, the websites of educational institutes provide a large user base which could be used to place the banner advertisements regarding educational programs.
3. **Extraction of APs from a website cluster:** In this step, the web pages and click stream data set of the websites of the cluster is processed, and the ad slot patterns are extracted with the expected number of views.
4. **Scheduling and allocation of APs:** Similar to the step 2 of the existing framework, the publisher follows appropriate scheduling and allocation strategy to maximize the revenue by allocating APs to advertisers.

4   Design Issues

We discuss the design issues by considering each step of the proposed framework. In the first step, the clusters of websites are formed. It requires the investigation of approaches for efficient clustering of websites such that each website cluster contains ad slots with a business potential so that a publisher could market advertisement space to advertisers with appropriate pricing strategy. The websites can be clustered based on the topics, demography, locality, types of business, profile of the users and so on. In the literature, research efforts are on to cluster the websites [12], associate a group of users to a set of websites [28] and identify clusters of similar home pages [18]. Scalable approaches are to be investigated to cluster millions of websites in an efficient manner.

Also, so far, publishers manage the advertisement space and provide services to advertisers. As, dividing a broad category of websites into several clusters and assigning the advertisement space of each cluster to different publishers is another kind of advertisement management task. The enterprises which carry out such task can be called as Ad Cluster Managers (ACMs).

The second step is the allocation of website clusters to publishers. Based on the demand from several publishers, ACM should allocate website clusters by meeting the demands of as many publishers as possible. In the existing framework, several approaches have been employed to help the publisher to schedule and allocate the ad slots by meeting the demands of as many advertisers as possible. For the proposed framework, similar approaches have to be investigated to allow ACM to allocate website clusters to as many publishers as possible.

The third step is to extract APs by processing the clickstream data of websites of the cluster so that the APs could be used by publishers to meet the demands of the maximum number of advertisers. Web usage mining [27], is an active area of research, which is being used extract interesting patterns from clickstream data of e-Commerce website to understand the user behaviour and recommend the products to users. Currently, APs are extracted by processing click stream data of single website. For the proposed framework, appropriate approaches have to be investigated to extract APs by processing the clickstream data of several websites of the cluster.

The fourth step is to allocate APs. This step is similar to the step 2 of the existing framework. The approaches employed to schedule and allocate APs of the existing framework can be used. In the literature, efforts have been made to generate ad schedules using traditional linear optimization techniques [5,20,21], greedy techniques [13] and pattern mining techniques [24–26,29].

The issues regarding privacy are the major aspect in the proposed framework. In the existing framework, developing approaches to protect the privacy of user is an important research issue [17]. However, in the proposed framework, the clickstream data of several websites is available to ACMs. The websites clusters and APs are to be managed by protecting the privacy and business interests of individual websites.

5   Summary and Conclusions

In this paper, we have proposed a framework to harvest page views of Web for banner advertising. It is proposed that the advertisement space of several websites could be aggregated by clustering similar websites to provide banner advertisement services. The publisher manages the advertising space of a cluster of websites. As a result, in principle, the expanded advertisement space of all websites in the web could be harvested to reach customers. It will provide wider opportunity for the sellers to reach the potential buyers. Also, the proposed framework will provide opportunity to a large number of publishers to play a role in managing the advertising space which will balance the management of banner advertisement market.

The proposed framework opens-up several research problems. Approaches have to be developed to cluster the websites having similar target customers.

It has to be demonstrated that the page views of users who are accessing multiple websites could be aggregated to form a potential banner advertisement space which could be marketed to potential advertisers with appropriate pricing strategy. Efficient allocation of website clusters to publishers is another issue. Also, efficient approaches have to be developed for extracting ad slot patterns by processing click stream data of the multiple websites of the cluster. Efficient scheduling of advertisers' requests and efficient allocation of ad slot patterns extracted from cluster to advertisers are also research issues. Also, most important, the advertising space of multiple websites have to be managed by protecting the privacy and the business interests of the website owner.

References

1. Interactive Advertising Bureau. http://www.iab.net
2. Internet Live Stats (2015). http://www.internetlivestats.com/total-number-of-websites
3. Online advertising (2015). https://en.wikipedia.org/wiki/Onlineadvertising
4. Right Media (2015). https://en.wikipedia.org/wiki/Right_Media
5. Adler, M., Gibbons, P.B., Matias, Y.: Scheduling space-sharing for internet advertising. J. Sched. **5**(2), 103–119 (2002)
6. Amiri, A., Menon, S.: Efficient scheduling of internet banner advertisements. ACM Trans. Internet Technol. (TOIT) **3**(4), 334–346 (2003)
7. Bleier, A., Eisenbeiss, M.: Personalized online advertising effectiveness: the interplay of what, when, and where. Mark. Sci. **34**(5), 669–688 (2015)
8. Budhiraja, A., Reddy, P.K.: An approach to cover more advitisers in adwords. In: 2015 International Conference on Data Science and Advanced Analytics (DSAA) (accepted: to be published, 2015)
9. Caruso, F., Giuffrida, G., Zarba, C.: Heuristic Bayesian targeting of banner advertising. Optim. Eng. **16**(1), 247–257 (2015). doi:10.1007/s11081-014-9248-8
10. Claessens, J., Díaz, C., Faustinelli, R., Preneel, B.: A secure and privacy-preserving web banner system for targeted advertising. Electronic Commerce Research (2003)
11. Contantin, R., Feldman, J., Muthukrishnan, S., Pal, M.: Online ad slotting with cancellations. In: Fourth Workshop on Ad Auctions; Symposium on Discrete Algorithms (SODA) (2009)
12. Ester, M., Kriegel, H.P., Schubert, M.: Web site mining: a new way to spot competitors, customers and suppliers in the world wide web. In: Proceedings of the Eighth ACM SIGKDD International Conference on Knowledge Discovery and Data Mining, pp. 249–258. ACM (2002)
13. Feige, U., Immorlica, N., Mirrokni, V., Nazerzadeh, H.: A combinatorial allocation mechanism with penalties for banner advertising. In: Proceedings of the 17th International Conference on World Wide Web, pp. 169–178. ACM (2008)
14. Gallagher, K., Parsons, J.: A framework for targeting banner advertising on the internet. In: 1997 Proceedings of the Thirtieth Hawaii International Conference on System Sciences, vol. 4, pp. 265–274. IEEE (1997)
15. Ghosh, A., McAfee, P., Papineni, K., Vassilvitskii, S.: Bidding for representative allocations for display advertising. In: Leonardi, S. (ed.) WINE 2009. LNCS, vol. 5929, pp. 208–219. Springer, Heidelberg (2009)

16. Kazienko, P., Adamski, M.: Personalized web advertising method. In: De Bra, P.M.E., Nejdl, W. (eds.) AH 2004. LNCS, vol. 3137, pp. 146–155. Springer, Heidelberg (2004)

17. Kazienko, P., Adamski, M.: Adrosa–adaptive personalization of web advertising. Inf. Sci. **177**(11), 2269–2295 (2007)

18. Kenekayoro, P., Buckley, K., Thelwall, M.: Clustering research group website homepages. Scientometrics **102**(3), 2023–2039 (2015)

19. Kumar, S., Dawande, M., Mookerjee, V.S.: Optimal scheduling and placement of internet banner advertisements. IEEE Transactions on Knowledge and Data Engineering **19**(11), 1571–1584 (2007)

20. Kumar, S., Jacob, V.S., Sriskandarajah, C.: Scheduling advertisements on a web page to maximize revenue. Eur. J. Oper. Res. **173**(3), 1067–1089 (2006)

21. Nakamura, A., Abe, N.: Improvements to the linear programming based scheduling of web advertisements. Electron. Commer. Res. **5**(1), 75–98 (2005)

22. Nazerzadeh, H., Saberi, A., Vohra, R.: Dynamic cost-per-action mechanisms and applications to online advertising. In: Proceedings of the 17th International Conference on World Wide Web, pp. 179–188. ACM (2008)

23. Rogers, A., David, E., Payne, T.R., Jennings, N.R.: An advanced bidding agent for advertisement selection on public displays. In: Proceedings of the 6th International Joint Conference on Autonomous Agents and Multiagent Systems, AAMAS 2007, pp. 51:1–51:8. ACM, New York (2007). http://doi.acm.org/10.1145/1329125.1329186

24. Srinivas, P.G., Reddy, P.K., Bhargav, S., Kiran, R.U., Kumar, D.S.: Discovering coverage patterns for banner advertisement placement. In: Chawla, S., Ho, C.K., Bailey, J., Tan, P.-N. (eds.) PAKDD 2012, Part II. LNCS, vol. 7302, pp. 133–144. Springer, Heidelberg (2012)

25. Srinivas, P.G., Reddy, P.K., Trinath, A.V.: CPPG: efficient mining of coverage patterns using projected pattern growth technique. In: Li, J., Cao, L., Wang, C., Tan, K.C., Liu, B., Pei, J., Tseng, V.S. (eds.) PAKDD 2013 Workshops. LNCS, vol. 7867, pp. 319–329. Springer, Heidelberg (2013)

26. Srinivas, P.G., Reddy, P.K., Trinath, A., Bhargav, S., Kiran, R.U.: Mining coverage patterns from transactional databases. J. Intell. Inf. Syst., 1–17 (2014)

27. Su, Q., Chen, L.: A method for discovering clusters of e-commerce interest patterns using click-stream data. Electron. Commer. Res. Appl. **14**(1), 1–13 (2015)

28. Trainor, D., Choc, T.N., Ainslie, A.N.: Automatically grouping resources accessed by a user. US Patent 9,043,464, 26 May 2015

29. Trinath, A., Gowtham Srinivas, P., Krishna Reddy, P.: Content specific coverage patterns for banner advertisement placement. In: 2014 International Conference on Data Science and Advanced Analytics (DSAA), pp. 263–269. IEEE (2014)

30. Wu, C.: Matching markets in online advertising networks: The tao of taobao and the sense of adsense (2012). Accessed 18 October 2012

Utility-Based Control Flow Discovery from Business Process Event Logs

Kritika Anand[1], Nisha Gupta[1], and Ashish Sureka[2(✉)]

[1] Indraprastha Institute of Information Technology, Delhi (IIITDU),
New Delhi, India
http://www.iiitd.ac.in/
[2] Software Analytics Research Lab (SARL), New Delhi, India
ashish@iiitd.ac.in
http://www.software-analytics.in/

Abstract. Process Aware Information Systems (PAIS) are IT systems which support business processes and generate event-logs as a result of execution of the supported business processes. Fuzzy-Miner (FM) is a popular algorithm within Process Mining which consists of discovering a process model from the event-logs. In traditional FM algorithm, the extracted process model consists of nodes and edges of equal value (in terms of the economic utility and objectives). However, in real-world applications, the actors, activities and transition between activities may not be of equal value. In this paper, we propose a Utility-Based Fuzzy Miner (UBFM) algorithm to efficiently mine a process model driven by a utility threshold. The term utility can be measured in terms of profit, value, quantity or other expressions of user's preference. The focus of the work presented in this paper is to incorporate the statistical (based on frequency) and semantic (based on user's objective) aspects while driving a process model. We conduct experiments on real-world dataset and synthetic dataset to demonstrate the effectiveness of our approach.

Keywords: Fuzzy-Miner (FM) · Process aware information systems (PAIS) · Process mining · Utility based process mining

1 Research Motivation and Aim

Process Mining consists of analyzing event-logs generated by Process Aware Information Systems (PAIS) for the purpose of discovering run-time process models, checking conformance between design-time and run-time process maps, analyzing the process from control flow and organizational perspective for the purpose of process improvement and enhancement [1]. FM algorithm [5] is one of the fundamental algorithms in Process Mining consisting of discovering a process model (reconstructing causality and work flow between activities) from an event-log consisting of process instances or traces. Several real-world run-time process models can be quite complex (spaghetti-like) due to the large number of variations and flexibility in process flow allowed by the PAIS. Filters are used by the

© Springer International Publishing Switzerland 2015
N. Kumar and V. Bhatnagar (Eds.): BDA 2015, LNCS 9498, pp. 69–83, 2015.
DOI: 10.1007/978-3-319-27057-9_5

process analyst or owner to focus on the important and interesting aspects of the process model and remove nodes and edges which are not important. Node and edge filters in traditional process discovery algorithms like FM are based on frequency of events and precedence relationships (captured as one aspect under metric called as significance). Increasing the value of node and edge filters removes events and relationships which have low significance and low correlation [5]. However, the output display behaviour and the abstraction level of the process model in traditional process discovery algorithms such as FM are not driven by utility or economic objectives or value [5].

The concept of economic utility of events, activities and relationships is not captured in traditional FM algorithm. Real life event logs often contain activities and precedence relations which are: (1) very frequent but of low utility to the organization and (2) less frequent but of high utility to the organization. Considering these two cases, we believe that frequency alone should not be the only driving factor for process simplification. We believe that the concept of utility of events and precedence relations should also be taken into account while simplifying and discovering process models. Utility-Based Data Mining is an area that has attracted several researchers attention dealing with cost-sensitive learning, economic factors and utility considerations [9]. A popular example in Utility-Based Association Rule or Frequent Pattern Mining is of lipstick and perfume which falls into the class of High-Utility Rare Itemset (HURI) rather than bread and butter which can be categorized as high-frequency but low utility itemset. Utility Based Process Mining (UBPM) is a relatively unexplored area and the work presented in this paper is motivated by the need to investigate efficient Utility-Based Process Mining (in particular process discovery which is the focus of this paper) approaches which do not capture only statistical correlations but also semantic significance of events, activities and relations.

We present real-life scenarios to demonstrate the importance of utility based control flow discovery:

1. **ITIL Service Change:** Figure 1 represents a small subset of activities and edges in an ITIL service change request. The number above the edges in Fig. 1 represents the frequency whereas the thickness of the edge represents the utility of transition. The process map in Fig. 1 reveals that in 7 cases, change is implemented without analyzing its impact on the system. The transition from 'Request for Change' and 'Change Implemented' is of High Utility and Low Frequency (HULF). The change may lead to implementation of an unfavourable modification. The FM process discovery may miss this flow at a user-defined high value of edge and node filter. However, Utility Based Process Discovery will retain the edge between the 'Request for Change' and 'Change Implemented' due to its high utility.

2. **Purchasing Process Example from SAP:** The example dataset of SAP has been taken from Fluxicon Disco[1]. Figure 2 shows the subset of a process model constructed using DISCO tool at activity resolution set to 50 % and

---

[1] https://fluxicon.com/disco/.

edge resolution set to 50 %. Low percentage value of resolution in DISCO corresponds to the high value of edge and node filter. Increase in the resolution value on slider in DISCO lowers the value of edge and node filter. 100 % resolution represents that all of the activities and paths are included in the process model. The red oval in Fig. 3 depicts 10 transitions from activity 'Send Invoice' to activity 'Authorize Supplier Invoice Payment'. Figure 3 depicts that at activity resolution 30 % and edge resolution 20 % these transitions which are important from security perspective remains undetected. The Purchasing Process example shows High Utility and Low Frequency (HULF) case.

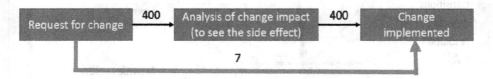

Fig. 1. Subset of Information Technology Infrastructure Library (ITIL) service change flow

Real life event logs can contain nodes and edges which are of low utility to the organization but are highly frequent. The Low Utility and High Frequency (LUHF) cases can make a process model more complex and hard to analyze due to presence of several nodes and transitions which may not be important from the perspective of economic utility and objective. For example, an activity which is responsible for saving the process state after every five activities [5]. In such situations, frequency plays a less significant role. Therefore, it is important to take into account both HULF and LUHF cases while simplifying the process model. This motivated us to investigate UBFM.

The research aim of the work presented in this paper is the following:

1. To propose the concept of utility based process model discovery in process mining.
2. To transform the spaghetti like process model to comprehensible process model, taking into account both the statistical (based on frequency) and semantic (based on user's goal) aspects.
3. To demonstrate the effectiveness of our proposed approach by conducting experiments on a large and real-world incident management data of an enterprise (Rabobank Group[2]) and synthetic dataset (Airport data[3]).

2   Related Work and Research Contributions

Our work falls at the intersection of Process Mining and High Utility Itemset Mining. In this Section, we discuss closely related work (to the research presented

---

[2] http://data.3tu.nl/repository/uuid:c3e5d162-0cfd-4bb0-bd82-af5268819c35.
[3] https://dl.dropboxusercontent.com/u/48972351/AFDATASET.csv.

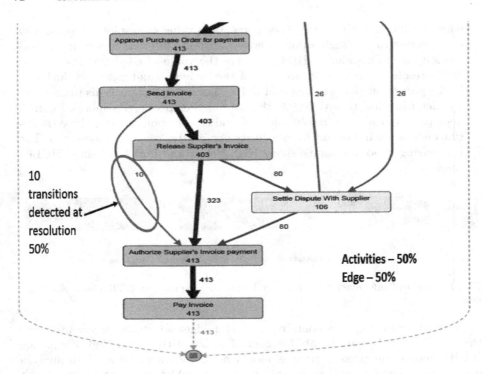

Fig. 2. Subset of process model build using purchasing example from SAP (Color figure online)

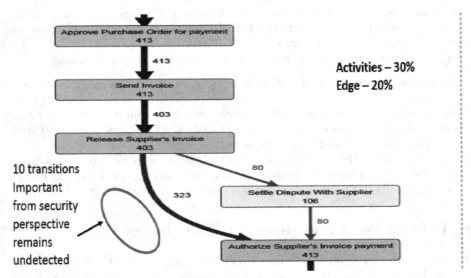

Fig. 3. Subset of process model build using purchasing example from SAP (Color figure online)

in this paper). Cook et al. [3] were the first ones to work on process mining. They explored the techniques that can use basic event data captured from an on-going process to generate process model. Weijters et al. propose Heuristics Miner [8], an algorithm which deals with noise and presents the main behavior of the event log. The algorithm includes constructing the dependency graph, constructing the input output expression for each activity in the graph and search for longest distance dependency relation [8]. Günther and Van der Aalst [5] propose FM, an adaptive simplification and visualization technique based on significance and correlation measures to visualize the behavior in event logs at various levels of abstraction. Utility is a concept from economics and is important for decision making by consumers [4]. Wang et al. propose that items or transactions may be of varying importance to the user. For example, the itemset (Perfume, Diamond) may suggest higher potential profits to a sales manager than the itemset (Perfume, Lipstick) [7]. Chan et al. propose high utility mining (HUM) approach that assumes that items in a database have different utility values [2]. Liu et al. in [6] propose a Two-phase algorithm for finding high utility itemsets. In Phase I, only the combinations of high transaction weighted utilization itemsets are added into the candidate set at each level during the level-wise search. In phase II, only one extra database scan is performed to filter the overestimated itemsets. In [10], Yao et al. propose a theoretical model of utility mining, which finds all itemsets in a transaction database with utility values higher than the minimum utility threshold.

3 Research Framework and Solution Approach

In this Section, we describe our proposed UBFM algorithm to efficiently mine a process model driven by utility thresholds. As an input to Algorithm, a business process analyst or a process owner provides external values to activities (Node Utility (nu)) and precedence relations (Edge Utility (eu)) in event log on the basis of benefit or usefulness to the organization in terms of profit, time, cost, security, etc. We introduce two terminologies:

1. **Utility Value of a Single Activity** - It is the product of frequency of activity and its nu value.
2. **Utility Value of a Single Edge** - It is the product of frequency of an edge and its eu value.

Node Filter (nf) and Edge Filter (ef) remove activities and edges according to their utility values. Higher the filter values, lesser activities and edges will be included in the process model.

UBFM uses same fundamental metrics [5] as FM but with different semantic meaning: (1) **Significance** - It measures the relative importance of behaviour of activities (events) and edges. It uses the concept of utility values rather than frequency of events and edges and (2) **Correlation** - It measures how much two events following one another are closely related.

UBFM takes two additional inputs: Node Utility (nu) and Edge Utility (eu) and the same set of following initial parameters as traditional FM [5]:

1. **Preserve Threshold** (λ_p) - It specifies how significant two conflicting relations need to be in order to both be preserved. Two relations are said to be in conflict when two events in the process model are connected by the edges in both directions.
2. **Ratio Threshold** (λ_r) - If set to a high value, conflicting relations will rather be resolved by removing both relations from the graph. If set to a low value, conflicting relations will rather be preserved by removing only the weaker relation.
3. **Edge Filter** (ef) - Higher the ef value, lesser edges will be included in the process model.
4. **Node Filter** (nf) - All event classes with significance measure lower than nf value will be subjected to filtering.
5. **Utility Ratio** (ur) - ur specifies the weightage given to significance and correlation. ur value of 0.75 specifies that 75% significance and 25 % correlation is taken into account.
6. **Attenuation** (*attenuation*) - It ensures that longer distance relationship affect the measurement less than the direct following relationship.
7. **Maximum Distance** (*distance*) - It measures the number of hops considered while detecting the edges within each trace.

UBFM consists of 3 phases: Phase 1 involves calculation of unary significance for activities and binary significance and correlation for precedence relations taking into consideration the statistical (based on frequency) and semantic (based on user's objective) aspects. Phase 2 involves edge removal and node aggregation and abstraction. Phase 3 involves the construction of process model using the GraphViz[4] API. We make some changes to the traditional FM algorithm so as to come up with UBFM algorithm. The pseudocode for UBFM is shown in Algorithm 1. The input to the algorithm is data comprising of Event Log, ef, nf, eu, nu, λ_p, λ_r, ur, *attenuation* and *distance*. The algorithm returns process model as output.

Steps 1–17 represent Phase 1. We calculate *unaryUtilitySignificance*, *binaryUtilitySignificane* and *binaryCorrelation* in Steps 4–8 for each trace within Event Log. *binaryCorrelation* is sum of Proximity, Originator, Data Value, Data Type and End Point correlations. We calculate *routingSignificance* and *distanceSignificance* in Step 11 and 13. Step 15 calculates *binarySignificance* metric as sum of *binaryUtilitySignificance* metric and *distanceSignificance* metric. Step 17 calculates *unarySignificance* metric as sum of *unaryUtilitySignificance* metric and *routingSignificance* metric.

Steps 18–32 represent Phase 2. Steps 19–22 perform conflict resolution for each precedence relation. *conflictResolution()* calculates the relative importance of edge in both the directions based on their *binarySignificance* values. If importance of both edges are greater than λ_p then both the edges are categorized as length-2 loop and signifies that both relations are important and thus need to be preserved, else they are categorized as exception or concurrency based on λ_r.

---

[4] http://graphviz.org/.

Step 24 calculates *sigCor* of each edge using *binarySignificance* and *binaryCorrelation* based on *ur*. Edge filtering is done in Step 26 for each node. For every incoming edge to that node, we normalize edge *sigCor* value. If the normalized *sigCor* value of edge is greater than *inLimit* then that precedence relation is preserved, else the relation is pruned. Same procedure is repeated for every outgoing edge from that node. We identify nodes for aggregation or abstraction by calling *findClusters()* in Step 27. The nodes whose *unarySignificance* is less than *nf* are either aggregated or abstracted. Nodes who are less significant but highly correlated are the candidates for clustering. Node aggregation occurs in Step 28 by calling the function *merge()*. The function call *merge()* checks all the predecessors of candidate cluster generated in Step 27. If all of the predecessors are clusters then the candidate cluster is merged with the most correlated one. Similarly, we check for all the successors. Node abstraction involves removal of isolated and singular clusters in Steps 29–30. Significance of clusters is average of significance of nodes contained in it. We remove the low utility clusters by calling the Function *removeLowUtilityClusters()* in Step 31. Steps 33–36 represent Phase 3. We save the edges to be included in the process model in 'Graph.dot' file. Then, we construct the process model using GraphViz API. The UBFM differs from traditional FM in following aspects:

1. UBFM uses the utility values of activities and edges instead of frequency to calculate the metrics in Phase 1.
2. We add an additional function *removeLowUtilityClusters()*. Low utility cluster means the cluster in which the sum of significance of nodes present in cluster is less than the node filter value. *removeLowUtilityClusters()* removes low utility clusters from the process model by making a connection between predecessors and successors. The low utility clusters are highly correlated but unimportant from organizational perspective. This helps in further simplification of process model.
3. We extend the function *findClusters()* in UBFM to reduce the complexity. We calculate the sum of significance of all nodes contained in all the candidate clusters, if the sum is less than *nf*, then there is no need to perform the Steps 29–31 in Algorithm 1.
4. UBFM takes into account the HULF and LUHF cases if the utility values of edges and activities are above threshold values while constructing the process model.

4   Experimental Analysis and Results

4.1   Experimental Dataset

We conduct our experiment on 2 datasets : (1) Small synthetic Airport dataset depicting the behavior of passenger at airport (2) Large real world BPI 2014 dataset from Rabobank Group Information and Communication Technology (ICT). The large real world BPI 2014 data is related to the Information Technology Infrastructure Library (ITIL) process implemented in the bank. The dataset is provided in the CSV format. It contains the event logs from interactions records, incidents records, incident activities and change records. The provided dataset is of six month duration from October 2013 – March 2014. We choose Incident Activity event log to build process models as it has information regarding the type of activities performed on a particular incident id and also the timestamp when this incident activity type started. 'Incident Activity' event log contains 46,606 traces, 466,737 events and 242 originators. There are 39 unique activities. Some of the examples are: Assignment, Status Change, Update and OOResponse. We order the activities according to increasing order of DateTime Stamp for each unique IncidentID. We add a start and end node at the beginning and at the end of each trace.

Algorithm 1. Utility Based Fuzzy Miner Algorithm(Event Log, ef, nf, eu, nu, λ_p, λ_r, ur, *attenuation*, *distance*)

Data: Event Log
Result: A Process Model

1 create an empty 2-D arrayList binarySignificance, binaryCorrelation
2 create an empty 1-D arrayList unarySignificance
3 **foreach** Trace t in Event Log **do**
4   **foreach** Activity A in t **do**
5    $\lfloor$ unaryUtilitySignificance(A) += nu[A]

6   **foreach** pair (A, B) where $(A, B) \in$ Activity &noOfHops$(A, B) < 4$ **do**
7   binaryUtilitySignificance(A, B) += eu[A][B] * attenuation
8   binaryCorrelation(A,B) = Proximity(A,B) + Endpoint(A,B)+Datavalue(A,B) + Datatypve(A,B) + Originator(A,B)

9 Normalize the metrics unaryUtilitySignificance, binaryCorrelation, binaryUtilitySignificance
10 **foreach** distinct Activity A in Event Log **do**
11   $\lfloor$ calculateRoutingSignificance(A, binaryUtilitySignificance, binaryCorrelation)

12 **foreach** pair (A, B) where $(A, B) \in$ Activity **do**
13   $\lfloor$ calculateDistanceSignificance(A, B, binaryUtilitySignificance, unaryUtilitySignificance)

14 **foreach** pair (A,B) where $(A, B) \in$ Activity **do**
15   $\lfloor$ binarySignificance(A, B) = binaryUtilitySignificance(A, B) + DistanceSignificance(A, B)

16 **foreach** Activity A in Event Log **do**
17   $\lfloor$ unarySignificance(A) = unaryUtilitySignificance(A) ++ routingSignificance(A)

18 **foreach** pair (A, B) where $(A, B) \in$ Activity **do**
19   sigFwd = binarySignificance(A, B)
20   sigRwd = binarySignificance(B, A)
21   **if** sigFwd>0 &sigRwd>0 **then**
22    $\lfloor$ conflictResolution(A, B, λ_r, λ_p, binarySignificance, binaryCorrelation)

23 **foreach** pair (A,B) where $(A, B) \in$ Activity **do**
24   $\lfloor$ sigCor(A, B) = ur * binarySignificance(A, B) + (1-ur) * binaryCorrelation(A,B)

25 **foreach** Activity A in EventLog **do**
26   $\lfloor$ edgeFiltering(A, ef, sigCor ,binarySignificance, binaryCorrelation)

27 clusters = findClusters(nf, unarySignificance, binaryCorrelation)
28 clusters = merge(clusters)
29 clusters = removeIsolatedClusters(clusters)
30 clusters = removeSingularClusters(clusters)
31 clusters = removeLowUtiltyClusters(clusters)
32 setSignificance(clusters)
33 Construct a Graph.dot file
34 **foreach** pair $(A, B)$where $(A, B) \in$ Activity &normalizedBinarysignficance(A, B) != 0 &normalizedBinaryCorrelation(A, B) != 0 **do**
35   $\lfloor$ Add the edge A -¿ B in Dot file

36 Make process model from Graph.dot using the GraphViz API

The Airport dataset contains 47 events, 7 activities, 8 unique traces and 7 originators. The 7 unique activities are: Show Identification Proof, Luggage Check, Collect Boarding Pass, Security Check, Wait, Board Flight and Enquiry. Table 1 shows the sequence of activities performed during one of the traces Trace3.0.

Table 1. Snapshot of airport dataset for Trace3.0

TraceID	DateStamp	ActivityName	Originator
Trace3.0	04-06-2009 17:21:03	Show Identification Proof	John
Trace3.0	04-06-2009 17:22:03	Luggage Check	Peter
Trace3.0	04-06-2009 17:23:03	Collect Boarding Pass	Katty
Trace3.0	04-06-2009 17:24:03	Security Check	Radha
Trace3.0	04-06-2009 17:25:03	Wait	Adolf
Trace3.0	04-06-2009 17:25:03	Board Flight	Om

4.2 Experimental Results

We perform experiment on 2 datasets using UBFM and FM. We choose λ_p = 0.6, λ_r = 0.7, ur = 0.75, $attenuation$ = linear and $distance$ = 4 for our experiment. Two of the inputs to UBFM is edge utility and node utility. We give default utility for all activities and precedence relation between activities as 5. We assign external utility to some of activities and relations as shown in Table 2 for Airport dataset and Table 3 for BPI dataset.

Table 2. External Utility of Activties and Precendence Realtions

Activity / Precedence Relation	Utility
Enquiry	20
Wait	0
Luggage Check ->Enquiry	20
Luggage Check ->Board Flight	19
Show Identification Proof ->Security Check	1
Collect Boarding Pass ->Board Flight	20

4.3 Airport Dataset Results

We create process models at distinct values of edge and node filter after applying UBFM to the Airport dataset. The value inside the nodes represents the significance and the value on edges represents the *util* value. Process models are described as follows:

Table 3. External utility provided by business process analyst

Activities / Precedence Relation	Frequency	Per-unit external utility
Quality Indicator Fixed	7,791	25
Status Change	50,914	0.5
Update	35,969	0.5
Assignment ->Closed	8,082	1.0

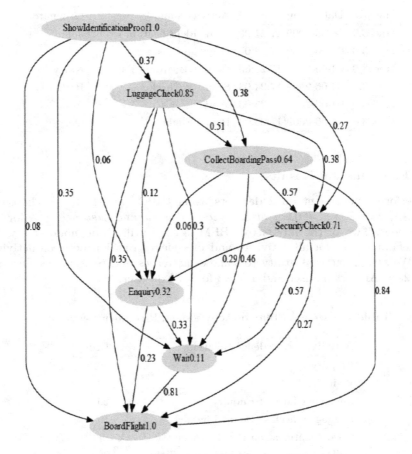

Fig. 4. Process model created using UBFM at edge filter = 0.0 and node filter = 0.0

1. Figure 4 depicts the process model at node filter = 0.0 and edge filter = 0.0. The process model includes all activities and relations of the event log.
2. Figure 5 shows the process model at node filter = 0.25 and edge filter = 0.25.
3. Figure 6 shows the process model at node filter = 0.75 and edge filter = 0.75.

4.4   BPI 2014 Dataset Results

The process model created by UBFM and traditional FM differs. Some of the points are as follows:

1. Node 'Wait' gets pruned in UBFM but it is there in FM at node filter = 0.25 and edge filter = 0.25 as shown in Figs. 5 and 7 respectively. The reason for removal of node is that 'Wait' is a LUHF node. Unary significance of 'Wait' in UBFM is 0.11 whereas, its unary significance in FM is 0.61.
2. Node 'Enquiry' gets pruned in FM at node filter = 0.25 and edge filter = 0.25 but it is present in UBFM as shown in Figs. 7 and 5 respectively. The reason is that 'Enquiry' is a HULF node,it occurs only 1 time in full dataset. Unary significance of 'Enquiry' in UBFM is 0.32 whereas, its unary significance in FM is 0.14.
3. Edge 'Luggage Check' ->'Board Flight' gets pruned in FM at node filter = 0.25 and edge filter = 0.25 as shown in Fig. 7 respectively. The distance from 'Luggage Check' to 'Board Flight' is high as compared to other edges. Due to low attenuation its binary frequency significance is less. Therefore, it is pruned by FM but it is present in UBFM as shown in Fig. 5 due to its high utility.
4. Edge 'Show Identification Proof' ->'Security Check' has utility value of 1. The edge is present at edge filter = 0.25 and node filter = 0.25 but gets pruned at edge filter = 0.75 and node filter = 0.75 in UBFM as shown in Figs. 5 and 6 respectively. Despite of having low utility, edge is still present in the process model because of its very high utility value. It depicts that the edge is of high importance to the organization. For example, utility threshold is defined by vendor as Rs 40. A supermarket vendor sells 100 breads at a profit of Rs 1/bread. Utility value of bread or total profit to the vendor by selling bread is Rs 100. Despite of having low per unit utility, it is still categorized as a profitable item.

UBFM discovers a complex spaghetti like process model at node filter = 0.0 and edge filter = 0.0 as shown in Fig. 8. The process models in Figs. 9 and 10 reveals that as we increase node filter to 0.25 and edge filter to 0.5 in UBFM and FM respectively, spaghetti like model transforms to a comprehensible model. Figures 9 and 10 differs in following perspectives:

1. Activity 'Quality Indicator Fixed' (QIF) has relatively less frequency (1.39% of activities present in event log) and high economic utility (HULF case) as shown in Table 3. At $nf = 0.25$ and $ef = 0.5$, QIF is not present in Fig. 10 but appears in process model discovered using UBFM in Fig. 9.
2. Activity 'Status Change' (SC) and 'Update' (UPD) has high frequency (50,914 and 35,969 respectively), but low utility from business perspective (LUHF case). Figure 9 reveals that SC and UPD disappears in process model discovered using UBFM. Here, process model simplification is driven by utility threshold and objectives.

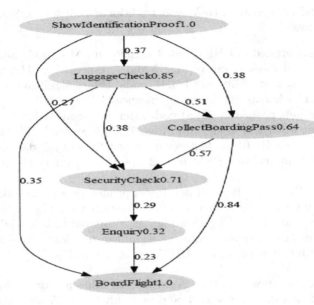

Fig. 5. Process model created using UBFM at edge filter = 0.25 and node filter = 0.25

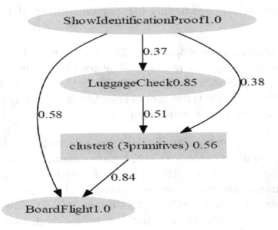

Fig. 6. Process model created using UBFM at edge filter = 0.75 and node filter = 0.75

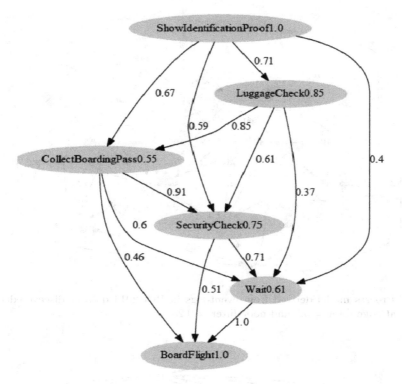

Fig. 7. Process model created using FM at edge filter = 0.25 and node filter = 0.25

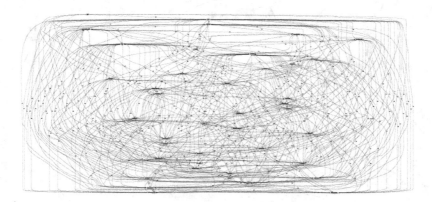

Fig. 8. Process model derived from event-logs in BPI 2014 dataset discovered using UBFM at edge filter = 0.0 and node filter = 0.0

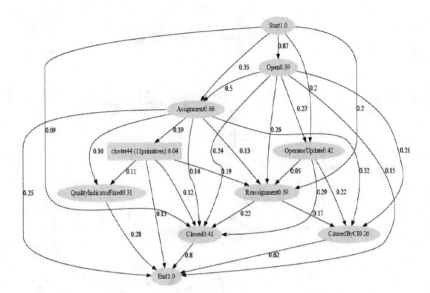

Fig. 9. Process model derived from event-logs in BPI 2014 dataset discovered using UBFM at edge filter = 0.5 and node filter = 0.25

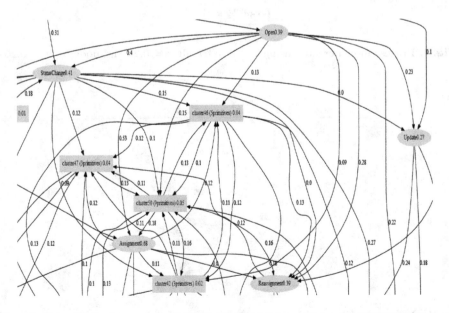

Fig. 10. Snapshot of process model derived from event-logs in BPI 2014 dataset discovered using FM at edge filter = 0.5 and node filter = 0.25

3. There is a decrease in number of clusters from process model discovered using FM in Fig. 10 to the model discovered using UBFM in Fig. 9. Function *removeLowUtilityclusters()* removes low utility clusters from process model which further simplifies process model based on economic utility in Fig. 9.

5   Conclusion

In traditional FM algorithm, the extracted process model consists of nodes and edges of equal value. However, real life event logs often contain activities and precedence relations which are HULF and LUHF. Therefore, the concept of utility of activities and precedence relations should also be taken into account while simplifying process models. We incorporate the utility concept in traditional FM algorithm, so as to come up with a new UBFM algorithm. We conduct a series of experiments on real-world dataset to demonstrate that the proposed approach is effective. We observe that UBFM mines successfully the high utility activities and precedence relations within utility threshold.

References

1. van der Aalst, W.M.P.: Process-aware information systems: lessons to be learned from process mining. In: Jensen, K., Aalst, W.M.P. (eds.) Transactions on Petri Nets and Other Models of Concurrency II. LNCS, vol. 5460, pp. 1–26. Springer, Heidelberg (2009)
2. Chan, R., Yang, Q., Shen, Y.D.: Mining high utility itemsets. In: Third IEEE International Conference on Data Mining, ICDM 2003, pp. 19–26. IEEE (2003)
3. Cook, J.E., Wolf, A.L.: Automating process discovery through event-data analysis. In: 17th International Conference on Software Engineering, ICSE 1995, pp. 73–73. IEEE (1995)
4. Edwards, W.: The theory of decision making. Psychol. Bull. **51**(4), 380 (1954)
5. Günther, C.W., van der Aalst, W.M.P.: Fuzzy mining – adaptive process simplification based on multi-perspective metrics. In: Alonso, G., Dadam, P., Rosemann, M. (eds.) BPM 2007. LNCS, vol. 4714, pp. 328–343. Springer, Heidelberg (2007)
6. Liu, Y., Liao, W.k., Choudhary, A.: A fast high utility itemsets mining algorithm. In: Proceedings of the 1st international workshop on Utility-based data mining, pp. 90–99. ACM (2005)
7. Wang, K., Zhou, S., Han, J.: Profit mining: from patterns to actions. In: Jensen, C.S., Jeffery, K., Pokorný, J., Šaltenis, S., Bertino, E., Böhm, K., Jarke, M. (eds.) EDBT 2002. LNCS, vol. 2287, pp. 70–87. Springer, Heidelberg (2002)
8. Weijters, A., van Der Aalst, W.M., De Medeiros, A.A.: Process mining with the heuristics miner-algorithm. Technische Universiteit Eindhoven, Technical report WP 166, pp. 1–34 (2006)
9. Weiss, G.M., Zadrozny, B., Saar-Tsechansky, M.: Guest editorial: special issue on utility-based data mining. Data Min. Knowl. Discov. **17**(2), 129–135 (2008)
10. Yao, H., Hamilton, H.J., Butz, C.J.: A foundational approach to mining itemset utilities from databases. In: SDM. vol. 4, pp. 215–221. SIAM (2004)

An Efficient Algorithm for Mining High-Utility Itemsets with Discount Notion

Ruchita Bansal, Siddharth Dawar[✉], and Vikram Goyal

Indraprastha Institute of Information Technology-Delhi (IIIT-D), New Delhi, India
{ruchita13104,siddharthd,vikram}@iiitd.ac.in

Abstract. High-utility itemset mining has attracted significant attention from the research community. Identifying high-utility itemsets from a transaction database can help business owners to earn a better profit by promoting the sales of high-utility itemsets. The technique also finds applications in web-click stream analysis, biomedical data analysis, mobile E-commerce etc. Several algorithms have been proposed to mine high-utility itemsets from a transaction database. However, these algorithms assume that items have a constant profit associated with them and don't embed the notion of discount into the utility-mining framework. In this paper, we integrate the notion of discount in state-of-the-art utility-mining algorithms and propose an algorithm for efficiently mining high-utility itemsets. We conduct extensive experiments on real and synthetic datasets and our results show that our proposed algorithm outperforms the state-of-the-art algorithms in terms of total execution time and number of itemsets that need to be explored.

1 Introduction

High-utility itemset mining finds patterns from a database which have their utility value no less than a given minimum utility-threshold. In utility-itemset mining, a utility function is generally defined to measure the importance of an itemset and varies according to an application domain. For example, in a retail store, a utility function can measure the profit made by the store by selling the items in the itemset together over a period of time. Recently, the high-utility itemset mining research has up-surged due to its wide applicability to different applications such as identifying fraudulent credit card transactions, network intrusions, medicine [1], molecular biology etc. Utility-mining has also been applied with other mining techniques like sequential-pattern mining [2] and episode-pattern mining [3]. One of the main reason of interest in the topic is due to its model expressiveness in terms of capturing the relevance and multiplicity of individual items within a transaction, which were the shortcomings in the case of frequent itemset mining (FIM). The FIM considers the frequency of itemsets to define the importance of an itemset and works on the model of presence and absence of an item only.

The majority of the utility mining algorithms consider that the items have constant profits associated them and do not take into account various discount

© Springer International Publishing Switzerland 2015
N. Kumar and V. Bhatnagar (Eds.): BDA 2015, LNCS 9498, pp. 84–98, 2015.
DOI: 10.1007/978-3-319-27057-9_6

schemes prevalent in the retail-market domain. However, in real life scenarios, shopkeepers often give discounts on the bulk purchase of items to improve their sales and earn a better profit. Discounts are also given on items which are close to being expired. Online shopping sites like Flipkart and Snapdeal provide discounts on the bulk purchase of items which varies for different items. Discounts are also given on the supply side of the retail chain. For example, Wal-Mart is able to offer low prices in part because it buys large volumes of goods from suppliers at cheaper rates. Suppliers often bid low prices in order to get a large amount of business which Wal-Mart promises. Mining of high-utility itemsets may result in the generation of false positives if the discount notion is not included. We propose to integrate the discount notion in the process of high-utility mining so as to get the correct high-utility itemsets as the output. Specifically, algorithms proposed by Dawar et al. [4] and Viger et al. [5] are two state-of-the-art algorithms for mining high-utility itemsets. We show how to embed the notion of discount in these algorithms and avoid false positives in the result set.

The algorithms on high-utility itemset mining can be classified into two different paradigms, tree-based algorithms [4,6] and vertical mining algorithms [7]. The tree-based algorithms mainly work in two phases. In the first phase, they find candidate high-utility itemsets, which are then verified in the second phase. The advantage of tree-based approaches is that the tree data structure is a compact representation of the complete transaction database and allows mining of candidate high-utility itemsets quickly. However, the verification time taken by these algorithms increases with the number of candidates generated. The vertical mining algorithms use an Inverted-list like data structure for its working. The algorithms in this category basically work similar to Apriori [8] and generate k-length high-utility itemsets by intersecting (joining) the $k-1$ itemsets. Basically, these algorithms first generate all the singleton high-utility itemsets and then proceed to the generation of pairs, triplets and so on. However, solutions based on vertical mining approach are simple and have shown to perform better as compared to tree-based approaches. But, the join operation cost is generally higher for small-size itemsets as compared to join operation cost for large-size itemsets. It is due to the size of lists associated with small itemsets being more than size of lists associated with large itemsets. On the other hand, it is efficient to perform join for itemsets with small size Inverted-list.

In order to avoid the costly join operation for short itemsets in the case of Inverted-list based approaches and avoid the costly operation of verifying the candidates in the case of tree-based approaches, we propose an algorithm which generates high-utility patterns without generating any candidate. Basically, our proposed approach combines the techniques used in tree-based and vertical mining based algorithm. The idea is to start with a tree-based recursive algorithm and traverse the tree until there is a possibility of high-utility itemset being generated. The algorithm then switches to vertical mining algorithm. We, in this case, study the performance gained by combining UP-Hist tree and FHM approaches.

Our research contributions can be summarized as follows:

- We show how the notion of discount can be embedded in the state-of-the-art high-utility itemsets mining algorithms to efficiently retrieve the correct set of patterns.
- We propose an algorithm, namely UP-Hist FHM discount, which combines two state-of-the-art algorithms, UP-Hist Growth and FHM.
- We conduct extensive experiments on real as well as synthetic datasets and the results demonstrate that our proposed algorithm outperforms the state-of-the-art algorithms individually in terms of total execution time and the number of itemsets explored.

2 Related Work

Frequent-itemset mining [8,9] has been studied extensively in the literature. Agrawal et al. [8] proposed an algorithm named Apriori, for mining association rules from market-basket data. Their algorithm was based on the downward closure property [8]. The downward closure property states that every subset of a frequent itemset is also frequent. Park et al. [10] proposed a hash-based algorithm for mining association rules which generates less number of candidates compared to Apriori algorithm. Zaki et al. [11] proposed an algorithm, namely ECLAT, for mining association rules which used itemset clustering to find the set of potentially maximal frequent itemsets. Han et al. [9] proposed a pattern-growth algorithm to find frequent itemsets by using FP-tree data structure. Vu et al. [12] proposed an algorithm namely FEM, which combined the FP-Growth and ECLAT algorithm for mining frequent patterns. However, frequent-itemset mining algorithms can't be used to find high-utility itemsets as it is not necessarily true that a frequent itemset is also a high-utility itemset in the database. On the other hand, mining high-utility patterns is challenging compared to the frequent-itemset mining, as there is no downward closure property [8] like we have in frequent-itemset mining scenario.

Several algorithms have also been proposed to find high-utility itemsets. Liu et al. [13] proposed a two-phase algorithm which generates candidate high-utility itemsets in the first phase and verification is done in the second phase. Ahmed et al. [14] proposed another two-phase algorithm, which uses a data structure named IHUP-Tree, to mine high-utility patterns incrementally from dynamic databases. The problem with the above-mentioned algorithms is the generation of a huge amount of candidates in the first phase which leads to longer execution times. In order to reduce the number of candidates, Tseng et al. [6] proposed a new data structure called UP-Tree and algorithms, namely UP-Growth [6] and UP-Growth+ [15]. The authors proposed effective strategies like DGU, DGN, DLU and DLN to compute better utility estimates. In order to reduce the number of candidates generated in the first phase by UP-tree based algorithms, Dawar et al. [4] proposed another data structure UP-Hist tree and better utility estimates. Liu et al. [7] proposed a new data structure named utility-lists and an algorithm *HUI-Miner* for mining high-utility itemsets. The algorithm avoids the costly generation and verification of candidates. However, the joining of utility-lists of an itemset to produce a new itemset is a costly operation. In order to reduce the number of join operations, Viger et al. [5] proposed a novel strategy EUCP(Estimated Utility Co-occurrence Pruning) to prune itemsets without performing the join operation. Recently, Li et al. [16] proposed several strategies to embed discount notion in the utility mining framework. Discount strategies like "buy 2 get 1 free", "buy 1 get the second at 70 % discount" were considered. They proposed a three-phase level-wise algorithm to mine high-utility itemsets. In this paper, we propose an algorithm, which is efficient compared to the state-of-the-art algorithm for mining high-utility itemsets with discount strategies.

3   Background

In this section, we present some definitions given in the earlier works and describe the problem statement formally. We also discuss the data structures and state-of-the-art algorithms for mining high-utility itemsets briefly.

3.1   Preliminary

We have a set of m distinct items $I = \{i_1, i_2, ..., i_m\}$, where each item has a profit $pr(i_p)$ (*external utility*) with respect to number of quantities. An itemset X of length k is a set of k items $X = \{i_1, i_2, ..., i_k\}$, where for $j \in 1.....k$, $i_j \in I$. A transaction database $D = \{T_1, T_2, ..., T_n\}$ consists of a set of n transactions, where every transaction has a subset of items belonging to I. Every item i_p in a transaction T_d has a quantity $q(i_p, T_d)$ associated with it. Below we define how utility of an item, an itemset can be computed in the context of a transaction.

Definition 1 *(Utility of an item in a transaction). The utility of an item i_p in a transaction T_d is denoted as $u(i_p, T_d)$ and defined as the product of the profit of the item and its quantity in the transaction i.e. $u(i_p, T_d) = q(i_p, T_d) * pr(i_p)$.*

Definition 2 *(Utility of an itemset in a transaction). The utility of an itemset X in a transaction T_d is denoted as $u(X, T_d)$ and defined as $\sum_{X \subseteq T_d \wedge i_p \in X} u(i_p, T_d)$.*

We also define a utility of a transaction as similar to an itemset over a transaction as given below.

Definition 3 *(Utility of transaction). The utility of a transaction T_d is denoted as $TU(T_d)$ and defined as $\sum_{i_p \in T_d} u(i_p, T_d)$.*

Let us consider the example database shown in Table 1 and the profit associated with each item in Table 2. The utility of item $\{A\}$ in $T_3 = 5$ and the utility of itemset $\{A, B\}$ in T_3 denoted by $u(\{A, B\}, T_3) = u(A, T_3) + u(B, T_3) = 5 + 6 = 11$. The transaction utility of every transaction is shown in Table 1.

Table 1. Example Database

TID	Transaction	TU
T_1	$(A:1)(C:1)(D:1)$	9
T_2	$(A:2)(C:6)(E:2)(G:5)$	67
T_3	$(A:1)(B:2)(C:1)(D:6)(E:1)(F:5)$	40
T_4	$(B:4)(C:3)(D:3)(E:1)$	29
T_5	$(B:2)(C:2)(E:1)(G:2)$	29

Table 2. Profit Table

Item	Profit
A	5
B	3
C	2
D	2
E	5
F	2
G	7

Definition 4 (*Utility of an itemset in Database*). *The utility of an itemset* X *in database* D *is denoted as* $u(X)$ *and defined as* $\sum_{X \subseteq T_d \wedge T_d \in D} u(X, T_d)$.

For example, $u(B, C) = u(\{B, C\}, T_3) + u(\{B, C\}, T_4) + u(\{B, C\}, T_5) = 8 + 18 + 10 = 36$.

Definition 5 (*High-utility itemset*). *An itemset is called a high-utility itemset if its utility is no less than a user-specified minimum threshold denoted by* min_util.

For example, $u(C, E) = u(\{C, E\}, T_2) + u(\{C, E\}, T_3) + u(\{C, E\}, T_4) + u(\{C, E\}, T_5) = 22 + 7 + 11 + 9 = 49$. If $min\_util = 40$, then $\{C, E\}$ is a high-utility itemset. However, if $min\_util = 50$, then $\{C, E\}$ is a low-utility itemset.

Definition 6 (*Problem Statement*). *Given a transaction database* D *and a minimum utility threshold* min_util, *the aim is to find all the itemsets which have high-utility.*

The high-utility itemsets at minimum utility threshold 50 are $\{CG\}$:65, $\{EG\}$:64, $\{ACG\}$:57, $\{AEG\}$:55, $\{BCE\}$:51, $\{CEG\}$:80, $\{ACEG\}$:67 and $\{BCDE\}$:54. We now describe the concept of transaction utility and transaction weighted downward closure (TWDC) [17].

Definition 7 (*TWU of an itemset*). *Transaction-weighted utility of an itemset* X *is the sum of the transaction utilities of all the transactions containing* X, *which is denoted as* $TWU(X)$ *and defined as* $\sum_{X \subseteq T_d \wedge T_d \in D} TU(T_d)$.

Definition 8 (*High TWU itemset*). *An itemset* X *is called a high-transaction-weighted utility itemset (HTWUI), if* $TWU(X)$ *is no less than* min_util.

Property 1 (Transaction-weighted downward closure). For any itemset X, if X is not a (HTWUI), any superset of X is not a HTWUI.

For example, $TU(T_1) = u(\{ACD\}, T_1) = 9; TWU(\{A\}) = TU(T_1) + TU(T_2) + TU(T_3) = 116$. If $min\_util = 110$, $\{A\}$ is a HTWUI. However, if $min\_util = 120$, $\{A\}$ and any of its supersets are not HTWUIs.

3.2   UP-Hist Tree and UP-Hist Algorithm

UP-Hist Growth is a tree-based algorithm that uses the UP-Hist tree for mining high-utility itemsets. The UP-Hist tree is created in two database scans. In the first scan of the database, TWU of individual items is computed. Items which have their TWU values less than the minimum threshold are identified and removed. The remaining items in the transactions are sorted in descending order of their TWU value and inserted to construct a global UP-Hist tree in the second scan. The root of the tree is a special empty node which points to its child nodes. Every other node N in UP-Hist tree [4] consists of a name $N.item$, overestimated utility $N.nu$, support count $N.count$, a histogram of item quantities (explained later), a pointer to the parent node $N.parent$ and a pointer $N.hlink$ to the node which has the same name as $N.name$. The support count of a node N along a path is the number of transactions in the database that contain the itemset consisting of items on the path from the root to that node. In order to facilitate efficient traversal of the tree, a header table is also maintained. The header table has three columns, *Item*, TWU and *Link*. The nodes in a UP-Hist tree along a path are maintained in descending order of their TWU values in the header table. All nodes with the same label are stored in a linked list and the link pointer in the header table points to the head of the list. The histogram associated with every node of the UP-Hist tree is defined below.

Definition 9 (Histogram). *A histogram h is a set of pairs $\langle q_i, num_i \rangle$, where q_i is an item quantity and num_i is the number of transactions that contain q_i copies of an item.*

The histogram associated with each node helps in computing the minimum and maximum quantity estimates of the node as defined below.

Definition 10 (minC). *Let h be a histogram, associated with an item-node N_i, consisting of n, $(1 \leq i \leq n)$ pairs $< q_i, num_i >$, sorted in **ascending order** of q_i. $minC(N_i, s)$ returns the sum of item-copies of k entries of h, i.e., $minC(N_i, s) = \sum_1^k q_i$, such that k is the minimal number fulfilling $k \leq \sum_1^k num_i$.*

Definition 11 (maxC). *Let h be a histogram, associated with an item-node N_i, consisting of n, $(1 \leq i \leq n)$ pairs $< q_i, num_i >$, sorted in **descending order** of q_i. $maxC(N_i, s)$ returns the sum of item-copies of k entries of h, i.e., $maxC(N_i, s) = \sum_1^k q_i$, such that k is the minimal number fulfilling $k \leq \sum_1^k num_i$.*

For example, the histogram of item C is $h = \{< 1, 2 >, < 2, 1 >, < 3, 1 >, < 6, 1 >\}$ and let support be 3. $minC(C, 3)$ and $maxC(C, 3)$ is 3 and 11 respectively. These quantity estimates are used by the algorithm to finally compute better estimates for the lower-bound and upper-bound value of any itemset. The readers can refer to [4] for more details of the algorithm.

3.3 Utility-List Data Structure and FHM Algorithm

FHM [5] is a vertical data mining algorithm that uses a utility-list data structure for mining high-utility itemsets. A utility-list associated with an itemset I is a list of triples storing three columns of information: TID, Iutils and Rutils. TID is a transaction identifier. Iutils(I, T_i) is the exact utility of itemset I in the transaction T_i. Rutils(I, T_i) is the aggregate utility value of items which occur after itemset I in transaction T_i. FHM algorithm assumes that items in a transaction are sorted in ascending order of their TWU values. For example, the utility-list of items $\{A\}$ and $\{B\}$ for our example database is shown in Fig. 1. FHM works similar to HUI-Miner algorithm in a level-wise manner. The algorithm joins two $\{k-1\}$-length itemsets to get a $\{k\}$-length itemset. For example, the utility-list of itemset $\{AB\}$ constructed from the intersection of utility-list of item $\{A\}$ and $\{B\}$ consists of single tuple $< 3, 11, 30 >$ only.

TID	Iutils	Rutils
1	5	2
2	10	22
3	5	7

TID	Iutils	Rutils
3	6	12
4	12	11
5	6	23

Fig. 1. Utility-list of item $\{A\}$ and $\{B\}$

3.4 Three-Phase Algorithm for Mining High-Utility Itemsets with Discount Strategies

Recently, Li et al. [16] proposed a three-phase algorithm for mining high-utility itemsets from a transaction database by applying several discount strategies. They propose to use rules to specify discount strategies and discussed four rules; "buy 1 with 50 % discount", "buy 2 get 1 free", "buy 1 get the second at 70 % discount" and "zero discount or no discount".

To mine correct set of high-utility itemsets with a discount notion, they incorporate all applicable discounts while computing of TWU of singleton itemsets. The $\{1\}$-itemset with their TWU less than the threshold are pruned immediately. In the second phase, a level-wise search is performed to find all the candidate high-utility itemsets. However, they do not consider any discount related information afterwards and their utility estimates are very loose. Due to which, their approach ends up in the generation of many candidate itemsets. In the third phase, the exact utility of candidate-itemsets is computed to find the actual high-utility itemsets.

4 Integration of Discount Notion in State-of-the-art Algorithms

In this section, we will discuss how trivial it is to introduce the discount notion in state-of-the-art algorithms, UP-Hist Growth and FHM.

4.1   UP-Hist Discount Algorithm

The utility value estimates are the places where if the discount notion is incorporated then it may help to compute better utility estimates. The tight estimates will result into improved pruning of useless search space. The UP-Hist algorithm computes TWU, Lower-bound and Upper-bound utility values of itemsets while exploring the search space for finding high-utility itemsets. The incorporation of various discounts schemes on items while computing the TWU value of singleton itemsets is straight forward, i.e., apply discount rules while computing the TU value of a transaction. We embed the notion of discount by assuming that different profits are associated with different quantities of an item x in the database. The discount strategies specified by Li et al. [16] can also be represented by a quantity-profit table as shown in Table 3.

Table 3. Quantity Profit Table

Item	1	2	3	4	5	6
A	5	7	11	13	13	13
B	3	4	5	6	10	10
C	2	3	4	6	8	10
D	2	3	4	6	8	10
E	5	8	13	17	21	21
F	2	3	4	7	9	9
G	7	8	18	25	30	30

Definition 12 *(Maximum and Minimum profit per unit item of an item x). Let x be an item in database D. Let $minq(x)$ and $maxq(x)$ be the minimum and maximum quantity associated with item x in D. The minimum quantity of item x in the database. Maximum profit per unit item of x denoted by $max\_pr(x)$ is defined as*

$$max\_pr(x) = pr_x(minq(x))/minq(x)$$

$pr_x(minq(x))$ is the profit of item x at $minq(x)$ quantity from the quantity profit table. Similarly, $min\_pr(x)$ is defined as

$$min\_pr(x) = pr_x(maxq(x))/maxq(x)$$

We now show how discounts rules can be considered to compute lower-bound and upper-bound estimates.

Definition 13 *(Maximum utility of an item in a set of transactions with support s). Let x be an item with support $total\_support(x)$, utility $u(x)$ in database D. $minq(x)$ is the minimum quantity of item x in the database. The maximum utility of x for s transactions is denoted by $MaxU(x, s)$ is defined as*

$$MaxU(x, s) = u(x) - (minq(x) * min\_pr(x)).$$

Definition 14 *(**Minimum utility of an item in a set of transactions with support s**). Let x be an item with support $total\_support(x)$, utility $u(x)$ in database D. $maxq(x)$ is the maximum quantity of item x in the database. The minimum utility of x for s transactions is denoted by $MinU(x, s)$ is defined as*

$$MinU(x, s) = u(x) - (maxq(x) * max\_pr(x))$$

Using the upper-bound and lower-bound utility values of individual items, we can compute the lower-bound and upper-bound utility value of an itemset as given below.

Definition 15 *(**Upper-bound utility**). Given an itemset $I = < a_1, a_2, ..., a_k >$ corresponding to a path in UP-Hist tree , with support count s, the upper-bound utility of itemset I denoted by $ub(I)$ is defined as*

$$ub(I) = \sum_{i=1}^{k} min(maxC(a_i, s) * max\_lpr(a_i), MaxU(a_i, s))$$

$max\_lpr(a_i)$ is the maximum profit per unit item of a_i.

Definition 16 *(**Lower-bound utility**). Given an itemset $I = < a_1, a_2, ..., a_k >$ corresponding to a path in UP-Hist tree , with support count s, the lower bound utility value of itemset I denoted by $lb(I)$ is defined as*

$$lb(I) = \sum_{i=1}^{k} max(minC(a_i, s) * min\_lpr(a_i), MinU(a_i, s))$$

$min\_lpr(a_i)$ is the minimum profit per unit item of a_i.

Claim 1. *The utility values of an itemset I are correct lower bound and upper bound estimates of the exact utility of I.*

4.2 FHM Discount Algorithm

The FHM algorithm constructs the utility-list of singleton items and explores the search-space in a level-wise manner. The utility-list data structure keeps the information of utility of an itemset transaction-wise. Therefore, once discount rules are applied for individual items that information remains in the utility list for each transaction. During join of two $\{k-1\}$ length itemsets, computation of exact-utility and remaining-utility uses utility value of each node (transaction) in the intersection list. Therefore, discount rules once applied over each transaction are carried forward in the case of a vertical mining-based approach like FHM.

5 Mining High-Utility Itemsets

In this section, we present our algorithm, UP-Hist FHM discount, that mines high-utility itemsets from a transaction database and incorporates discount notion. We will also illustrate the working of our algorithm with an example.

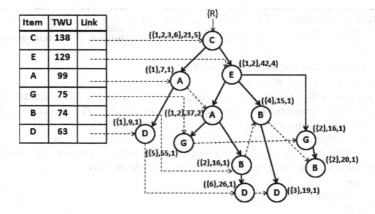

Fig. 2. Global UP-Hist Tree

Our algorithm is recursive and requires two scans of the database. In the first scan, transactions are scanned to compute the *TWU* values of each item. Items which have their *TWU* less than the utility threshold parameter are called as unpromising items and removed from further consideration. In the next scan of the database, items in every transaction are sorted in decreasing order of their *TWU* values. The transactions are then inserted one-by-one to construct the global UP-Hist tree. The utility-list of singleton items is also created in this step.

Each item i is picked from the header table in a bottom-up manner. The sum of node utility is computed by traversing the linked list associated with item i and if the sum is no less than the utility threshold, the upper-bound utility of the itemset including item i is computed. However, if the sum value for the node is less, the current itemset including item i as well as any superset itemset can not be of high-utility. Therefore, no processing is done further for the itemset. In the other case, the upper-bound utility is checked with respect to the threshold parameter. The algorithm switches to FHM strategy if the estimate of the itemset is no less than the threshold, i.e., the utility-list of the itemset is created and FHM algorithm is invoked. Else, the local tree is created and the UP-Hist algorithm is called recursively. We now present an example to illustrate the working of our proposed algorithm. We consider the example database shown in Table 1 with a quantity profit table as shown in Table 3. Let the utility threshold be 36. The global UP-Hist tree is shown in Fig. 2. Since, the header table is processed in a bottom-up manner, item $\{D\}$ is processed first.

The linked list associated with item $\{D\}$ is traversed and the sum of node utilities will be computed. The sum of node utilities is greater than the threshold. Therefore, item D is processed further. The upper-bound utility of item D is 16. Since, the upper bound utility value is less than threshold, a local tree for prefix D is created using paths $< CA >$: 9, $< CEAB >$: 26 and $< CEB >$: 19. The set of these paths is called Conditional Pattern Base (CPB). The *TWU* of each item

---

Algorithm 1. UP-Hist FHM discount(T_x, H_x, X)

Input: A UP-Hist tree T_x, a header table H_x, an itemset X, a minimum utility threshold min_util.
Output: All candidate high-utility itemsets in T_x.

1: **for** each entry $\{i\}$ in H_x **do**
2:     Compute $node.nu\_sum$ by following the links from the header table for each item $\{i\}$. Also, compute the upper bound utility of item $\{i\}$ denoted by $UB(\{i\})$
3:     **if** (**then** $node.nu\_sum(i) \geq min\_util$)
4:         **if** (**then** $UB_{sum}(a\_i) \geq min\_util$)
5:             Construct $I = prefix \cup i$ and its utility-list. Construct the utility-list of I-1 extensions (ULs) and call FHM(Y,item,ULs,threshold)
6:         **else**
7:             Construct the CPB of $I = X \cup i$.
8:         **end if**
9:         Put local promising items in $\{I\} - CPB$ into H_I and apply DLU, DLN. Insert every reorganized path into T_I.
10:         **if** $T\_I \neq null$ **then**
11:             Call UP-Hist FHM discount(T_I, H_I, I)
12:         **end if**
13:     **end if**
14: **end for**

---

in the CPB is computed similar to original database and unpromising items are removed. For our example, Item A is an unpromising item and hence removed. The transactions are reorganized and inserted to form the local tree of item $\{D\}$. In the next recursive invocation, item $\{B\}$ from the local header of $\{D\}$ is processed. Like the previous step, the sum of node-utility for item $\{B\}$ is greater than the threshold and the upper bound utility of itemset $\{BD\}$ is 25, which is less than the minimum threshold. The local tree of item $\{BD\}$ prefix is created and the algorithm is called recursively. Next item in the header table is $\{E\}$. The upper-bound utility value of itemset $\{EBD\}$ is 40, which is greater than the threshold. Therefore, the algorithm now constructs a utility-list for itemset $\{BED\}$ and switches to FHM strategy. The FHM algorithm computes the exact utility of itemset $\{BED\}$, which is 34. The algorithm explores the supersets of $\{EBD\}$ to find high-utility itemsets. After FHM completes its execution, the execution proceeds with the UP-Hist Growth algorithm. The complete set of high-utility itemsets returned by the algorithm is: $\{BCDE\}$:40, $\{BCE\}$:38, $\{G\}$:38, $\{AG\}$:37, $\{AEG\}$:45, $\{ACEG\}$:55, $\{ACG\}$:47, $\{EG\}$:51, $\{CEG\}$:64, $\{CG\}$:51, $\{ACE\}$:37 and $\{CE\}$:42.

6   Experiments and Results

In this section, we compare the performance of our proposed algorithm against the state-of-the-art algorithms UP-Hist Growth [4] and FHM [5]. We integrated our model in FHM and UP-Hist Growth to make them comparable with our

Table 4. Characteristics of Real Datasets

Dataset	#T_x	Avg. length	#Items	Type
Kosarak	9,90,002	8.1	41270	Sparse
Retail	88,162	10.3	16470	Sparse
Accidents	3,40,183	33.8	468	Dense
Connect	67,557	43	129	Dense

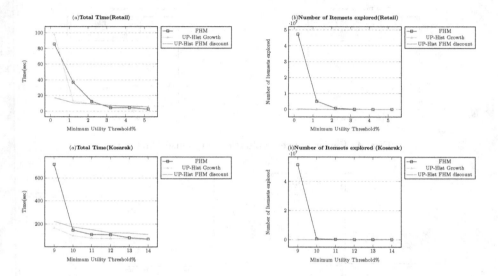

Fig. 3. Performance Evaluation on Sparse Datasets

proposed algorithm. We also implemented the three-phase algorithm integrating discount strategies [16]. However, we don't report the results of the three-phase algorithm as the execution didn't stop for three days on dense datasets. The algorithm gave out of memory error when executed on sparse datasets. We conduct experiments on various real and synthetic datasets. The description of the real datasets is shown in Table 4. We implemented all the algorithms in Java with JDK 1.7 on a Windows 8 platform. The experiments were performed on an Intel Xeon(R) CPU=26500@2.00 GHz with 64 GB RAM. All real datasets were obtained from FIMI Repository [18]. The quantity information for items was chosen randomly from 1 to 5. The external utility values were generated between 1 to 1000 using log-normal distribution. We compared the performance of the algorithms on the basis of total execution time as well as the number of itemsets explored. In our experiments, the utility values are expressed in terms of percentage. For each dataset, we find the utility threshold above which there are no high-utility itemsets and use it as a reference to express other threshold values in percentage. The results on sparse datasets are shown in Fig. 3.

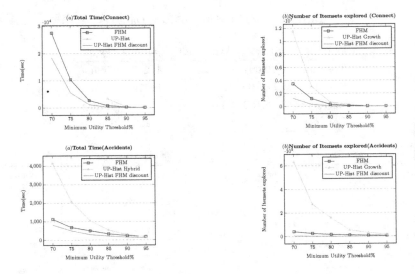

Fig. 4. Performance Evaluation on Dense Datasets

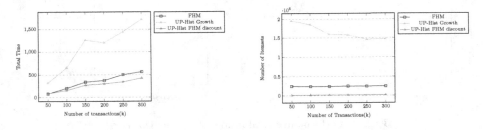

Fig. 5. Scalability on Accidents Dataset

The results show that our proposed algorithm beats FHM in terms of total execution time and number of itemsets explored. We observe that the difference between the runtime of the algorithms becomes marginal at high threshold value.

The results on dense datasets are shown in Fig. 4. The results show the better performance of our algorithm at lower threshold values, especially on Connect and Accidents dataset. UP-Hist performs worst on dense datasets as it generates a lot of candidate itemsets which need to be verified later. We are unable to report the execution time on Connect dataset at lower threshold values as UP-Hist algorithm didn't stop execution for more than 10 h.

We also conduct experiments to evaluate the scalability of our algorithm on Accidents dataset by varying the number of transactions in the dataset and the result is shown in Fig. 5. The result shows that performance of our algorithm improves with an increase in the number of transactions.

7 Conclusion and Future Work

In this paper, we integrate the notion of discount in the state-of-the-art algorithms and propose an algorithm to mine high-utility itemsets. We conduct extensive experiments on various real and synthetic datasets and the results confirm the superior performance of our algorithm compared to the state-of-the-art algorithms in terms of total execution time and the number of itemsets explored.

Acknowledgement. Third author will like to acknowledge the support provided by ITRA project, funded by DeITy, Government of India, under grant with Ref. No. ITRA/15(57)/Mobile/HumanSense/01.

References

1. Medici, F., Hawa, M.I., Giorgini, A., Panelo, A., Solfelix, C.M., Leslie, R.D., Pozzilli, P.: Antibodies to gad65 and a tyrosine phosphatase-like molecule ia-2ic in filipino type 1 diabetic patients. Diabetes Care **22**(9), 1458–1461 (1999)
2. Yin, J., Zheng, Z., Cao, L.: Uspan: an efficient algorithm for mining high utility sequential patterns. In: Proceedings of the 18th ACM SIGKDD, pp. 660–668 (2012)
3. Wu, C.-W., Lin, Y.-F., Yu, P.S., Tseng, V.S.: Mining high utility episodes in complex event sequences. In: Proceedings of the 19th ACM SIGKDD, pp. 536–544 (2013)
4. Dawar, S., Goyal, V.: Up-hist tree: An efficient data structure for high utility pattern mining from transaction databases. In: International Database Engineering and Applications Symposium (2015)
5. Fournier-Viger, P., Wu, C.-W., Zida, S., Tseng, V.S.: FHM: faster high-utility itemset mining using estimated utility co-occurrence pruning. In: Andreasen, T., Christiansen, H., Cubero, J.-C., Raś, Z.W. (eds.) ISMIS 2014. LNCS, vol. 8502, pp. 83–92. Springer, Heidelberg (2014)
6. Tseng, V.S., Wu, C.-W., Shie, B.-E., Yu, P.S.: Up-growth: an efficient algorithm for high utility itemset mining. In: ACM SIGKDD, pp. 253–262 (2010)
7. Liu, M., Qu, J.: Mining high utility itemsets without candidate generation. In: Proceedings of the 21st ACM International Conference on Information and Knowledge Management, pp. 55–64 (2012)
8. Agrawal, R., Srikant, R., et al.: Fast algorithms for mining association rules. In: Proc. 20th VLDB, vol. 1215, pp. 487–499 (1994)
9. Han, J., Pei, J., Yin, Y.: Mining frequent patterns without candidate generation. ACM SIGMOD **29**, 1–12 (2000)
10. Park, J.S., Chen, M.-S., Yu, P.S.: An effective hash-based algorithm for mining association rules, vol. 24 (1995)
11. Zaki, M.J., Parthasarathy, S., Ogihara, M., Li, W., et al.: New algorithms for fast discovery of association rules. In: KDD, vol. 97, pp. 283–286 (1997)
12. Vu, L., Alaghband, G.: A fast algorithm combining fp-tree and tid-list for frequent pattern mining. In: Proceedings of Information and Knowledge Engineering, pp. 472–477 (2011)
13. Liu, Y., Liao, W., Choudhary, A.K.: A two-phase algorithm for fast discovery of high utility itemsets. In: Ho, T.-B., Cheung, D., Liu, H. (eds.) PAKDD 2005. LNCS (LNAI), vol. 3518, pp. 689–695. Springer, Heidelberg (2005)

14. Ahmed, C.F., Tanbeer, S.K., Jeong, B.-S., Lee, Y.-K.: Efficient tree structures for high utility pattern mining in incremental databases. IEEE TKDE **21**(12), 1708–1721 (2009)
15. Tseng, V.S., Shie, B.-N., Wu, C.-W., Yu, P.S.: Efficient algorithms for mining high utility itemsets from transactional databases. IEEE TKDE **25**(8), 1772–1786 (2013)
16. Li, Y., Zhang, Z.H., Chen, W.B., Min, F.: Mining high utility itemsets with discount strategies. Inf. Comput. Sci. **11**, 6297–6307 (2014)
17. Liu, Y., Liao, W.-K., Choudhary, A.: A fast high utility itemsets mining algorithm. In: International Workshop on Utility-Based Data Mining, pp. 90–99 (2005)
18. Goethals, B., Zaki, M.J.: The fimi repository (2012)

Big Data: Models and Algorithms

Design of Algorithms for Big Data Analytics

Raj Bhatnagar[✉]

Department of Electrical Engineering and Computing Systems,
University of Cincinnati, Cincinnati, OH, USA
raj.bhatnagar@uc.edu

Abstract. Processing of high volume and high velocity datasets requires design of algorithms that can exploit the availability of multiple servers configured for asynchronous and simultaneous processing of smaller chunks of large datasets. The Map-Reduce paradigm provides a very effective mechanism for designing efficient algorithms for processing high volume datasets. Sometimes a simple adaptation of a sequential solution of a problem to design Map-Reduce algorithms doesn't draw the full potential of the paradigm. A completely new rethink of the solution from the perspective of the powers of Map-Reduce paradigm can provide very large gains. We present here an example to show that the simple adaptation does not perform as well as a completely new Map-Reduce compatible solution. We do this using the problem of finding all formal concepts from a binary dataset. The problem of handling very high volume data is another important problem and requires newer thinking when designing solutions. We present here an example of the design of a model learning solution from a very high volume monitoring data from a manufacturing environment.

1 Introduction

Dataset sizes in all domains are growing at a pace that is faster than the pace at which the CPU speeds and the hardware performance metrics are growing. Most of the data analytics algorithms have high computational complexity and are rarely bounded within the polynomial time and space limits. Therefore, for analyzing these very large datasets the only viable alternative is to harness the power of multiple processors working in parallel, preferably working on different chunks of the large dataset. Traditional paradigms for parallel processing are too restrictive for the current scales of data. The flexibility in deployment and asynchronous operation of multiple independent servers expected to participate in these computations require an equally flexible and adaptable operating system structure and also a programming paradigm. Map-Reduce is an algorithms design formalism that working within the hadoop kinds of environments is very suitable for processing large datasets. This paradigm can deploy a flexible number of asynchronously working servers without requiring extensive message-passing or requiring shared memory among the processors. Design of data analytics algorithms using the Map-Reduce algorithms requires one to understand the nature, the strengths, and the weaknesses of this programming paradigm.

N. Kumar and V. Bhatnagar (Eds.): BDA 2015, LNCS 9498, pp. 101–107, 2015.
DOI: 10.1007/978-3-319-27057-9_7

Most analytics algorithms are designed as iterative algorithms that assume the large original dataset to persist across iterations and use some transient data that stays in dynamic memory. The Map-Reduce paradigm, as typically supported by hadoop type of environments, is not suitable for multi-iteration algorithms.

We illustrate below an example problem, that of finding all formal concepts from a large binary dataset. On single processor systems this problem is typically solved using an iterative formulation that processes the nodes of a Depth-first search tree. We illustrate a completely new formulation that can be performed in a single iteration and is facilitated by the power of Mapper and Reducer Operations. The second example we illustrate relates to a monitored data stream in which very large amounts of data is generated continuously. We need to use this data to predict the health related parameters of the underlying system. A model of the system also needs to be extracted from the same data stream. All of the data does not need to be retained for any long term record but enough information and features must be extracted to enable our model-building and prognostics tasks.

2   Building FCA Lattice

Let us consider the problem of building a lattice of formal concepts from a binary database. This is an important problem from a large number of knowledge extraction perspectives.

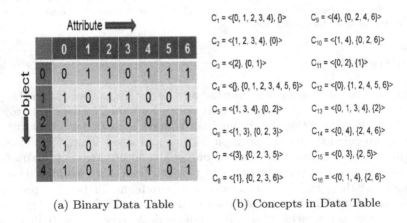

(a) Binary Data Table   (b) Concepts in Data Table

Fig. 1. Example binary dataset and its concepts

The binary dataset in Fig. 1a shows a dataset that is typically encountered in many application domains. The objects along the rows may be genes and the columns may correspond to diseases. The objects may also correspond to documents and the columns may correspond to words that occur in these documents. An entry of '1' in the table means that the column entry is related to row object and a '0' entry means that the column entry is not related to the row objects. In many applications binary datasets typically have about 50,000 rows and 1,000 columns. A "concept" existing in such a binary dataset is defined to be a rectangle of only '1' entries that can be formed by arbitrary shuffling of rows and columns of the binary dataset, such that the rectangle is the largest possible in the following sense. A rectangle of '1's corresponding to a "concept" should not be extendable by adding any additional row or column while still meeting the condition of containing only the '1's in the rectangle. These concepts found a database are very meaningful and concise representation of co-occurrence or associational knowledge embedded in the dataset. Figure 1b shows all the concepts embedded in the binary dataset of Fig. 1a.

All the concepts of a binary dataset can also be organized in the form of a lattice as shown in Fig. 2. The parent-child relationships of this lattice are defined using the subset/superset relation between their object sets and between their itemsets. The theory of formal concept analysis [2].

2.1 Inefficient Map-Reduce Based Design

Most of the existing algorithms for finding the concepts are not scalable to very large datasets. A dataset of 5000 rows and 60 columns takes more than twelve hours of CPU time on standard desktop computers. We need scalable algorithms that can process much larger datasets in reasonable time. Power of parallel computing using Map-Reduce paradigm can be employed for designing algorithms that are much more scalable than the

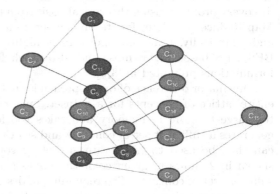

Fig. 2. Example binary dataset and its concepts

existing ones. There are various ways in which the concept-discovery problem can be formulated using the Map-Reduce paradigm and one such formulation has been presented in [3]. This parallel formulation takes the traditional Depth First Search (DFS) based algorithm for finding the concepts, uses the Map-Reduce formulation, and seeks to parallelize the processing of various branches at each node of the corresponding Breadth First Search tree. This formulation is not very efficient because it needs to run as many iterations of Map-Reduce as there are nodes in the DFS/BFS search tree. Multiple iterations of Map-Reduce make the algorithm computationally very expensive. Inherently, the search for concepts remains structured as DFS or BFS-based and therefore, at core, a serial processing of different nodes in the search tree takes place.

Map-Reduce paradigm has been employed to develop faster concept-discovery algorithms. The first such algorithm was presented in [3] and is a close Map-Reduce adaptation of the ClosebyOne algorithm [4]. The authors of [5] present two more algorithms called *MRGanter* and *MRGanter+* that are Map-Reduce adaptations of the basic DFS based algorithm presented by Ganter in [2]. The latter of these implementations is shown to perform the best among all possible algorithms, but the algorithms are run on Twister system that facilitates iterations of Map-Reduce operations. This is facilitated by splitting the data into static and dynamic parts and the static parts consisting the large volumes of the data, are not removed from the servers between the iterations. On the Mushrooms dataset having 125 attributes and 8124 objects the best of these algorithms requires 14 Map-Reduce iterations. On a commonly available hadoop implementations these iterations will become extremely expensive. Our algorithms has abandoned the DFS skeleton for finding the concepts and is using a different approach better suited to the Map-reduce paradigm. This proposed algorithms performs the tasks in less than tenth of the time required by the above mentioned algorithms.

2.2 Efficient Map-Reduce Based Design

We have developed and presented a completely new formulation for the concept discovery problem, using theoretical basis from the FCA theory and adapting the Map-Reduce paradigm for its implementation [1]. We show in [1] theoretically and empirically, that our algorithm is highly efficient when compared to the BFS/DFS based algorithms, and also much faster compared to Map-Reduce formulations presented in [3,5].

One major difference of our approach is that we do not seek to enumerate the entire lattice of concepts for a dataset. Such exhaustive enumeration is always too large to store in memory and takes too long to compute. Our algorithm generates a sufficient set of concepts and stores it. This sufficient set of concepts can then be used to enumerate any other concept in the lattice. The lattice shown in 2 shows in green color the nodes generated by our algorithm as the sufficient set of concepts. The remaining nodes of a lattice can then be generated by simple set union and intersection operations on the concepts in the sufficient set. This example shows a large number of concepts in the sufficient set, but for very large datasets typically the sufficient set of concepts is a very small fraction of the number of all the concepts in the lattice. The process for generating the sufficient set of is driven in part by a Map-Reduce formulation. This formulation looks at the problem of finding the rows or columns corresponding to a set of columns or rows in one single operation. That is, given a set of items, we should find all those rows for which all the item-columns contain '1's. And then, given a set of row ids, we should find all those columns such that the given rows have all '1's in them. For very large datasets these two mapping operations cannot be easily done as single step macro operations. But map-Reduce enables us to achieve this and that helps us design a very efficient algorithm. The process of merging the concept's components that appear in different regions of rows or columns can only be partially merged within the map-reduce based formulation. The final merging of concept components is much less complex problem because the problem size has been reduced from that of the whole big original data to only the size of the sufficient set of concepts. This last merging of concept components is done on a single processor machine by our algorithm Table 1.

Table 1. Time (Seconds) enumerating sufficient set and of complete lattice

Dataset	Mushroom	Anon-Web	CensusIncome
# of concepts	219010	129009	86532
NextClosure *Sequential*	618	14671	18230
CloseByOne *Sequential*	2543	656	7465
MRGanter map-red	20269 (5 nodes)	20110 (3 nodes)	9654 (11 nodes)
MRCbO map-red	241 (11 nodes)	693 (11 nodes)	803 (11 nodes)
MRGanter+ map-red	198 (9 nodes)	496 (9 nodes)	358 (9 nodes)
Our algorithm suffic. set only map-red	42 (10 nodes)	26 (10 nodes)	69 (10 nodes)
Our algorithm enumeration on single processor	OutOfMemory	361	OutOfMemory
Number of concepts in sufficient set	117	365	147

Exhaustive enumeration from the sufficient set may then be performed by a non-parallelized algorithm on a single processor. It is efficient to create and store only the sufficient set of concepts. This set implicitly contains information about all the other concepts in the lattice but we don't need to keep them in an enumerated form.

One primary idea underlying a Map-Reduce formulation of an algorithm is to split the table horizontally into a number of partitions. Each partition is then processed on an independent server by a *Mapper* function. The outputs from the mapper functions are gathered at a central location, sorted, and then split again among a number of independent servers that run the *Reducer* function. The outputs of the reducer function from different servers are then collected at a central location and form the output of a Map-Reduce iteration. One last step of the algorithm of merging of concepts' components is then performed on a single processor system.

A comparison of two different formulations as reported in [1] can be seen in the table here.

3 High Velocity Datasets

There are many situations in which a large amount of data is being generated as a result of monitoring some physical or social system. Storing all the data is neither useful nor feasible. However, we want to learn from this high volume stream of data all the essential details about the monitored system and discard the data. There is some buffer available for storing all monitored data for some limited window. We consider the case of a spindle from a manufacturing domain as shown in Fig. 3.

The problem to be addressed is that the bearings of these spindles wear out over time and crash during a manufacturing operation. Such disruptive crashes cause a lot of loss by first damaging the piece being manufactured and second by holding up the pipeline of operations on the shop floor. It is therefore very valuable to predict the remaining life of the bearings installed within a spindle. We installed an angular acceleration sensor on the spindle and this continuously monitors the acceleration and stores the data. In order to detect the

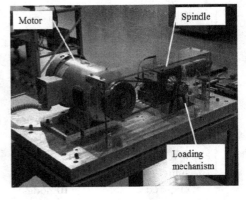

Fig. 3. Spindle testbed

vibrations that indicate deteriorating health we need to sample the acceleration at a rate of 25,000 samples per second. In addition to predicting the remaining life of the bearings we need to find out the characteristics of the operating mode in which the spindle is running at any time. We would also like to detect any slow of rapid drifts in the operating modes of the bearings.

The above can be achieved by learning a model of the current mode of operation and then using this model to perform the above two tasks. The model of current operating mode can be compared to some pre-existing models in a library to characterize its current mode. However, it turns out that there is so much uncertainty and continuous evolution in the models of operation that no one model come very close to any one other model learned in the past. Predictions based on the closest models from the past did not work very well. Our models were constructed using the frequency domain features derived from the sensor data.

We used these features to build regression models to predict the remaining life of a spindle's bearings. The plots in Fig. 4 show the results of predicting the health of the bearings based on the features derived from a 72 h window immediately preceding the time at which the prediction is made.

In this plot the light blue points show the actual time to failure (TTF) for the spindle at any point of time. The three other curves show the prediction results of three different types of regression models constructed by using different types of features. All these models seem to have an acceptable performance in predicting

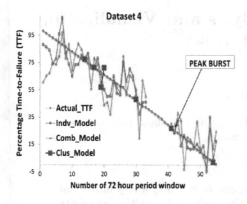

Fig. 4. Prediction results based on 72 h window

the remaining life of the bearings. However, the biggest drawback is that we need to store data for the preceding 72 h and use it to generate features to make these predictions. This is very long time window given that we need to collect 25,000 samples per second, and also generate Fourier transform signatures from 0.5 s time slices as the streaming data comes in. Any window size smaller than 72 h does not perform well enough to predict the remaining life of a spindle. From practical shop-floor perspective it is impractical to leave a machine unused for 72 h just so that it can be monitored for remaining life prediction. The challenge of using and exploiting the very high volume data still remains. Solutions that we are considering including monitoring the spindle for few minutes every couple of hours. Such data may not be able to generate the rich and informative features that help predict the remaining life of the bearings.

4   Conclusions

In the discussion above we have presented some challenges that are faced while designing systems for analytics of Big Data. We have presented the example of finding formal concepts from a large binary dataset and have shown that designing Map-reduce compatible algorithms must be attempted and this can result in significantly enhanced performance. We have also presented an example of a high volume data stream situation and described the challenges that need to be faced in exploiting the data stream effectively.

References

1. Bhatnagar, R., Kumar, L.: An efficient map-reduce algorithm for computing formal concepts from binary data. In: 2015 IEEE International Conference on Big Data, Big Data 2015, Santa Clara (to appear, 2015)
2. Ganter, B., Wille, R.: Formal Concept Analysis: Mathematical Foundations. Springer, Heidelberg (2012)
3. Krajca, P., Vychodil, V.: Distributed algorithm for computing formal concepts using map-reduce framework. In: Adams, N.M., Robardet, C., Siebes, A., Boulicaut, J.-F. (eds.) IDA 2009. LNCS, vol. 5772, pp. 333–344. Springer, Heidelberg (2009)
4. Kuznetsov, S.O.: A fast algorithm for computing all intersections of objects in a finite semi-lattice. Autom. Documentation Math. Linguist. **27**(5), 11–21 (1993)
5. Xu, B., de Fréin, R., Robson, E., Ó Foghlú, M.: Distributed formal concept analysis algorithms based on an iterative mapreduce framework. In: Domenach, F., Ignatov, D.I., Poelmans, J. (eds.) ICFCA 2012. LNCS, vol. 7278, pp. 292–308. Springer, Heidelberg (2012)

Mobility Big Data Analysis and Visualization (Invited Talk)

Masashi Toyoda[✉]

Institute of Industrial Science, The University of Tokyo, Tokyo, Japan
mtoyoda@acm.org

Abstract. Transportation systems in mega-cities play a very important role in social and economic activities. Especially in Japan, the Tokyo city is strongly required to increase resiliency and safety of its transportation systems, because of the 2020 Olympic games and big earthquakes predicted to occur. Our research group is trying to address those challenges utilizing mobility big data. We have been archiving several mobility data sets, such as smart card data and vehicle recorder data, and developed platforms for processing, analyzing, and visualizing them. In this paper I briefly introduce our analysis and visualization of passenger flows in public transportation systems and behaviors of vehicle drivers.

Keywords: Mobility big data · Smart card data · Vehicle recordar data

1 Introduction

Transportation systems in mega-cities play a very important role in maximizing efficiency of social and economic activities. In Japan, the Tokyo city has one of the most complex train systems in the world, and it is often suffered by various events, such as accidents, public gatherings, and natural disasters. Once a major disruptive event occurs, it can cause delay and congestion over a wide area. Although road and driver safety in Japan has been improved over the years, numerous traffic accidents still suffer our society. Now Tokyo is strongly required to increase resiliency and safety of transportation systems, because of the 2020 Olympic games, and big earthquakes predicted to occur.

Our research group is trying to address those challenges utilizing mobility big data. We have been archiving several mobility data sets, such as smart card data and vehicle recorder data, and developed platforms for processing, analyzing, and visualizing them.

One of our goals is building a platform for real-time analysis and prediction of passengers' behaviors in a complex public transportation system based on smart card data and social media streams. As the first step to this goal, we have been

---

This paper includes joint work with Daisaku Yokoyama, Masahiko Itoh, and Masaru Kitsuregawa (Institute of Industrial Science, the University of Tokyo). Yoshimitsu Tomita and Satoshi Kawamura (Tokyo Metro Co. Ltd.).

© Springer International Publishing Switzerland 2015
N. Kumar and V. Bhatnagar (Eds.): BDA 2015, LNCS 9498, pp. 108–120, 2015.
DOI: 10.1007/978-3-319-27057-9_8

developing a system for off-line analysis and visualization of passenger flows in a metro network in Tokyo based on a large-scale trip records extracted from smart card data [2,3].

The other goal is building a vehicle data analysis platform for driver centric services, such as safety support and fleet driver management. In [4], we proposed a method for analyzing relationships between vehicle drivers' properties and their driving behaviors based on large-scale and long-term vehicle recorder data. In [1], we proposed a visual interface for exploring spatio-temporal caution spots from large-scale vehicle recorder data.

In the following sections, I introduce those research on mobility big data. In Sect. 2, I will describe our research on public transportation data analysis utilizing the smart card data. In Sect. 3, our research on vehicle recorder data analysis will be explained.

2   Public Transportation Data Analysis

In this section, I introduce our framework for analyzing large-scale smart card data, and a method for predicting passenger behaviors after a train accident [3]. Then, I will show our visual fusion analysis environment [2] supporting ex post evaluations of troubles using the smart card data and social media data from Twitter.

2.1   Framework for Analyzing Smart Card Data

In [3], we proposed a framework for analyzing large-scale smart card data. It included a method for deriving passenger flows from the origin-destination records, and a method for predicting how passengers behave after an accident.

The smart card data is collected from entrance/exit gates (wicket) on each station. The information is aggregated on a central server each night. From the orign-destination records in the data, our framework calculates trip routes (start, transfer, and end points), and estimates passenger flows (the number of passengers traveled each section at a certain time). Based on the estimated flow, passenger behaviors are predicted.

Smart Card Data. We used two years' worth of smart card data from the Tokyo Metro subway system. As shown in Fig. 1, the Tokyo Metro has a complicated route structure connecting with lines of various railway companies such as Japan Railway (JR), Toei Subway, and other private railroads. We analyzed the Tokyo Metro trip records over almost all of the Tokyo business area, covering 28 lines, 540 stations, and about 300 million trips. We used records from anonymous smart cards without personal identity information, such as name, address, age, and gender. Each record consisted of the origin, destination, and exit time. Since transfer information was not included, we had to estimate the probable route for each trip.

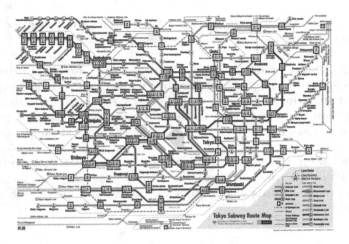

Fig. 1. Tokyo subway map (http://www.tokyometro.jp/en/subwaymap/index.html.)

Estimation of Passengers' Flow. From the trip records, we could determine how many passengers exited from each station at each time period. Since the data did not include the entrance time, we could not determine how many passengers entered each station at each time period. Moreover, the origin-destination pair information was not enough for estimating the crowdedness of each train or the effects of a disruptive incident at a certain location. We need the trip route for each passenger.

There are usually several possible routes for traveling from an origin station to a destination station. A smart card log contains information about where a passenger touched in and where and when he/she touched out at a station gate. It does not include the entrance time and transfer station information. We therefore assumed that the most probable route for each trip (origin and destination pair) was the one with the shortest total trip time.

We defined total trip time $t = T + C + W$, where

- T is the time spent riding, as defined by the timetable,
- C is the walking time when transferring, as determined by the layout of each station and roughly defined using information provided by the train company, and
- W is the time waiting for a train to arrive, as defined by the timetable (average train interval / 2).

Using this definition, we calculated the estimated time for every possible trip route for each origin-destination pair. We then used the Dijkstra algorithm to find the fastest route.

Predicting Passengers' Behaviors After Train Accidents. Passenger flows after train accidents are predicted using the demand and behavior models.

To predict the number of passengers at the time of an accident without using real-time data, we estimate how many passengers will want to travel during or after the time of the accident by using the demand model. We then estimate how these passengers will change their route by using the behavior model.

Our prediction method requires two kinds of information as input: average passenger demand in the past, and the expected time to recover from the accident. The proposed method can predict passenger flows after an accident from this information, without real-time data.

As the passenger demand, we estimated each passenger's entrance time by using the trip time estimation method as described above. We then calculated the number of passengers starting a trip, for every origin-destination pair, for every 10 min. The results reflected the passenger demand during a certain time period. We calculated the average demand for each time slot over one year (Apr. 1, 2012, to Mar. 31, 2013). Data for weekdays and weekends were treated independently.

In the passenger behavior model, each passenger has an origin and a destination, and the route is calculated as explained above. Example spatio-temporal behaviors of passengers, when a section of a line is suspended, is illustrated in Fig. 2.

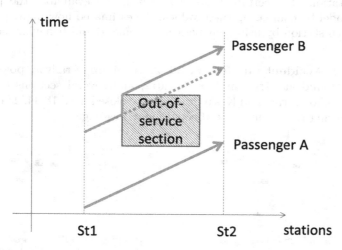

Fig. 2. Model of passenger behavior following an unusual event; red arrows indicate passenger trajectories (Color figure online).

Two passengers (A and B) want to travel from Station 1 (St1) to St2. We assume that we know about the service suspension and the begin and end times of the suspension (represented in the figure as "out-of-service section"). Passenger A completes passage through that section before service is suspended and is thus not affected. Passenger B is affected and thus must change his route or time of travel:

- If there is another route from St1 to St2 that does not use the out-of-service section, he can change his route, which will likely change the arrival time.
- If there is no such route, he must wait until service is restored (as illustrated in Fig. 2).

Since passengers often change their travel method in such situations, such as by switching to travel by bus or taxi, we use the "Abandonment Rate" to capture this behavior. When N passengers are affected by the out-of-service section, we assume only $N \times (1 - AbandonmentRate)$ passengers continue to use the train system. The Abandonment Rate should be based on historical data.

Evaluation. For evaluation, we focused on one of the busiest lines (the "Tozai Line" in Tokyo Metro) in order to examine the parameter of our model under the simplest conditions. We found that six disruptive events occurred on the Tozai Line during the year. They caused service suspensions on several sections, and it took several hours to restore service.

Since each trip record contained each passenger's arrival time and not the departure time, we could only determine how many passengers had left from a certain station at a certain time ($Exitnum$). We evaluated the passenger behavior model by comparing these values. We estimated how many passengers left from each station by using our passenger demand and behavior models.

Test Case – Accident on Nov. 6, 2012. A failure of railway power supply system was found at 17:11 on Nov. 6, 2012, and several sections of the line between Toyocho Station and Kasai Station were closed until 18:34. The accident happened during rush hour, so it affected many passengers.

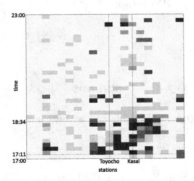

Fig. 3. Difference in number of passengers after accident on Nov. 6, with no out-of-service information (Color figure online)

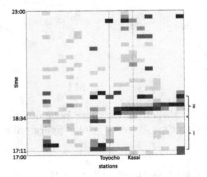

Fig. 4. Difference in number of passengers after accident on Nov. 6, with out-of-service information and Abandonment Rate (AR) = 0.0 (Color figure online)

Figure 3 shows the difference in *Exitnum* between the estimation obtained using the demand model and the actual trip record data. The estimation was made without considering the accident information. Colors are used in the figure to represent the difference in *Exitnum* normalized by the value in the trip record data. Blue represents the situation in which the actual number of passengers was lower than the estimated one, and red represents the opposite case. The large blue area indicates that many passengers were unable to travel as they normally did.

We also estimated *Exitnum* for all the other stations in the metro system. Since the difference was at the highest for stations on the Tozai Line, we focused on that line in our evaluation.

The estimation results when the out-of-service information was considered, with Abandonment Rate = 0, are shown in Fig. 4. Most of the blue area (labeled i) disappeared. However, a new large blue area (labeled ii) appeared around 18:50, after the accident.

We adjusted the Abandonment Rate to find the most appropriate setting. We computed the sum of the absolute number of difference in this sections and timespan to estimate the correctness of our model. Figure 6 shows this value normalized by the average number of passengers who used the Tozai Line at this time of the day. The difference for Abandonment Rate = 0 was larger than the case of no information about the service suspension (green line). We can see that the best setting of the Abandonment Rate was 0.9. With the out-of-service information, the difference improved by about 9 %. Figure 5 shows the best case, with Abandonment Rate = 0.9. The large problematic blue area (ii) disappeared with this setting.

Even in the best case (Fig. 5), we can see several chunks of blue area (iii and iv). We obtained train operation information for that date from the railway company and determined that most of the decrease in the number of passengers is understandable: the entire Tozai Line was stopped twice for a short time, from 17:11 to 17:28 (iii), and from 19:19 to 19:29 (iv). The blue chunk in Fig. 5 is reasonably explained by this information.

2.2   Visual Fusion Analysis Environment

In [2], we developed a visual fusion analysis environment supporting ex post evaluation of anomalous events using the analysis framework for smart card data, and social media stream from Twitter. The environment was designed for discovering unusual phenomena such as events and troubles, understanding changes in passenger flows after the phenomena, and exploring reasons of the phenomena from social media.

Figure 7 shows the overview of the environment integrating three information visualization techniques.

HeatMap view provides a temporal overview of passenger flows in metro lines. The color in each (section, time) shows the crowdedness and emptiness compared with the average flow. Red represents crowded flow, green represents

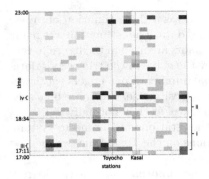

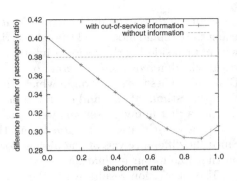

Fig. 5. Difference in number of passengers after accident on Nov. 6, with out-of-service information and $AR = 0.9$ (Color figure online)

Fig. 6. Difference in number of passengers after accident on Nov. 6 (Color figure online)

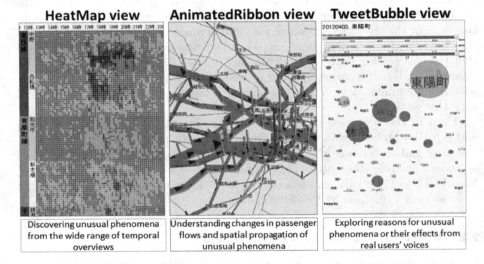

HeatMap view	AnimatedRibbon view	TweetBubble view
Discovering unusual phenomena from the wide range of temporal overviews	Understanding changes in passenger flows and spatial propagation of unusual phenomena	Exploring reasons for unusual phenomena or their effects from real users' voices

Fig. 7. Overview of the visual fusion analysis environment (Color figure online)

average flow, and blue represents sparse flow. We can find unusual phenomena from increase or decrease of passenger flows.

AnimatedRibbon view visualizes spatio-temporal changes in passenger flows using animated 3D ribbons on the metro network map representing the absolute number of passengers by their height. The color of the ribbon shows the deviation from the average as same as the HeatMap view.

TweetBubble view shows an overview of occurring words in tweets relevant to a specified time period and a station/line, which is selected in the HeatMap or AnimatedRibbon view. We can see passengers' situations, complaints, and decisions.

Case Study: The Great East Japan Earthquake. Figure 8 visualizes passenger flows on 11 Mar. 2011, the day of the Great East Japan Earthquake. The earthquake struck off the northeastern coast of Japan at 14:46. Since many

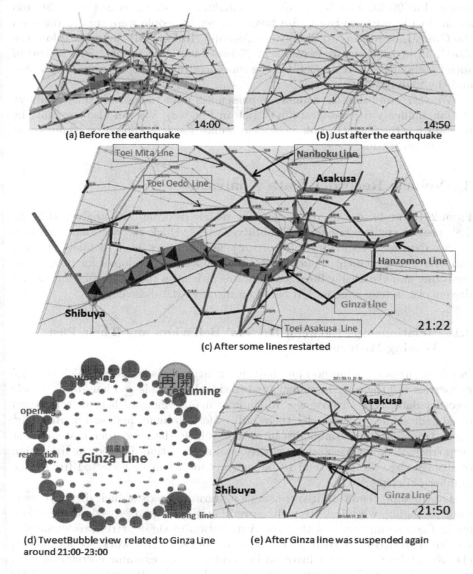

Fig. 8. Passenger flows and tweets on 11 Mar. 2011

public transportation systems suspended operation just after the earthquake, many people could not go back to their home until midnight or the next morning.

Figure 8(a) shows the situation just before the earthquake, in which most of lines were normally operated. In Fig. 8(b), we can see almost all lines suspended their operation after the earthquake.

The Tokyo Metro Ginza Line and a part of the Tokyo Metro Hanzomon Line resumed at 20:40. The Tokyo Metro Nanboku Line also resumed at 21:20, and so on. In Fig. 8(c), we can find a huge number of people were concentrated on the Ginza Line moving to Shibuya or Asakusa. In Fig. 8(d), we can explore the situation, in which many tweets said "Ginza Line is resuming". The spread of such tweets might have accelerated the concentration of people to the Ginza Line and the Shibuya station.

We also found that the number of passengers went to and exited the Shibuya station suddenly decreased around 21:50 in Fig. 8(e). We can also see that the reason from the TweetBubble view, and found that it is caused by confusion at the Shibuya station.

3   Vehicle Recorder Data Analysis

From 2014, we have started a project for vehicle recorder data analysis (Fig. 9). This project archives big data in mobility, such as vehicle recorder data, and provides a data analysis platform for driver centric services, such as safety support and driver management. Fundamental techniques are developed for processing, analyzing and visualizing huge scale data records from thousands of vehicles and drivers over a long time period based on ultrafast database engine.

3.1   Relationships Between Drivers' Behaviors and Their Past Driving Histories

In [4], we proposed a method for analyzing relationships between vehicle drivers' properties and their driving behaviors based on large-scale and long-term vehicle recorder data. Our purpose was to support management of fleet drivers based on classification of drivers by their skill, safety, fatigue, and so on. Recently, many transportation companies introduce vehicle data recorder systems that keep track of GPS trajectories, velocity, and acceleration. Due to the limitation of storage size, the data tend to be sparse, but it can be collected from large number of drivers.

Our method classified drivers using long-term recoreds of their driving operations (breaking, wheeling, etc.) with several attributes (max speed, acceleration, etc.). The assumption was that the distribution of these attributes would differ driver to driver by their past driving histories. In this work, we focused on classifying drivers recently involved in accidents, and examine correlation with driving behaviors. The results could be useful for education of drivers, and for preventing further accidents.

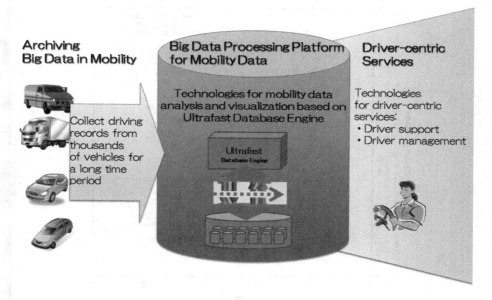

Fig. 9. Overview of the vehicle big data platform

Dataset. We use a large-scale vehicle recorder data collected by one of the largest door-to-door delivery service company in Japan. It consisted of around 1400 drivers assigned in Tokyo prefecture, worth about 10 months (from July 2014 to June 2015). The data was recorded by a multi-functional vehicle data recorder with longitudinal accelerometer, lateral accelerometer, gyro compass, and GPS.

The vehicle data recorder automatically detects four basic driving operations; breaking, wheeling, turning, and stopping operations. Several attributes such as maximum speed or acceleration during the operations are recorded.

With the help of the delivery company, we could access to the drivers' history about their accidents from 10 years before. We split drivers into two groups, drivers who experienced accidents within 5 years, or not.

Classification of Drivers. We designed several features using frequency of the quantized attributes, and try to evaluate their ability to classify drivers by using Support Vector Machine (SVM). We first chose 6 basic attributes related to velocity, and combine them with other properties such as acceleration, jerk, yaw velocity, and so on. These attributes were binned into several intervals, and driving operations are accumulated for each bin. The total number of bins were 540. Then, each driver had 540 features of operation frequency. We used the occurrence probabilities of operations in each bin for each driver, and also used the difference from the average probability for all drivers. We examined several models to represent that difference. The details will be published soon.

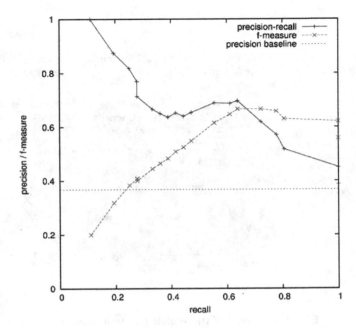

Fig. 10. Classification result

Evaluation. We evaluated the performance of these features by 10-fold cross validation using SVM with feature selection. The Fig. 10 shows the precision-recall curve that overwhelms the precision of the random classification for all recall values. It means that the selected features have certain information to explain drivers' past accident histories. We are now examining details of these features, and how these behaviors relate to actual accidents.

3.2   Visual Exploration of Caution Spots

In [1], we proposed a visual interface for exploring spatio-temporal caution spots from large-scale vehicle recorder data. Although road and driver safety in Japan has been improved over the years, numerous traffic accidents still suffer our society. Local governments provide potential risk maps based on accident statistics and questionnaires from drivers and pedestrians. They however lack accuracy and comprehensiveness. Time and weather information are not included in most of those maps, and questionnaires tend to be biased by vague human impressions.

Visual Exploration Interface. We designed a flexible interface to explore large-scale driving operations occurred in a spatio-temporal space by zooming and filtering by their attributes in a 3D information visualization environment (Fig. 11). It provided an exploration interface to design caution degrees from correlation between attribute values of driving operations (Fig. 11(a)). A dynamic query interface based on parallel coordinates view was provided for filtering driving operations (Fig. 11(b)). Results were displayed in a 3D spatio-temporal space to discover caution spots (Fig. 11(c–e)). To investigate details in caution spots, the exploration interface visualized trajectory paths around the spots (Fig. 11(f)).

Case Studies. We performed case studies using a vehicle recorder dataset consisting of about 80 drivers assigned to the Bunkyo district in Tokyo worth about one month. We first compared extracted caution spots with the risk map provided by the government of Bunkyo, and confirmed that we could extract almost the same spots with our interface. We could also discover several caution spots in areas not covered by the risk map. As an instance, we found a gate of an apartments that was hard to see from drivers.

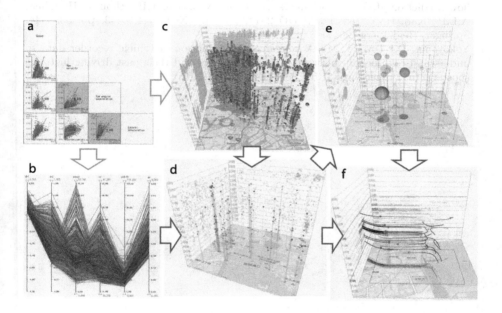

Fig. 11. Overview of caution spots exploration in our visual interface

4   Conclusions

In this paper, I introduced our recent research on mobility big data analysis and visualization. For public transportation, we utilized the large-scale smart card data from the Tokyo Metro subway system. Our analysis framework estimates passenger flows, predicts changes in the flows after accidents, and visualize traffics with social media streams. To improve road and driver safety, we utilized the large-scale vehicle recorder data. For fleet driver management, we tried to classify drivers with potential risks. For road safety, we built a visual interface to discover spatio-temporal caution spots. We plan to integrate various big data such as weather and infrastructure data for approaching wider application areas.

References

1. Itoh, M., Yokoyama, D., Toyoda, M., Kitsuregawa, M.: Visual interface for exploring caution spots from vehicle recorder big data. In: Proceedings of the IEEE BigData 2015 (2015)
2. Itoh, M., Yokoyama, D., Toyoda, M., Tomita, Y., Kawamura, S., Kitsuregawa, M.: Visual fusion of mega-city big data: an application to traffic and tweets data analysis of metro passengers. In: Proceedings of the IEEE BigData 2014, pp. 431–440 (2014)
3. Yokoyama, D., Itoh, M., Toyoda, M., Tomita, Y., Kawamura, S., Kitsuregawa, M.: A framework for large-scale train trip record analysis and its application to passengers' flow prediction after train accidents. In: Tseng, V.S., Ho, T.B., Zhou, Z.-H., Chen, A.L.P., Kao, H.-Y. (eds.) PAKDD 2014, Part I. LNCS, vol. 8443, pp. 533–544. Springer, Heidelberg (2014)
4. Yokoyama, D., Toyoda, M.: A large scale examination of vehicle recorder data to understand relationship between drivers behaviors and their past driving histories (poster). In: Proceedings of IEEE BigData 2015 (2015)

Finding Periodic Patterns in Big Data

R. Uday Kiran[1]([envelope]) and Masaru Kitsuregawa[1,2]

[1] University of Tokyo, Tokyo, Japan
{uday_rage,kitsure}@tkl.iis.u-tokyo.ac.jp
[2] National Institute of Informatics, Tokyo, Japan

Abstract. Periodic pattern mining is an important model in data mining. It typically involves discovering all patterns that are exhibiting either complete or partial cyclic repetitions in a dataset. The problem of finding these patterns has been widely studied in time series and (temporally ordered) transactional databases. This paper contains these studies along with their advantages and disadvantages. This paper also discusses the usefulness of periodic patterns with two real-world case studies. The first case study describes the useful information discovered by periodic patterns in an aviation dataset. The second case study describes the useful information discovered by periodic patterns pertaining to users' browsing behavior in an eCommerce site.

The tutorial will start by describing the frequent pattern model and the importance of enhancing this model with respect to time dimension. Next, we discuss the basic model of finding periodic patterns in time series, describe its limitations, and the approaches suggested to address these limitations. We next discuss the basic model of finding periodic patterns in a transactional database, describe its limitations, and the approaches suggested to address them. Finally, we end this tutorial with the real-world case studies that demonstrate the usefulness of these patterns.

Keywords: Data mining · Knowledge discovery in databases · Frequent patterns and periodic patterns

1 Introduction

Time and frequency are two most important dimensions to determine the interestingness of a pattern in a given data set. Periodic patterns are an important class of regularities that exist in a data set with respect to these two dimensions. Periodic pattern mining involves discovering all patterns that are exhibiting either complete or partial cyclic repetitions in a data set [1,2]. Finding these patterns is a significant task with many real-world applications. Examples include finding co-occurring genes in biological data sets [3], improving the performance of recommender systems [4], intrusion detection in computer networks [5], and finding events in Twitter [6]. A classic application to illustrate the usefulness of these patterns is market-basket analysis. It analyzes how regularly the sets of items are being purchased by the customers. An example of a periodic pattern is as follows:

© Springer International Publishing Switzerland 2015
N. Kumar and V. Bhatnagar (Eds.): BDA 2015, LNCS 9498, pp. 121–133, 2015.
DOI: 10.1007/978-3-319-27057-9_9

$$\{Bed, \ Pillow\} \quad [support = 10\%, \ period = 1 \ h].$$

The above pattern says that 10 % of customers have purchased the items '*Bed*' and '*Pillow*' at least once in every hour.

The problem of finding periodic patterns has been studied in [1–3,7–16]. Some of these approaches consider input data as time series [2,3,7–11], while others consider data as an enhanced transactional database having time attribute [1,12–16]. In this paper, we study all of these approaches with respect to the following topics:

1. **Data Representation.** How a periodic pattern model considers input data? What are the implicit assumptions pertaining to the frequency and periodic behavior of the items within the data?
2. **Computational Expensiveness.** What is the size of search space? What properties are used to reduce the search space efficiently?
3. **Mining Rarity.** In many real-world databases, some items appear very frequently in the data, while others appear rarely. The knowledge pertaining to rare items is often of great interest and high value. However, finding this knowledge is challenging due to infrequent appearances of rare items. This problem is known as the *rare item problem*. We discuss how some of the periodic pattern models are trying to address this problem.

The rest of the paper is organized as follows. Section 2 describes the approaches for finding periodic patterns in time series. Section 3 describes the approaches for finding periodically occurring frequent patterns in a transactional database. Sections 4 reports on the experimental results. Finally, Sect. 5 concludes the paper.

2   Periodic Pattern Mining in Time Series

In this section, we first describe the basic model of periodic patterns. We next discuss the limitations of this model. Finally, we describe the approaches that try to address these limitations.

2.1   The Basic Model of Periodic Patterns

Time series is a collection of events obtained from sequential measurements over time. Han et al. [2] have studied the periodic behavior of patterns in a series, and discussed a model to find periodic patterns. The model is as follows:

Let I be the set of items and D be a set of transactions (or a database), where each transaction t is a set of items such that $t \subseteq I$. The time series S represents the gathering of n timestamped databases into a single database, i.e., $S = D_1, D_2, \cdots, D_n, 1 \leq n$. Let the symbol * denote a wild (or do not care) character, which can match any single set of items. The pattern $s = s_1, \cdots, s_p$ is a non-empty sequence over $(2^I - \{\emptyset\}) \cup \{*\}$. Let $|s|$ denote the length (or *period*) of the pattern s. Let the I-length of $s = s_1 \cdots s_p$ be the number of s_i which contains letters from I. A pattern with I-length k is also called a k-pattern.

Moreover, a subpattern of a pattern $s = s_1 \cdots s_p$ is a pattern $s' = s'_1 \cdots s'_p$ such that s and s' have the same length, and $s'_i \subseteq s_i$ for every position i where $s'_i \neq *$. The *support* of a pattern s in S is denoted as $Sup(x) = |\{i|0 \leq i < m, \text{ and the string } s \text{ is true in } D_{i|s|+1} \cdots D_{i|s|+|s|}\}|$, where m is the maximum number of *periods* of length s. Each segments of the form $D_{i|s|+1} \cdots D_{i|s|+|s|}$, where $0 \leq i < m$, is called a period segment. The pattern s is said to be a periodic pattern if $Sup(s) \geq minSup$, where $minSup$ represents the user-defined minimum support threshold value.

Example 1. Given the time series $S = a\{bc\}baebace$, $I = \{a, b, c, e\}$. If the user-defined *period* is 3, S is divided into three periodic-segments: $D_1 = a\{bc\}b$, $D_2 = aeb$ and $D_3 = ace$. Let $a * b$ be a pattern. The length of this pattern is 3, and its I-length is 2 (i.e., it contains only two items within this pattern). Therefore, we represent this pattern as 2-pattern. This pattern appears in the periodic-segments of D_1 and D_2. Therefore, its *support* count is 2. If the user-defined $minSup$ is 2, then $a * b$ represents a periodic pattern.

2.2   The Limitations of Basic Model

Aref et al. [17] have extended the Han's model to incremental mining of periodic patterns. Yang et al. [11] have studied the change in periodic behavior of a pattern due to the influence of noise, and enhanced the basic model to discover a class of periodic patterns known as asynchronous periodic patterns. Zhang et al. [3] have enhanced the basic model to discover periodic patterns in character sequences like protein data. The popular adoption and successful industrial application of this basic periodic pattern model suffers from the following obstacles:

1. **Computationally Expensive Model:**
   - In the basic periodic pattern model, a pattern represents sets of items. Therefore, the search space of this model is $\sum_{i=1}^{p} n^p$, where n and p represent the total number of items in a series and the user-defined *period*, respectively. This search space is typically much higher than the frequent pattern model that has the search space of $2^n - 1$.
   - Periodic patterns satisfy the *anti-monotonic property* [18]. That is, all non-empty subsets of a periodic pattern are also periodic patterns. However, this property is insufficient to make the periodic pattern mining practical or computationally inexpensive in real-life. The reason is that number of frequent i-patterns shrink slowly (when $i > 1$) as i increases in time series data. The slow speed of decrease in the number of frequent i-patterns is due to a strong correlation between frequencies of patterns and their sub-patterns [19].
   - Overall, the huge search space followed by the inability to reduce the search space using *anti-monotonic property* makes the model computationally expensive or impractical in real-world applications.
2. **Sparsity Problem:** The basic model of periodic patterns uses the wild character '$*$' to represent an event within a pattern. This leads to the sparsity

problem, which involves many discovered patterns having a large number of wild characters with very few events. For example, $a \star\star\star\star\star\star\star\star\star\star\star\star\star\star\star$ $bc \star\star\star\star\star\star\star\star\star a \star\star\star\star\star\star\star\star b$. This problem makes the discovered patterns impracticable in applications.

3. **The Rare Item Problem:** Since only a single *period* and *minSup* are used for the whole data, the model implicitly assumes that all items in the data have same periodic behavior and uniform frequency. However, this is seldom not the case in many real-world data sets. In many data sets, some items appear very frequently in the data, while others rarely appear. Moreover, rare items typically occur with long *periods* (i.e., inter-arrival times) as compared against the frequent items. Henceforth, finding periodic patterns with a single *period* and *minSup* leads to the following two problems:
   - If the *period* is set too short and/or the *minSup* is set too high, we will miss the periodic patterns involving rare items.
   - In order to find the periodic patterns involving both frequent and rare items, we have to set a long *period* and a low *minSup*. However, this may result in combinatorial explosion, producing too many patterns, because frequent items can combine with one another in all possible ways and many of them may be meaningless.

4. **Methodology to Specify Period:** An open problem of this model is the methodology to specify *period* that can capture the heterogeneous temporal behavior of all items in a series effectively.

5. **Inability to Consider Temporal Information of Events:** Han's model considers time series as a symbolic sequence. As a result, this model does not take into account the actual temporal information of events within a sequence [5].

2.3   Research Efforts to Address the Limitations

Han et al. [19] have introduced "maximum sub-pattern hit set property" to reduce the computational cost of finding these patterns. Based on this property, a tree-based algorithm, called max-subpattern tree, has been proposed to discovered periodic patterns effectively. A max-subpattern tree takes the candidate max-pattern, C_{max}, as the root node. Each subpattern of C_{max} with one non-* letter missing is a direct child node of the root. The tree expands recursively according to the following rules. A node w may have a set of children if it contains more 2 non-* letters. Then the tree from the root of the tree is constructed and the missing non-* letters are checked in order to find the corresponding node. The count increases by 1 if the node w is found. Otherwise, a new node w (with count 1) and its missing ancestor nodes (only those on the path to w, with count 0) are created. If one exists, it (or them) is (or are) inserted into the corresponding place(s) of the tree. After a max-subpattern tree has been built, the tree is scanned to find frequency counts of the candidate patterns and eliminate the non-frequent ones. Notice that the frequency count of a node is the sum of the count of itself and those of all of the reachable ancestors. If the derived frequent pattern set is empty, then return. For more details, refer to the study by [19].

Zhang et al. [3] have tried to address the sparsity problem by limiting the gap (i.e., number of wild characters allowed between two itemsets) within a pattern. Yang et al. [7] have used *"information gain"* to address the rare item problem in periodic pattern mining. The discovered patterns are known as *surprising patterns*. Alternatively, Chen et al. [8] have tried to address this problem by finding periodic patterns using multiple *minSups* [20]. In this approach, each item in the series is specified with a *support* constraint known as *minimum item support (MIS)*. The *minSup* for a pattern is represented with the lowest *MIS* value of its items. That is,

$$minSup(s) = minmum(MIS(i_j)|\forall i_j \in s)$$

where, $MIS(i_j)$ represents the user-specified minimum item support for an item $i_j \in s$. The usage of *minimum item support* enables us to achieve the goal of having higher *minSup* for patterns that only involve frequent items, and having lower *minSup* for patterns that involve rare items.

Berberidis et al. [9] have discussed a methodology to specify approximate *period* using Fast Fourier Transformations and auto-correlation. Unfortunately, this method may miss some frequent periods and it requires a separate pass to scan the data sequence to compute the periods. Moreover, for each item, it needs to compute, at a high cost, the circular auto-correlation value for different periods in order to determine whether the period is frequent or not. Cao et al. [10] have proposed a computationally inexpensive approach to determine *period* with an implicit assumption that periodic pattern can be approximately expressed by an arithmetic series together with a support indicate about its frequency.

All of the above mentioned approaches consider time series as a symbolic sequence, and therefore, do not take into account the actual temporal information of the items in the data. In the next section, we discuss the approaches that take into account the temporal information of the items in the data.

3   Periodic Pattern Mining in Transactional Databases

In this section, we first describe the basic model of periodic-frequent patterns. We next discuss the limitations of this model, and describe the efforts made in the literature to address these limitations.

3.1   The Basic Model of Periodic-Frequent Patterns

Ozden et al. [1] have enhanced the transactional database by a time attribute that describes the time when a transaction has appeared, investigated the periodic behavior of the patterns to discover cyclic association rules. In this study, a database is fragmented into non-overlapping subsets with respect to time. The association rules that are appearing in at least a certain number of subsets are discovered as cyclic association rules. By fragmenting the data and counting the number of subsets in which a pattern occurs greatly simplifies the design of the mining algorithm. However, the drawback is that patterns (or association rules) that span multiple windows cannot be discovered.

Tanbeer et al. [12] have discussed a simplified model to discover periodically occurring frequent patterns, i.e., periodic-frequent patterns, in a transactional database. The model is as follows:

Let I be a set of items. Let $X \subseteq I$ be a pattern (or an itemset). A pattern containing k number of items is known as a k-pattern. A **transaction**, $tr = (ts, Y)$, is a tuple, where $ts \in R$ represents the timestamp and Y is a pattern. A **transactional database** TDB over I is a set of transactions, $TDB = \{tr_1, \cdots, tr_m\}$, $m = |TDB|$, where $|TDB|$ is the size of the TDB in total number of transactions. For a transaction $tr = (ts, Y)$, such that $X \subseteq Y$, it is said that X occurs in tr and such a timestamp is denoted as ts^X. Let $TS^X = \{ts_k^X, \cdots, ts_l^X\}$, where $1 \leq k \leq l \leq m$, denote an **ordered set of timestamps** at which X has occurred in TDB.

Example 2. Table 1 shows the transactional database with each transaction uniquely identifiable with a timestamp (ts). All transactions in this database have been ordered with respect to their timestamps. This database do not contain any transaction with timestamps 6 and 9. However, it has to be noted that these two timestamps still contribute in determining the periodic interestingness of a pattern. The set of all items in this database, $I = \{a, b, c, d, e, f, g, h\}$. The set of items '$a$' and '$b$', i.e., '$ab$' is a pattern. This pattern contains only two items. Therefore, this is a 2-pattern. This pattern appears at the timestamps of $1, 2, 5, 7$ and 10. Therefore, $TS^{ab} = \{1, 2, 5, 7, 10\}$.

The above measures, *support* and *all-confidence*, determine the interestingness of a pattern in frequency dimension. We now describe the measures to determine the interestingness of a pattern in time dimension.

Table 1. A transactional database

ts	Items	ts	Items	ts	Items	ts	Items	ts	Items
1	ab	3	$cdgh$	5	ab	8	cd	11	cdg
2	abd	4	cef	7	$abce$	10	$abdef$	12	aef

Definition 1 *(Support of a Pattern X). The number of transactions containing X in TDB (i.e., the size of TS^X) is defined as the support of X and denoted as $sup(X)$. That is, $sup(X) = |TS^X|$.*

Example 3 The support of 'ab' in Table 1 is the size of TS^{ab}. Therefore, $sup(ab) = |TS^{ab}| = |1, 2, 5, 7, 10| = 5$.

Definition 2 *(A frequent Pattern X).* *The pattern X is said to be frequent if its support satisfies the user-specified* **minimum support** *(minSup) constraint. That is, if $SUP(X) \geq minSup$, then X is a frequent pattern.*

Example 4 Continuing with the previous example, if the user-specified $minSup = 3$, then ab is a frequent pattern as $sup(ab) \geq minSup$.

Definition 3 *(A period of X).* *Given $TS^X = \{ts_a^X, ts_b^X, \cdots, ts_c^X\}$, $1 \leq a \leq b \leq c \leq |TDB|$, a period of X, denoted as p_k^X, is calculated as follows:*

- $p_1^X = ts_a^X - ts_{ini}$, *where $ts_{ini} = 0$ denotes the initial timestamp of all transactions in TDB.*
- $p_k^X = ts_q^X - ts_p^X$, $1 < k < Sup(X) + 1$, *where ts_p^X and ts_q^X, $a \leq p < q \leq c$, denote any two consecutive timestamps in TS^X.*
- $p_{sup(X)+1}^X = ts_{fin} - ts_c^X$, *where ts_{fin} denotes the final timestamp of all transactions in TDB.*

Example 5 In Table 1, the pattern ab has initially appeared at the timestamp of 1. Therefore, the initial period of ab, i.e., $p_1^{ab} = 1$ $(= 1 - ts_{ini})$. Similarly, other periods of this pattern are: $p_2^{ab} = 1$ $(= 2-1)$, $p_3^{ab} = 3$ $(= 5-2)$, $p_4^{ab} = 2$ $(= 7-5)$, $p_5^{ab} = 3$ $(= 10 - 7)$ and $p_6^{ab} = 2$ $(= ts_{fin} - 10)$.

The terms 'ts_{ini}' and 'ts_{fin}' play a key role in determining the periodic appearance of X in the entire database. Let $P^X = \{p_1^X, p_2^X, \cdots, p_k^X\}$, $k = Sup(X) + 1$, denote the set of all periods of X in TDB. The first *period* in P^X (i.e., p_1^X) provides useful information pertaining to time taken for initial appearance of X in TDB. The last *period* in P^X (i.e., p_k^X) provides useful information pertaining to time elapsed after the final appearance of X in TDB. Other periods in P^X provide information pertaining to inter-arrival times of X in TDB.

The occurrence intervals, defined as above, gives information of appearance behavior of a pattern. The largest occurrence period of a pattern provides the upper limit of its periodic occurrence characteristic. Hence, the measure of the characteristic of a pattern of being periodic in a TDB can be defined as follows.

Definition 4 *(Periodicity of X).* *Let P^X denote the set of all periods of X in TDB. The maximum period in P^X is defined as the* **periodicity** *of X and is denoted as $per(X)$, i.e., $per(X) = max(p_i^X | \forall p_i^X \in P^X)$.*

Example 6. Continuing with the previous example, $P^{ab} = \{1, 1, 3, 2, 3, 2\}$. Therefore, the *periodicity* of ab, i.e., $per(ab) = max(1, 1, 3, 2, 3, 2) = 3$.

Definition 5 *(A Periodic-Frequent Pattern X).* *The pattern X is said to be periodic-frequent if $sup(X) \geq minSup$ and $per(x) \leq maxPer$.*

Example 7. Continuing with the previous example, if the user-specified $maxPer = 3$, then ab is a periodic-frequent pattern as $sup(ab) \geq minSup$ and $per(ab) \leq maxPer$.

3.2   The Performance Issues of the Periodic-Frequent Pattern Model

Unlike the periodic pattern mining models in time series, periodic-frequent pattern mining model takes into account the temporal information of the items within the data. Moreover, the latter model do not suffer from the *sparsity problem*. This model is also computationally inexpensive than the periodic pattern model, because its search space of $2^n - 1$, where n is the total number of items within the database, is much less than search space of periodic pattern model. However, this model still suffers from the following performance issues:

1. **The Rare Item Problem.** The usage of single *minSup* and *maxPer* leads to the rare item problem.
2. **Inability to Discover Partial Periodic-Frequent Patterns.** Since *maxPrd* controls the maximum inter-arrival time of a pattern in the entire database, this model discovers only full periodic-frequent patterns (i.e., only those frequent patterns that have exhibited complete cyclic repetitions in a database). As the real-world is imperfect, partial periodic patterns are ubiquitous in real-world databases. This model fails to discover these patterns.

3.3   Research Efforts to Address the Performance Issues

To address the rare item problem, Uday et al. [13] have proposed an enhanced model to discover periodic-frequent patterns using multiple *minSups* and *maxPrds*. In this model, the *minSup* and *maxPrd* for a pattern are represented as follows:

$$minSup(X) = min(minIS(i_j)|\forall i_j \in X)$$
$$and \tag{1}$$
$$maxPer(X) = max(maxIP(i_j)|\forall i_j \in X).$$

where $minIS(i_j)$ and $maxIP(i_j)$ respectively represent the user-specified *minimum item support* and *maximum item periodic* for an item $i_j \in X$. This model facilitates the user to specify a low *minSup* and a high *maxPrd* for a pattern containing rare items, and high *minSup* and a low *maxPrd* for a pattern containing only frequent items.

The periodic-frequent patterns discovered by [13] do not satisfy the anti-monotonic property. This increases the search space, which in turn increases the computational cost of finding the periodic-frequent patterns. In other words, this enhanced model is impracticable in real-world very large databases. Akshat et al. [21] have proposed another model using the notion of multiple *minSups* and *maxPrds*. In this model, the *minSup* and *maxPer* for a pattern are represented as follows:

$$minSup(X) = max(minIS(i_j)|\forall i_j \in X)$$
$$and \tag{2}$$
$$maxPer(X) = min(maxIP(i_j)|\forall i_j \in X)$$

The periodic-frequent patterns discovered by this model satisfy the anti-monotonic property. Therefore, this model is practicable in real-world databases.

Amphawan et al. [14] have used standard deviation of *periods* to determine the periodic interestingness of a pattern in the database. Uday et al. [22] have introduced a novel measure, called *periodic-ratio*, to discover partial periodic-frequent patterns in a database. The *periodic-ratio* of a pattern X is calculated as follows:

$$PR(x) = \frac{|IP^X|}{|P^X|}, \qquad (3)$$

where $IP^X \subseteq P^X$, such that $\forall p_i^X \in IP^X$, $p_i^X \leq maxPeriod$. The term $maxPeriod$ refers to the user-defined maximum period threshold value.

4   Experimental Results

In this section, we discuss the usefulness of periodic-frequent patterns using two real-world (**Shop-4** and **Accidents**) databases. We use periodic-frequent pattern-growth++ (PF-growth++) [16] to discover periodic-frequent patterns. In this paper, we do not discuss the usefulness of periodic patterns discovered in time series data. The reasons are as follows: (*i*) there exists no publicly available real-world time series data and (*ii*) current periodic pattern mining algorithms do not consider temporal information of the items within a series.

4.1   Experimental Setup

The PF-growth++ algorithm is written in GNU C++, and run on Ubuntu 14.04 machine having 16GB of RAM. The details of the databases are as follows:

1. **Shop-4 Database.** A Czech company has provided clickstream data of seven online stores in the ECML/PKDD 2005 Discovery challenge [23]. For our experiment, we have considered the click stream data of product categories visited by the users in "Shop 4" (www.shop4.cz), and created a transactional database with each transaction representing the set of web pages visited by the people at a particular *minute interval*. The transactional database contains 59,240 transactions (i.e., 41 days of page visits) and 155 distinct items (or product categories).

2. **Accidents Database.** The Federal Aviation Authority (FAA) has collected data pertaining to aircraft damages. In order to improve aviation safety, this data was made available in Aviation Safety Information Analysis and Sharing (ASIAS) system. The **Accidents** database is created from the data retrieved from ASIAS from 1-January-1978 to 31-December-2014 [24]. The raw data collected by FAA contains both numerical and categorical attributes. For our experiments, we have considered only categorical attributes, namely 'local event date,' 'event city,' 'event state,' 'event airport,' 'event type,' 'aircraft damage,' 'flight phase,' 'aircraft make,' 'aircraft model,' 'operator,' 'primary

flight type,' 'flight conduct code,' 'flight plan filed code' and 'PIC certificate type.' The missing values for these attributes are ignored while creating this database.

The statistical details of these two databases are provided in Table 2.

Table 2. Database statistics. The terms, T_{min}, T_{avg} and T_{max}, represent the minimum, average and maximum number of items within a transaction, respectively

Database	T_{min}	T_{avg}	T_{max}	Size	Items
Shop-4	1	2.4	82	59,240	155
Accidents	3	8.9	9	98,864	9,290

4.2   Generation of Periodic-Frequent Patterns

Figure 1(a) and (b) shows the number of periodic-frequent patterns discovered in Shop-4 and Accidents database, respectively. The X-axis represents the $maxPer$ values used to discover periodic-frequent patterns. The Y-axis represents the number of periodic-frequent patterns generated at a particular $maxPer$ value. Each line in this figure represents the number of periodic-frequent patterns generated at a particular $minSup$ value. The $minSup$ used in our experiments are 0.01 %, 0.06 % and 0.11 %. The reason for setting low $minSup$ values is to generate periodic-frequent patterns involving both frequent and rare items. The following observations can be drawn from these two figures:

1. The increase in $maxPrd$ results in the increase of periodic-frequent patterns. The reason is that increase in $maxPrd$ causes sporadically appearing patterns to be discovered as periodic-frequent patterns.
2. The increase in $minSup$ results in the decrease the periodic-frequent patterns, because it is difficult for the items to appear frequently with other items in the entire database.

4.3   Interesting Patterns Discovered in Accidents Database

We discuss the usefulness of periodic-frequent patterns discovered in Accidents database. Table 3 presents some of the interesting periodic-frequent patterns discovered in accidents database when $minSup = 0.11$ % and $maxPer = 4$ %. The first pattern in this table conveys the useful information that 'substantial' damages to an aircraft have happened during 'general operating rules.' The frequency of this event is 1,899 and the maximum inter-arrival time of this event is 110 days (i.e., almost 4 months). The second pattern conveys the information that 'substantial' damages to an aircraft with 'private pilot' have happened during 'general operating rules.' The frequency of this event is 750, while the *periodicity* of this event is 219 days (i.e., around 7 months). The third pattern

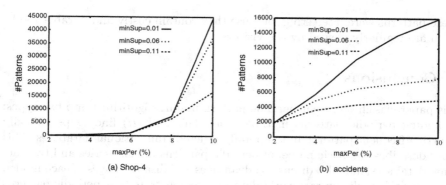

Fig. 1. Periodic-frequent patterns generated at different *minSup* and *maxPer* values

Table 3. Interesting patterns found in accidents database

S. No.	Patterns	Support	Periodicity
1	{General operating rules, Substantial}	1899	110
2	{General operating rules, private pilot, substantial}	750	219
3	{Cessna, Minor}	17,971	15
4	{California, Minor}	6,620	22
5	{General operating rules, Cessna, Minor}	16,154	15

conveys the crucial information that within every 15 days, aircrafts of 'Cessna' airlines undergo a 'minor' accident. The fourth pattern provides the information that within every 22 days, aircrafts in 'California' airport witness a 'minor' accident. The fifth pattern provides the information that with an interval of 15 days, 16154 'minor' aircraft accidents pertaining to 'Cessna' airlines have happened during 'general operating rules'.

4.4 Interesting Patterns Discovered in Shop-4 Database

We now discuss the useful information discovered by periodic-frequent patterns in Shop-4 database. Table 4 presents some of the interesting patterns discovered in Shop-4 database. The *periodicity* of a pattern is expressed in *minutes*.

Table 4. Interesting patterns discovered in Shop-4 database

S. No	Patterns	Support	Periodicity
1	{{Built-in ovens, hobs, grills}, {Washer dryers}}	4861	1353
2	{{Built-in ovens, hobs, grills}, {Microwave ovens}}	2134	2112
3	{{Refrigerators, freezers, show cases}, {washer dryers}}	5628	1288
4	{Washing machines, washer dryers}	8342	1114

These patterns were interesting, because they contain costly and durable goods, which are regularly viewed by the visitors.

5 Conclusions

This paper classifies current periodic pattern mining algorithms into two types: (*i*) finding periodic patterns in time series data and (*ii*) finding periodically occurring frequent patterns in temporally ordered transactional databases. This paper describes the basic model of periodic patterns in time series and transactional databases, and also discusses advantages and disadvantages of each model. Experimental results on real-world data sets demonstrate that periodic patterns can find useful information.

Acknowledgments. This work was supported by the Research and Development on Real World Big Data Integration and Analysis program of the Ministry of Education, Culture, Sports, Science, and Technology, JAPAN.

References

1. Özden, B., Ramaswamy, S., Silberschatz, A.: Cyclic association rules. In: ICDE, pp. 412–421 (1998)
2. Han, J., Gong, W., Yin, Y.: Mining segment-wise periodic patterns in time-related databases. In: KDD, pp. 214–218 (1998)
3. Zhang, M., Kao, B., Cheung, D.W., Yip, K.Y.: Mining periodic patterns with gap requirement from sequences. ACM Trans. Knowl. Discov. Data **1**(2) (2007)
4. Stormer, H.: Improving e-commerce recommender systems by the identification of seasonal products. In: Twenty Second Conference on Artificial Intelligence, pp. 92–99 (2007)
5. Ma, S., Hellerstein, J.: Mining partially periodic event patterns with unknown periods. In: ICDE, pp. 205–214 (2001)
6. Kiran, R.U., Shang, M.T., Kitsuregawa, M.: Discovering recurring patterns in time series. In: EDBT (2015, to be appeared)
7. Yang, R., Wang, W., Yu, P.: Infominer+: mining partial periodic patterns with gap penalties. In: ICDM, pp. 725–728 (2002)
8. Chen, S.-S., Huang, T.C.-K., Lin, Z.-M.: New and efficient knowledge discovery of partial periodic patterns with multiple minimum supports. J. Syst. Softw. **84**(10), 1638–1651 (2011)
9. Berberidis, C., Vlahavas, I.P., Aref, W.G., Atallah, M.J., Elmagarmid, A.K.: On the discovery of weak periodicities in large time series. In: Elomaa, T., Mannila, H., Toivonen, H. (eds.) PKDD 2002. LNCS (LNAI), vol. 2431, pp. 51–61. Springer, Heidelberg (2002)
10. Cao, H., Cheung, D.W., Mamoulis, N.: Discovering partial periodic patterns in discrete data sequences. In: Dai, H., Srikant, R., Zhang, C. (eds.) PAKDD 2004. LNCS (LNAI), vol. 3056, pp. 653–658. Springer, Heidelberg (2004)
11. Yang, J., Wang, W., Yu, P.S.: Mining asynchronous periodic patterns in time series data. IEEE Trans. Knowl. Data Eng. **15**(3), 613–628 (2003)

12. Tanbeer, S.K., Ahmed, C.F., Jeong, B.-S., Lee, Y.-K.: Discovering periodic-frequent patterns in transactional databases. In: Theeramunkong, T., Kijsirikul, B., Cercone, N., Ho, T.-B. (eds.) PAKDD 2009. LNCS, vol. 5476, pp. 242–253. Springer, Heidelberg (2009)

13. Uday Kiran, R., Krishna Reddy, P.: Towards efficient mining of periodic-frequent patterns in transactional databases. In: Bringas, P.G., Hameurlain, A., Quirchmayr, G. (eds.) DEXA 2010, Part II. LNCS, vol. 6262, pp. 194–208. Springer, Heidelberg (2010)

14. Amphawan, K., Lenca, P., Surarerks, A.: Mining top-k periodic-frequent pattern from transactional databases without support threshold. In: Papasratorn, B., Chutimaskul, W., Porkaew, K., Vanijja, V. (eds.) IAIT 2009. CCIS, vol. 55, pp. 18–29. Springer, Heidelberg (2009)

15. Kiran, R.U., Reddy, P.K.: An alternative interestingness measure for mining periodic-frequent patterns. In: Yu, J.X., Kim, M.H., Unland, R. (eds.) DASFAA 2011, Part I. LNCS, vol. 6587, pp. 183–192. Springer, Heidelberg (2011)

16. Kiran, R.U., Kitsuregawa, M.: Novel techniques to reduce search space in periodic-frequent pattern mining. In: Bhowmick, S.S., Dyreson, C.E., Jensen, C.S., Lee, M.L., Muliantara, A., Thalheim, B. (eds.) DASFAA 2014, Part II. LNCS, vol. 8422, pp. 377–391. Springer, Heidelberg (2014)

17. Aref, W.G., Elfeky, M.G., Elmagarmid, A.K.: Incremental, online, and merge mining of partial periodic patterns in time-series databases. IEEE TKDE 16(3), 332–342 (2004)

18. Agrawal, R., Imieliński, T., Swami, A.: Mining association rules between sets of items in large databases. In: SIGMOD, pp. 207–216 (1993)

19. Han, J., Dong, G., Yin, Y.: Efficient mining of partial periodic patterns in time series database. In: ICDE, pp. 106–115 (1999)

20. Liu, B., Hsu, W., Ma, Y.: Mining association rules with multiple minimum supports. In: KDD, pp. 337–341 (1999)

21. Surana, A., Kiran, R.U., Reddy, P.K.: An efficient approach to mine periodic-frequent patterns in transactional databases. In: Cao, L., Huang, J.Z., Bailey, J., Koh, Y.S., Luo, J. (eds.) PAKDD Workshops 2011. LNCS, vol. 7104, pp. 254–266. Springer, Heidelberg (2012)

22. Kiran, R.U., Kitsuregawa, M.: Discovering quasi-periodic-frequent patterns in transactional databases. In: Bhatnagar, V., Srinivasa, S. (eds.) BDA 2013. LNCS, vol. 8302, pp. 97–115. Springer, Heidelberg (2013)

23. Weblog dataset. http://web.archive.org/web/20070713202946rn_1/lisp.vse.cz/challenge/CURRENT/

24. Faa accidents dataset. http://www.asias.faa.gov/pls/apex/f?p=100:1:0::NO

VDMR-DBSCAN: Varied Density MapReduce DBSCAN

Surbhi Bhardwaj and Subrat Kumar Dash[✉]

Department of Computer Science and Engineering,
The LNM Institute of Information Technology, Jaipur, India
{surbhardwaj93,subrat.dash}@gmail.com

Abstract. DBSCAN is a well-known density based clustering algorithm, which can discover clusters of different shapes and sizes along with outliers. However, it suffers from major drawbacks like high computational cost, inability to find varied density clusters and dependency on user provided input density parameters. To address these issues, we propose a novel density based clustering algorithm titled, VDMR-DBSCAN (Varied Density MapReduce DBSCAN), a scalable DBSCAN algorithm using MapReduce which can detect varied density clusters with automatic computation of input density parameters. VDMR-DBSCAN divides the data into small partitions which are parallely processed on Hadoop platform. Thereafter, density variations in a partition are analyzed statistically to divide the data into groups of similar density called Density level sets (DLS). Input density parameters are estimated for each DLS, later DBSCAN is applied on each DLS using its corresponding density parameters. Most importantly, we propose a novel merging technique, which merges the similar density clusters present in different partitions and produces meaningful and compact clusters of varied density. We experimented on large and small synthetic datasets which well confirms the efficacy of our algorithm in terms of scalability and ability to find varied density clusters.

Keywords: Clustering · DBSCAN · Varied density · MapReduce · Hadoop · Scalable algorithm

1 Introduction

In today's era, the amount of data produced by different applications is increasing at a very fast pace. As of 2012, 90 % of the data in the world has been generated in the last two years alone [1]. There exists an immediate need to convert this huge data into some useful information and knowledge. Clustering is an important unsupervised learning technique in data mining which partitions the data objects into class of similar objects, based on the principle of maximizing intraclass similarity and minimizing interclass similarity [2]. For mining of huge data, clustering is well suited because unlike classification, it does not require labeling of large number of test tuples which is a very costly task. Clustering

© Springer International Publishing Switzerland 2015
N. Kumar and V. Bhatnagar (Eds.): BDA 2015, LNCS 9498, pp. 134–150, 2015.
DOI: 10.1007/978-3-319-27057-9_10

is broadly used for many applications like pattern recognition, data analysis, market research, image processing etc.

DBSCAN [3] is one of the popular density based clustering algorithm and has been widely used in past for various applications like land use detection, anomaly detection, spam identification, medical imaging, weather forecasting etc [4,5]. Unlike partitioning based clustering algorithms, DBSCAN does not require apriori knowledge regarding number of clusters to be formed. It has good noise handling abilities and can discover non-convex clusters of arbitrary shapes and sizes. However, DBSCAN has three major drawbacks. First, it is computationally very expensive due to iterative neighborhood querying and faces scalability problems while processing large data. Second, the input density parameters ε, $MinPts$, which directly influence the clustering results are specified by the user. Third, due to adoption of global ε value, it is unable to detect clusters of varied density.

To address these problems, many enhancements over DBSCAN have been proposed in literature, but they address only some of the limitations of DBSCAN, as discussed above. Today, the size of data is too huge that even a simple data analysis task faces scalability issues. Being no exception, DBSCAN also faces the scalability problem due to its high computational cost. Therefore, a need arises for parallelization of DBSCAN algorithm to reduce its processing time. Also, in huge data, it becomes a very challenging task to find good quality clusters with minimal domain knowledge. Poor quality clusters, even obtained in a very less time, are meaningless. Therefore, quality of clusters produced by a clustering algorithm are equally important as its processing time. Some parallel and distributed solutions for DBSCAN have been proposed in literature, but they are inefficient in dealing with varied density clusters. Hence, there arises a need of a density based clustering algorithm which is highly scalable and discovers varied density clusters with automatic computation of input parameters.

In this paper, we propose a density based clustering algorithm, titled *VDMR-DBSCAN (Varied Density Map Reduce DBSCAN)* which overcomes the major drawbacks of traditional DBSCAN and its various enhancements. VDMR-DBSCAN is designed on top of Hadoop [7] Platform and uses Google's MapReduce [6] paradigm for parallelization. Varied density clusters are obtained using the concept of Density Level Partitioning. Most importantly, we have proposed a novel merging technique, which merges the similar density clusters present in different partitions and tends to produce meaningful and compact clusters of varied density. We evaluated VDMR-DBSCAN on large and small synthetic datasets. The results reveal that the proposed algorithm is highly scalable and detects varied density clusters with minimal requirement of domain knowledge.

The rest of the paper is organized as follows. Section 2 presents related work, which discusses the traditional DBSCAN and its various enhancements. In Sect. 3, our proposed algorithm VDMR-DBSCAN is discussed in detail. Section 4 presents experimental settings and results, followed by Sect. 5 which concludes the paper.

2   Related Work

In 1996, Ester et al. proposed DBSCAN [3], a well known density based clustering algorithm. It defines the density in terms of two user provided input parameters: ε, $MinPts$. To find clusters, DBSCAN starts with an arbitrary unclassified point p_i and finds the points present in ε-neighborhood of p_i ($NEps(p_i)$). If $|NEps(p_i)|$ is greater than $MinPts$, then a cluster C is formed which includes all the points in $NEps(p_i)$, with p_i as a core point, otherwise p_i will be marked as a noise point. DBSCAN then iterates to expand the cluster C by collecting the density-reachable points from all core points present in C. This step repeats until no more points can be added to the cluster. The algorithm will continue until all the points in dataset are assigned to a cluster or labeled as noise point. DBSCAN has some drawbacks like unscalability, inability to find varied density clusters and dependency on user provided input density parameters.

In 1999, Ankerst et al. proposed OPTICS [8] to attack the varied density problem with DBSCAN by creating an augmented ordering of the data points, which represents its density based clustering structure. OPTICS does not produce clustering results explicitly and experimentally its runtime is almost constantly 1.6 times the run time of DBSCAN. Like DBSCAN, it also suffers from scalability problems. In 1999, Xu et al. proposed PDBSCAN [9], a master-slave-mode parallel implementation of DBSCAN. It works on shared nothing architecture where communication between nodes occur through message passing, thereby it leads to a large communication overhead while dealing with huge data. Also, it is unable to deal with clusters of varied density. In 2006, Uncu et al. proposed GRIDBSCAN [10] to solve the varied density problem with DBSCAN. Empirically, GRIDBSCAN is better than DBSCAN in terms of accuracy however, in terms of computational complexity, it is very expensive due to pairwise distance computations which makes it unsuitable for clustering of large data. In 2007, Liu et al. proposed VDBSCAN [11] to attack the varied density problem of DBSCAN. VDBSCAN is good at finding varied density clusters but it is not scalable and parameter k has to be subjectively chosen. In 2008, Mahran et al. proposed GriDBSCAN [12] to solve the scalability issues with DBSCAN. Data partitioning in GriDBSCAN generates a large number of redundant boundary points which degrades the execution efficiency of parallel algorithm and increases the merging time. Furthermore, it is unable to find varied density clusters and the input parameters for DBSCAN execution are provided by the user. In 2012, Xiong et al. proposed DBSCAN-DLP [13] to solve the varied density problem with DBSCAN using the concept of *Density level partitioning*. DBSCAN-DLP is computationally very expensive due to the computation of kth nearest neighbor distances and density variations values, which make it unsuitable for large datasets. To address the scalability problem of DBSCAN, Dai et al. proposed DBSCAN-MR [14] in 2012, which is a *MapReduce* based parallel DBSCAN and uses Hadoop platform for parallel processing. DBSCAN-MR is highly scalable, but it is unable to find varied density clusters and input density parameters are need to be provided by user.

None of the above stated clustering techniques, is efficient enough to tackle all the three issues of DBSCAN. Therefore, we attempt to provide a solution by proposing a novel density based clustering algorithm VDMR-DBSCAN, which overcomes all these limitations.

3   Proposed Work

VDMR-DBSCAN is designed on top of Hadoop platform and uses MapReduce paradigm for parallelization. MapReduce improves the scalability of our algorithm by dividing large data into small partitions and sending those partitions to different nodes in the Hadoop cluster, where they can be processed independently. Later, the results from different nodes are aggregated to obtain final results.

VDMR-DBSCAN framework consists of five different stages: Data Partitioning, Map, Reduce, Merge & Relabeling. In the first phase, input data is partitioned using PRBP (Partition with reduced boundary points) [14] partitioning, with an objective to minimize the boundary points. The data partitions are stored in *HDFS* (Hadoop Distributed File System) [7]. In the second phase, the partitions obtained are clustered independently using density level partitioning [13], to obtain clusters of varied density. Then, the local clusters present in different partitions are merged to obtain global clusters, followed by relabeling of data points. In the following subsections, we discuss different phases of VDMR-DBSCAN which is also shown in Fig. 1.

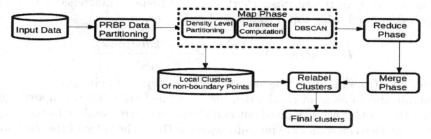

Fig. 1. Phases of VDMR-DBSCAN

3.1   Partitioning Phase

VDMR-DBSCAN uses PRBP partitioning [14] to divide the data into small partitions which can be easily handled by a single node in the Hadoop cluster. It partitions the data such that two adjacent partitions share a common region i.e. *split region*. The points lying in the split region are called *boundary points* which help in identifying connected clusters present in two adjacent partitions. PRBP mainly focuses on minimizing the boundary points. It works by dividing each dimension in slices of equal width, followed by calculation of data distribution in each slice. Further, the slice 's' with minimum points is selected to partition the data into two partitions. s being the common region (*split region*), is added to both the partitions. The data space is recursively split until the size of partition fits the node's memory. We are using PRBP as a data partitioning algorithm for VDMR-DBSCAN with an intuition that reduced number of boundary points will reduce the merging time as well as map reduce time, which in result will improve the execution efficiency of VDMR-DBSCAN. The partitions created by PRBP partitioning are stored in *HDFS* (Hadoop Distributed File System) [7] from where each partition is read by a mapper in map phase.

3.2   Map Phase

In Map phase, each mapper reads a complete partition from *HDFS* in the form of *(key, value)* pair, where *key* = NULL and *value* = Partition. Further, each mapper uses *Density level partitioning* [13] to find varied density clusters, based on statistical characteristics of data points present in a partition. Density level partitioning partitions the data into different density level sets such that points with similar density belongs to same density level set (DLS).

The data is partitioned into different density level sets based on their k^{th} nearest neighbor distance values (*kdist* value), where value of k is chosen from the range 3 to 10 [13]. *kdist* value of a point is the measure of how far is the kth nearest neighbor of that point, which gives an idea about the density around that point. Algorithm 1, shows the pseudocode for Map phase. Map phase proceeds by finding *kdist* values for all the points in a partition and stores them in *kdistlist*. The obtained *kdistlist* is sorted in ascending order. Further, for each adjacent points p_i and p_j in the *kdistlist*, $DenVar(p_i, p_j)$ (density difference between p_i &p_j) is computed using Eq. 1, to obtain *DenVarList*.

$$DenVar(p_i, p_j) = \frac{|kdist(p_j, k) - kdist(p_i, k)|}{kdist(p_i, k)}, \tag{1}$$

where, $kdist(p_j, k)$ is the kth nearest neighbor distance of point p_j.
To obtain the *DLS*s from *DenVarlist*, the values in *DenVarlist* which are larger than a threshold τ are separated out and the points corresponding to these separated out *DenVar* values are put into separate *DLS*. The value of the threshold τ is computed using the statistical characteristics of *DenVarlist*, as follows:

$$\tau = EX(DenVarlist) + \omega.SD(DenVarlist) \tag{2}$$

In Eq. 2, EX is the mathematical expectation, ω is the tuning coeffiecient and SD is the standard deviation of the *DenVarlist*. Value of ω is chosen from the range (0,3) [13]. The *DLS* so obtained are refined further by removing the *DLS*s of border and noise points and merging of *DLS*s with similar density levels. Based on the density characteristics of *DLS*, ε values are computed automatically for each DLS using Eq. 3 and stored in *EpsList*.

$$\varepsilon_i = maxkdist(DLS_i).\sqrt{\frac{mediankdist(DLS_i)}{meankdist(DLS_i)}} \tag{3}$$

Here, *maxkdist, meankdist* and *mediankdist* are the maximum, mean and the median *kdist* values of DLS_i respectively.

Algorithm 1. VDMR-DBSCAN Map phase (Mapper side)

Input: $key = Null, value = Partition, k$ ▷ value of k specified by user in range $[3, 10]$
Output: Local and boundary region outputs
1: D ← *value*   ▷ Whole partition is assigned to D
2: KD ← Build_ Kd_ Tree(D)   ▷ build KD tree spatial index
3: kdistlist ← Compute_ kdistlist(k, KD)   ▷ computation of *kdist* values
4: Sort_ in_ Asc(kdistlist)   ▷ Sort the kdistlist in ascending order
5: DenVarlist ← ComputeDenVar(kdistlist)
6: τ ← EX(DenVarlist) + ω . SD(DenVarlist)   ▷ computation of density variation
   threshold τ
7: DLS_ List ← Create_ DLS(DenVarlist, τ, D)   ▷ D is partitioned into DLS
8: Refine_ DLS(DLS_ List)
9: EpsList ← Compute_ Eps(DLS_ List, kdistlist)   ▷ ε values are computed for each
   DLS
10: **for** each ε_i in EpsList **do**   ▷ EpsList is ordered in acending order
11: $\quad$| DBSCAN(DLS_List_i , ε_i, k, D)
12: **end for**
13: **for** each point Pt in D **do**
14: $\quad$| **if** Pt.isBoundary = true **then**
15: $\quad$| $\quad$| output(Pt.index, Pt.cluster_ id + Pt.isCore_ point + Pt.Eps_ value +
   kdistvalues)
16: $\quad$| **else**
17: $\quad$| $\quad$| write_ to_ local(Pt.index, Pt.cluster_ id)   ▷ output written to local disk
18: $\quad$| **end if**
19: **end for**

Further, DBSCAN is applied on each DLS, using its corresponding ε values from *EpsList* and with $MinPts = k$. DBSCAN iterates by selecting the initial seed points from the DLS only, but the neighborhood counting is done over all the unprocessed data objects. VDMR-DBSCAN improves the efficiency of traditional DBSCAN from $O(n^2)$ to $O(nlogn)$ by using KD-Tree [15] spatial index. After all the iterations, final clusters of varied density are obtained and the non-marked points are considered as noise points in the dataset.

The clustering results obtained after applying DBSCAN are divided into two regions: *Boundary* and *local region*. The clustering results of boundary region are used in merging of similar density clusters, which are present in adjacent partitions. The results of boundary region are passed to the reducer in the form of *(key, value)* pairs as *(point_index, cluster_id + isCore_point + Eps_value + kdistvalues)*, where *point_index* is the index of the point, *cluster_id* is the cluster identification number for the point, *isCore_point* is a flag which indicates whether the point is core or not, *Eps_value* is the ε value of the cluster to which the point belongs. *kdistvalues* is the list of k nearest neighbor distances of a point in the partition. The clustering results of local region are stored in the local disk, in the form of key/value pair as *(point_index, cluster_id)*.

3.3   Reduce Phase

Reduce phase finds the pairs of clusters from adjacent partitions, which can be merged in Merge phase. It outputs a *Merge_Comb* list of mergable cluster pairs and ensures the merging of density similar clusters only. Reduce phase collects the boundary points from Map phase and gathers all the points with same point index from different partitions. Points with same point index (*key*) are executed at the same reducer. Based on boundary point values, Reduce phase decides whether the two clusters which share a boundary point can be merged or not. However, the final merging will take place in Merge phase only. If two clusters, say, *C1* and *C2* share a boundary point *b*, then *C1* and *C2* forms a merge combination (*MC*), if they satisfy the following two criterion:

- Boundary point should be a core point in at least one of the clusters.
- The difference in the ε values of the two clusters should be smaller than a threshold, α.

A core point in the boundary region helps in identifying, if a cluster can be extended upto a different partition. Difference in ε values of the two clusters gives a measure of density difference between the two clusters. To ensure merging of similar density clusters, it creates a *Merge_Comb* list of only those clusters whose ε difference is less than α. The value of α can be controlled, depending upon the quality of clusters required. Algorithm 2, gives a summary of steps involved in Reduce phase.

Algorithm 2. VDMR-DBSCAN Reduce phase (Reducer side)

Input: $key = Pt\_index, value = cluster\_id + isCore\_point + Eps\_value + kdistvalues$
Output: $key = Pt\_index, value = Merge\_Comb$ list
1: **for all** $C1, C2 \in l$ **do**   ▷ l is the list of clusters to which point_index belong
2:     **if** Pt_index is core point in $C1\|C2$ **then**
3:         $Eps\_dif \leftarrow$ compute difference in ε values of $C1$ &$C2$
4:         **if** $Eps\_dif < \alpha$ **then**
5:             $Merge\_Comb$.add($\{C1, C2\}$)
6:         **end if**
7:     **end if**
8: **end for**
9: **if** !$Merge\_Comb$.isEmpty() **then**
10:     write $Merge\_Comb$ to HDFS
11: **else**
12:     $kdistlist \leftarrow$ combine $kdistvalues$ from all partitions &sort
13:     $k\_dist \leftarrow kdistlist$.get(k-1)   ▷ Fetch the kth nearest neighbor value
14:     $cid \leftarrow$ find cluster with minimum absolute difference between its ε &k_dist
15:     output(key, cid);   ▷ The cluster-id of the point is written to the local disk
16: **end if**

Non-Merged Clusters: In cases where the clusters are found to be unsuitable for merging then the boundary point which is part of both the clusters, should only be assigned to either of the clusters.

VDMR-DBSCAN solves this issue by using the *kdistvalues* list which is a part of Mapper's output. *kdistvalues* contain the k nearest neighbor distances of a boundary point, in a partition. To find the global value of kth nearest neighbor distance for the boundary point, *kdistvalues* of the point are collected from all partitions, in Reducer. The *kdistvalues* collected for a point, are combined to form a single list (*kdistlist*) and sorted in ascending order where k^{th} value is picked from *kdistlist* to find k^{th} nearest neighbor distance for this boundary point. Further, difference between ε and *kdist* value is computed for all the clusters to which the point belongs. The point is assigned to the cluster with minimum absolute difference of ε and *kdist* values. Since, points belonging to same cluster are likely to have similar *kdist* values therefore, a point is more density similar to the cluster with minimum absolute difference of ε and *kdist* value. The cluster-id of such points are not part of *Merge_Comb* list and are written to the local disk with the output of local regions. At the end of Reduce phase, *Merge_Comb* list is written to the *HDFS* from where it is read by Merge phase for merging of clusters.

3.4   Merge Phase

Merge phase merges the *MC*s discovered by Reduce phase to identify the clusters which span over multiple partitions. It reads the input from *HDFS* as (*key*, *Merge_Comb* list), written by Reduce phase, where *key* is the point index and *Merge_Comb* list contains a list of *MC*s that can be merged. The output of this phase is a set of *MergeList*, where each *MergeList* represents the list of merged clusters. Assume, the output of reducer contains three *MC*s as {*P1C1*, *P2C2*}, {*P5C2*, *P2C2*}, {*P4C2*, *P1C1*} which can be further merged, like {*P1C1*, *P2C2*} can be merged with {*P2C2*, *P5C2*} to form a *MergeList* {*P1C1*, *P2C2*, *P5C2*}, which can be further merged with {*P4C2*, *P1C1*} to give a final *MergeList* as {*P1C1*, *P2C2*, *P5C2*, *P4C2*}. Merge phase identifies those *MC*s which can be merged further and merges them to produce a final set of *MergeList*.

Merge phase starts with finding difference between ε values of clusters, for all *MC*s in *Merge_Comb* list and sorts all of them in ascending order based on their ε difference value. Then, it first combines the one with the minimum ε difference i.e. the most density similar *MC* to form a *MergeList*. Further, all the *MC*s which have an intersection with this *MergeList* are found, where all *MC*s are already sorted in ascending order based on their ε difference values. The intersection pair with minimum ε difference is chosen and its ε difference is computed with all the clusters present in this *MergeList*. If the maximum ε difference is found to be less than the threshold α then this *MC* is merged with the existing *MergeList* to form a new *MergeList*. Further, Merge phase proceeds by iterating on remaining *MC*s, until no more clusters can be merged.

Mathematically, it can be formulated as,

$$eps\_diff(C_i, C_j) = |eps(C_i) - eps(C_j)|. \tag{4}$$

In Eq. 4, $eps\_diff(C_i, C_j)$ computes the dissimilarity in the density of clusters C_i & C_j, where $eps(C_i)$ is the ε value of cluster C_i. After merging of cluster C_i, C_j, the eps_diff of resulting cluster with another C_k is computed as:

$$eps\_diff((C_i \cup C_j), C_k) = max(eps\_diff(C_i, C_k), eps\_diff(C_j, C_k)). \tag{5}$$

For Merging, $eps\_diff((C_i \cup C_j), C_k) < \alpha$. Intuitively, this is similar to the complete link hierarchical clustering [2], where the distance between two clusters is determined by the most distant nodes in the two clusters. Similar to complete link hierarchical clustering, merge phase tends to produce compact (density compact) clusters and avoids long chain of clusters which would be meaningless.

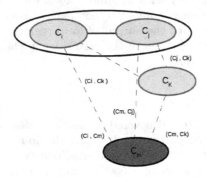

Fig. 2. Merging of clusters

For illustration of merging, consider Fig. 2 which represents six MCs namely, $\{C_i, C_j\}, \{C_j, C_k\}, \{C_k, C_m\}, \{C_i, C_k\}, \{C_m, C_j\}, \{C_i, C_m\}$, arranged in ascending order based on their eps_diff values. Here, lines between the clusters represent their eps_diff. Assuming, C_i and C_j has the least eps_diff, therefore, they are combined to form a *MergeList*. $\{C_j, C_k\}$ is the next most density similar MC (least value of eps_diff), which has an intersection with $\{C_i, C_j\}$ and its maximum eps_diff i.e. $eps\_diff(C_i, C_k)$ is less than α, therefore it is merged into *MergeList*. Now, the updated *MergeList* contains $\{C_i, C_j, C_k\}$. The next most density similar intersection pair for the *MergeList* is $\{C_k, C_m\}$ whereas, $eps\_diff(C_i, C_m)$ is greater than α, therefore C_m is not combined with the *MergeList*.

It can be observed from the above illustration, that a cluster can be combined to a list of clusters only if its eps_diff with all clusters in the list, is less than α, i.e. it is similar in density to all clusters in the list. In absence of this, it may lead to large variations of densities in a cluster and degrade the quality of cluster. Hence, it can be concluded that Merge phase avoids large variations in densities while merging of clusters and tends to provide compact clusters in terms of density.

3.5   Relabeling of Data Points

Once the clusters are combined in Merge phase, then all cluster-ids are sorted in ascending order and all clusters in the list are relabeled as the first one. For example, the clusters in the list {*P1C1, P2C2, P5C2, P4C2*} are relabeled as *P1C1*. Both boundary points and points in local output are relabeled to correct cluster-ids.

4   Results and Discussions

In this section, we evaluate the performance of VDMR-DBSCAN on synthetic datasets of different densities and sizes and compare its clustering results with DBSCAN-DLP [13] and DBSCAN-MR [14] which are found to be the best versions of DBSCAN clustering algorithm in the current state of art.

4.1   Experimental Settings

We conducted the experiments on Hadoop cluster with 4 DataNodes and 1 NameNode where NameNode contains 8 GB RAM with intel i5 CPU, running Ubuntu-14.04 Linux operating system. DataNodes contain intel i5 CPU and 4 GB RAM with Ubuntu-14.04. For MapReduce platform, we used Hadoop-1.2.1 version on all the nodes. Both JobTracker & NameNode are configured on same node. We have used three synthetic datasets, to illustrate the performance of our proposed algorithm. For intuitive illustration, we have restricted to the datasets in 2 dimensions only. No suitable cluster validity index is found in literature for validating varied density clusters, therefore we have verified the results visually with 2 dimensional data only. We have used two small synthetic datasets: Zahn_compound (DS1) and Spiral dataset (DS2) [16] of varied densities. Figure 3(a) and (b) shows the unclustured data points of dataset DS1 & DS2 respectively. Zahn_compound dataset contains 399 data points whereas spiral dataset contains 312 data points. We have generated, one large 2-dimensional synthetic dataset (DS3) to illustrate the efficiency of proposed algorithm in finding varied density clusters on large data.

4.2   Experimental Results

In this section, the clustering results of VDMR-DBSCAN on above metioned datasets and its comparison with DBSCAN-DLP and DBSCAN-MR are discussed. Clustering results are represented through points in different colors and markers which indicate the different clusters discovered whereas dashed lines represent the data partitions obtained. In VDMR-DBSCAN k, ω, α and σ are the user provided input parameters, whereas in DBSCAN-MR k, ε, $MinPts$ are provided by user. ρ is the number of partitions created by PRBP partitioning. Experimentally, $k = 4$ and $\omega = 2.5$ is found to be an ideal value for multi-density datasets [13].

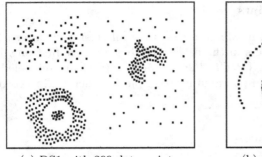
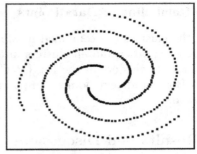

(a) DS1 with 399 data points   (b) DS2 with 312 data points

Fig. 3. Datasets

4.3   Clustering Results on Zahn_compound Dataset (DS1)

Figure 4(a) shows eight varied density clusters obtained after applying VDMR-DBSCAN whereas, Fig. 4(b), shows the clusters obtained by applying DBSCAN-MR, which clearly illustrates the inability of DBSCAN-MR to find varied density clusters. DBSCAN-MR is unable to identify the points around the cyan colored cluster (marked as red colored cross in Fig. 4(b)), as a cluster and treats them as noise points whereas these points are identified as a separate cluster by VDMR-DBSCAN (represented by black dots in Fig. 4(a)). In DBSCAN-MR, clusters in green and red are formed by merging of small density clusters into a single cluster, which is due to relatively larger ε value.

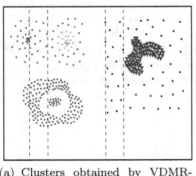
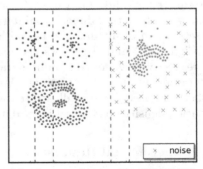

(a) Clusters obtained by VDMR-DBSCAN ($k = 4$, $\omega = 2.5$, $\alpha = 1.4790$, $\sigma = 3$, $\rho = 3$)

(b) Clusters obtained by DBSCAN-MR ($\varepsilon = 1.9$, $\sigma = 3.8$, $\rho = 3$, $MinPts = 4$)

Fig. 4. Clustering results on DS1 (Color figure online)

Through clustering and merging of two partitions *P1* & *P2* (Fig. 5), we demostrate the working of VDMR-DBSCAN. Figure 5(a) and (b) show the clusters obtained by VDMR-DBSCAN on *P1* and *P2* respectively. On applying

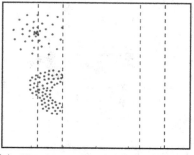 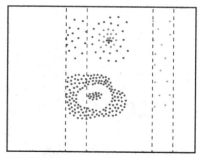

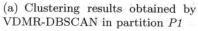

(a) Clustering results obtained by VDMR-DBSCAN in partition *P1*

(b) Clustering results obtained by VDMR-DBSCAN in partition *P2*

Fig. 5. Clustering results obtained on Partitions *P1* & *P2* (Color figure online)

VDMR-DBSCAN on *P1* (for $k = 4$ & $\omega = 2.5$), two ε values are generated. Cluster in blue points is generated by ε value of 0.40311 whereas red and green colored clusters are obtained by ε value of 2.20055 (Fig. 5(a)). In *P2*, four ε values are generated after applying VDMR-DBSCAN. The cluster in green is generated by ε value of 1.04209, cluster in magenta has an ε value of 2.00381, whereas yellow colored cluster which is formed in boundary region of partition *P2* & *P3* has an ε value of 2.84783 (Fig. 5(b)).

In Fig. 4(a), it is clearly visible that green colored cluster in *P2* is merged with green colored cluster in partition *P1*, this is because the ε difference between both the clusters is 1.1585 (2.20055 − 1.04209), which is less than α (merging threshold), (1.4790). Similarly, red colored cluster in *P1* is merged with magenta colored cluster in *P2* with an ε difference of 0.19674 (2.20055 − 2.00381) which is also less than α.

Varying Width of Partitioning Slice (σ): Change in σ value, changes the number of partitions, data points in each partition, boundary region and number of boundary points. We have experimented with σ value of 2.2, 3.4 and 3.8 respectively. Figure 6(a), (b) & Fig. 4(a) show the clustering results of VDMR-DBSCAN on partitions created by slice width of 3.4, 2.2 and 3.8 respectively and the results obtained for different slice widths are found to be almost similar.

Figure 7(a), shows the clustering results of DBSCAN-MR with 5 partitions created by $\sigma = 3.4$. In DBSCAN-MR, the ε value used should be half of σ, so a global ε value of 1.7 is used. As compared to the results obtained from VDMR-DBSCAN on the same partitions (Fig. 6(a)), DBSCAN-MR is able to discover only three clusters and rest are flagged as noise points. Due to a global ε value, DBSCAN-MR is unable to identify varied density clusters in the dataset. Figure 7(b) shows the clustering results of DBSCAN-MR on six partitions, created by $\sigma = 2.2$. It uses a global ε value of 1.1. Figure 4(b), shows the clustering results of DBSCAN-MR on three partitions created by $\sigma = 3.8$. From the above comparisons, we can clearly observe that VDMR-DBSCAN can efficiently find

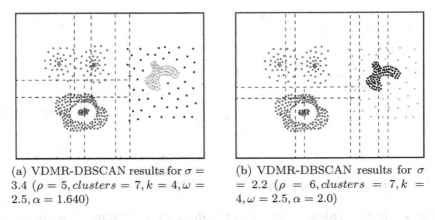

(a) VDMR-DBSCAN results for $\sigma =$ 3.4 ($\rho = 5, clusters = 7, k = 4, \omega = 2.5, \alpha = 1.640$)

(b) VDMR-DBSCAN results for $\sigma = 2.2$ ($\rho = 6, clusters = 7, k = 4, \omega = 2.5, \alpha = 2.0$)

Fig. 6. Clustering results of VDMR-DBSCAN for σ values of 3.4, 2.2 (Color figure online)

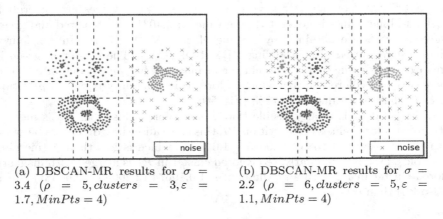

(a) DBSCAN-MR results for $\sigma = 3.4$ ($\rho = 5, clusters = 3, \varepsilon = 1.7, MinPts = 4$)

(b) DBSCAN-MR results for $\sigma = 2.2$ ($\rho = 6, clusters = 5, \varepsilon = 1.1, MinPts = 4$)

Fig. 7. Clustering results of DBSCAN-MR for σ values of 3.4, 2.2 (Color figure online)

varied density clusters in a dataset whereas DBSCAN-MR is unable to find, due to single ε value. Also, the results of DBSCAN-MR depends on the ε value used, as explained above.

4.4 Clustering Results on Spiral Dataset (DS2)

In Fig. 8(a) and (b), clustering results of VDMR-DBSCAN and DBSCAN-MR are compared on DS2 with four partitions, which are created by σ value of 3. It is clearly evident from the two figures, that VDMR-DBSCAN is able to capture the minute density change in yellow and black, magenta and green, also blue and cyan colored clusters, whereas DBSCAN-MR results in noise points and is unable to differentiate between the varied density clusters.

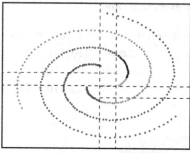 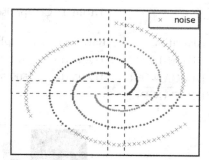

(a) Clustering result of VDMR-DBSCAN ($\rho = 4, \sigma = 3, clusters = 7, k = 4, \omega = 2.5, \alpha = 1.5$)

(b) Clustering result of DBSCAN-MR ($\rho = 4, \sigma = 3, clusters = 4, \varepsilon = 1.5, MinPts = 4$)

Fig. 8. Clustering results on DS2 (Color figure online)

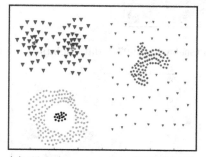 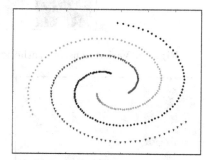

(a) Clustering results of DBSCAN-DLP on DS1 ($clusters = 9, k = 4, \omega = 2.5, MinPts = 4$)

(b) Clustering results of DBSCAN-DLP on DS2 ($clusters = 6, k = 4, \omega = 2.5, MinPts = 4$)

Fig. 9. Clustering results of DBSCAN-DLP on DS1 & DS2 (Color figure online)

Clustering Results of DBSCAN-DLP on Datasets DS1 & DS2: Results in Fig. 9(a) and (b) show the efficacy of DBSCAN-DLP in discovering varied density clusters. The results are comparable to that of VDMR-DBSCAN but the difference lies in scalability of the algorithm. As VDMR-DBSCAN partitions the data into p partitions and processes each partition parallelly before going for the merge phase, the time complexity is thus reduced by approximately a factor of p. Thus, VDMR-DBSCAN is scalable in comparison to DBSCAN-DLP which is partly evident from Table 1 also.

4.5 Large Synthetic Dataset (DS3)

In this section, clustering results of VDMR-DBSCAN on *DS3* are discussed. *DS3* consists of 499746 data points. It is synthetically generated to have four

Table 1. Comparison in execution time

Algorithm	Partition(sec)	MapReduce(sec)	Merge(sec)	Total time(sec)
VDMR-DBSCAN	412.95514	674.39250	3.73998	1091.08762
DBSCAN-MR	412.95514	509.50999	3.53355	925.99868
DBSCAN-DLP	–	–	–	165470.30148

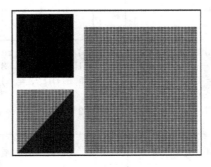

Fig. 10. Varied density synthetic dataset with 499746 data points

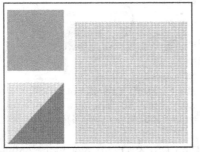
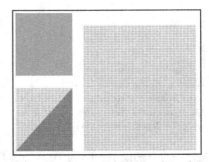

(a) Clusters discovered by VDMR-DBSCAN ($\rho = 117, \sigma = 0.02$, *clusters* $= 4, k = 5, \omega = 2.5, \alpha = 0.001$)

(b) Clusters discovered by DBSCAN-MR ($\rho = 117, \sigma = 0.02$, *clusters* $= 3, \varepsilon = 0.01$)

Fig. 11. Clustering results on DS3 (Color figure online)

clusters of three different densities. Figure 10 shows the data points of DS3 on a two-dimensional plot.

Figure 11(a) shows the result of VDMR-DBSCAN on *DS3*. Before applying VDMR-DBSCAN the dataset is partitioned using PRBP partitioning. We tried the partitioning with different slice width and out of them slice width of 0.02 is chosen because it produced least number of boundary points. As a result of partitioning, the dataset is divided into 117 partitions with 89459 boundary points. VDMR-DBSCAN is then applied on these 117 partitions and it discovered four varied density clusters in the dataset which are represented by yellow, cyan, red and green colored clusters in Fig. 11(a). Figure 11(b) shows the clusters obtained by DBSCAN-MR on *DS3*. DBSCAN-MR is run on the partitions obtained, using a global ε value of 0.01. As a result, it discovered only three different clusters in the dataset. DBSCAN-MR has merged two clusters of different densities into a single cluster, which is colored as red in Fig. 11(b), whereas VDMR-DBSCAN has discovered it as two clusters (Fig. 11(a)) of red and cyan color.

From Table 1, it can be observed that VDMR-DBSCAN has slightly higher execution time than DBSCAN-MR, which is due to extra computations done by VDMR-DBSCAN during map, reduce and merge phase to discover varied clusters. DBSCAN-DLP has a very high execution time as compared to VDMR-DBSCAN and DBSCAN-MR, because it is not scalable which makes it computationally very expensive while dealing with large datasets. Hence, in terms of execution time, DBSCAN-MR and VDMR-DBSCAN are much more efficient than DBSCAN-DLP. The execution time of DBSCAN-MR and VDMR-DBSCAN are comparable but VDMR-DBSCAN is far better than DBSCAN-MR in terms of finding varied density clusters with automatic computation of input density parameters. Therefore, from above results it can be concluded that VDMR-DBSCAN is better than existing versions of DBSCAN clustering algorithm because it can efficiently find varied density clusters of different shapes and sizes in small as well as large datasets, in a very less time.

5   Conclusions and Future Work

In this paper, we proposed a novel density based clustering algorithm VDMR-DBSCAN, which is highly scalable and finds clusters of varied-density with automatic computation of input density parameters in massive data. VDMR-DBSCAN is designed on top of Hadoop Platform and uses MapReduce paradigm for parallelization. We also proposed a novel merging technique, which merges the similar density clusters present in different partitions and ensures meaningful and compact clusters of varied density. We proved the efficiency of proposed algorithm by experimenting on large and small synthetic datasets. Experimental results revealed that our algorithm is highly scalable and detects varied density clusters with minimal requirement of domain knowledge. One of the future work is to use VDMR-DBSCAN with different existing data partitioning techniques like ESP, CBP [17], to see if they improve the execution efficiency of VDMR-DBSCAN.

References

1. IBM. http://www-01.ibm.com/software/data/bigdata/what-is-big-data.html
2. Han, J., Kamber, M., Pei, J.: Data Mining: Concepts and Techniques. Elsevier, Amterdam (2011)
3. Ester, M., et al.: A density-based algorithm for discovering clusters in large spatial databases with noise. Kdd **96**(34), 226–231 (1996)

4. Birant, D., Kut, A.: ST-DBSCAN: an algorithm for clustering spatial-temporal data. Data Knowl. Eng. **60**(1), 208–221 (2007)
5. Emre, C.M., Aslandogan, Y.A., Bergstresser, P.R.: Mining biomedical images with density-based clustering. In: 2005 International Conference on Information Technology: Coding and Computing, ITCC 2005, vol. 1. IEEE (2005)
6. Dean, J., Ghemawat, S.: MapReduce: simplified data processing on large clusters. Commun. ACM **51**(1), 107–113 (2008)
7. Hadoop, W.T.: The Definitive Guide, 1st edn. OReilly Media Inc., Sebastopol (2009)
8. Ankerst, M., et al.: OPTICS: ordering points to identify the clustering structure. ACM Sigmod Rec. **28**(2), 49–60 (1999)
9. Xu, X., Jger, J., Kriegel, H.-P.: A fast parallel clustering algorithm for large spatial databases. In: Guo, Y., Grossman, R. (eds.) High Performance Data Mining, pp. 263–290. Springer US, London (2002)
10. Uncu, O., et al.: GRIDBSCAN: grid density-based spatial clustering of applications with noise. In: 2006 IEEE International Conference on Systems, Man and Cybernetics, SMC 2006, vol. 4. IEEE (2006)
11. Liu, P., Zhou, D., Wu, N.: VDBSCAN: varied density based spatial clustering of applications with noise. In: 2007 International Conference on Service Systems and Service Management. IEEE (2007)
12. Mahran, S., Mahar, K.: Using grid for accelerating density-based clustering. In: 2008 8th IEEE International Conference on Computer and Information Technology, CIT 2008. IEEE (2008)
13. Xiong, Z., et al.: Multi-density DBSCAN algorithm based on density levels partitioning. J. Inf. Comput. Sci. **9**(10), 2739–2749 (2012)
14. Dai, B.-R., Lin, I.: Efficient map/reduce-based DBSCAN algorithm with optimized data partition. In: 2012 IEEE 5th International Conference on Cloud Computing (CLOUD). IEEE (2012)
15. Gaede, V., Gnther, O.: Multidimensional access methods. ACM Comput. Surv. (CSUR) **30**(2), 170–231 (1998)
16. University of Eastern Finland. http://cs.joensuu.fi/sipu/datasets/
17. He, Y., et al.: MR-DBSCAN: a scalable MapReduce-based DBSCAN algorithm for heavily skewed data. Front. Comput. Sci. **8**(1), 83–99 (2014)

Concept Discovery from Un-Constrained Distributed Context

Vishal Goel$^{(\boxtimes)}$ and B.D. Chaudhary

School of Computing and Electrical Engineering, IIT Mandi, Mandi, India
s13003@students.iitmandi.ac.in,
bdchaudhary@iitmandi.ac.in

Abstract. Formal Concept Analysis (FCA) is a method for analysing data set consisting of binary relation matrix between objects and their attributes to discover concepts that describe special kind of relationships between set of attributes and set of objects. These concepts are related to each other and are arranged in a hierarchy. FCA finds its application in several areas including data mining, machine learning and semantic web.

Few iterative MapReduce based algorithms have been proposed to mine concepts from a given data set. These algorithms either copy the entire data set (context) on each node or partition it in a specific manner. They assume that all attributes are known apriori and are ordered. These algorithms iterate based on the ordering of attributes. In some applications these assumptions will limit the scalability of algorithms.

In this paper, we present a concept mining algorithm which does not assume apriori knowledge of all attributes and permits the distribution of context on different nodes in an arbitrary manner. Our algorithm utilizes Apache Spark framework for discovering and eliminating redundant concepts in each iteration. When we aggregate data on attribute basis, we order the attributes based on the number of objects containing them. Our method relies on finding extents for combinations of attributes of particular size (say 'k'). An extent which is not regenerated in attribute combinations of size k + 1 corresponds to a valid concept. All concepts with particular intent size k are saved in one Resilient Distributed Data-set (RDD). We have tested our algorithms on two data sets and have compared its performance with earlier algorithm.

Keywords: Formal concept analysis · Distributed concept mining · Incremental mining

1 Introduction

FCA is a method for extracting all formal concepts from a given binary object-attribute relational database. A formal concept can be understood as a natural cluster of particular objects and particular attributes related to each other. For example if a query is made on an animal data-set to find all animals with certain attribute say '4 legs', the answer returned will contain a cluster or set of animals with '4 legs'. But a concept can give extended information about the same query such as every animal having '4 legs' also have 'tail' in the attributes. This is known as attribute implication. A data-set

© Springer International Publishing Switzerland 2015
N. Kumar and V. Bhatnagar (Eds.): BDA 2015, LNCS 9498, pp. 151–164, 2015.
DOI: 10.1007/978-3-319-27057-9_11

contains a number of formal concepts within it. These concepts mined have super-concept – sub-concept relationships among them. So if we find another concept containing '4 legs', 'tail' and 'long trunk' in attribute set, object set will probably contain only 'elephant'. As object set with single element 'elephant' is subset of object set of all animals with '4 legs', we say that the newly mined concept is a sub-concept of former concept. This type of super-concept – sub-concept relationship among all concepts can be visualized using a lattice structure, called concept lattice. Concept lattice provides an intuitive and powerful representation of data. For deeper understanding, related definitions and an example can be found in Sect. 2.

FCA finds its application in fields related to data mining and ontology engineering. FCA is proposed to be used in machine interpretable semantic web, association rule mining [9] and business application such as collaborative recommendation [10]. Several algorithms exist to mine formal concepts from a given data-set (also known as Context) on standalone systems. The applicability of such algorithms is restricted when the size of context is increased. These algorithms require scanning complete context to generate a new concept and thus when context is large, process of finding all concepts is time consuming. Each object or attribute can be present in a number of concepts, so the problem also demands high storage. This spurred interest in finding distributed solutions that would reduce the time for mining as well as enable distributed storage using low cost networked computing nodes.

The efforts in this direction exploited the MapReduce paradigm. Iterative MapReduce based solutions such as [3, 4, 12] were proposed to mine concepts. Two of the most popular algorithms are described in Sect. 3. These algorithms make certain assumptions that limit their ability to scale to large context size. One of them requires the entire context to be stored on every node whereas the other suffers from huge communication overhead at the end of each iteration. In practice we find large datasets that cannot be stored on a single machine. For example, dataset of emails sent by customers to a company might be used to find correlation between customers. Another example could be an e-commerce website that offers a number of products to its customers to categorize customers on specific product browsing habits.

In our approach context is neither stored on nodes statically nor is it scanned to compute concepts. Further, the context is aggregated on the lower dimension (either objects or attributes) as key-value pairs to create a distributed collection. In the processes of generating new key-value collection from an existing one and filtering concepts from parent collection, we efficiently utilize the MapReduce paradigm to scale well. Our approach is said to be unconstrained over the context because our algorithm does not use the context after generating the key-value pairs in the first iteration.

We have organized this paper in the following way. Basic definitions in formal concept analysis with an example can be found in Sect. 2. In Sect. 3 we briefly describe the two existing algorithms for distributed formal concept mining along with their drawbacks. In Sect. 4 we describe our concept mining algorithm in form of several steps. In Sect. 5 we describe our data processing pipeline and enlist the Spark functions we used for implementation. In Sect. 6 we demonstrate some experimental results. After discussing some facts about our algorithm in Sect. 7, we conclude our paper in Sect. 8.

2 Definitions and Properties in FCA

Formal Concept Analysis [1, 2] is a technique for knowledge discovery in databases (KDD). We adopt some notations as in [1]. Some of the basic definitions from [1] are reproduced below:

1. A formal context (G, M, I) consists of two sets G and M and of binary relation $I \subseteq G \times M$. The elements of G are called the objects, those of M the attributes of (G, M, I). If $g \in G$ and $m \in M$ are in relation I, we write $(g, m) \in I$ or $g\ I\ m$ and read this as "object g has attribute M".

2. Let $A \subseteq G$ and $B \subseteq M$, then: $A^{\uparrow} = \{m \in M \mid \forall g \in A, (g\ I\ m)\}$ and $B^{\downarrow} = \{g \in G \mid \forall m \in B, (g\ I\ m)\}$.
   $A^{\uparrow\downarrow}$ (precisely $(A^{\uparrow})^{\downarrow}$) and $B^{\downarrow\uparrow}$ (precisely $(B^{\downarrow})^{\uparrow}$) are closure operators. From context Table 1, consider a given object set $A = \{1, 2\}$, then $A^{\uparrow} = \{c, g\}$, also $A^{\uparrow\downarrow} = \{c, g\}^{\downarrow} = \{1, 2, 5\}$ and we can notice that $A \subseteq A^{\uparrow\downarrow}$. Similarly $B^{\downarrow\uparrow}$ gives complete set of attributes present in objects containing all attributes in B and $B \subseteq B^{\downarrow\uparrow}$. Also $\emptyset^{\uparrow} = M$, set of all attributes and $\emptyset^{\downarrow} = G$, set of all objects. The symbol '$\emptyset$' represents a null set.

3. (A, B) is formal concept of (G, M, I) iff, $A \subseteq G$, $B \subseteq M$, $A^{\uparrow} = B$, and $A = B^{\downarrow}$. The set A is called the extent and the set B is called the intent of the formal concept (A, B).

4. For a context (G, M, I), a concept (A1, B1) is sub-concept of a concept (A2, B2) (and equivalently (A2, B2) is super-concept of (A1, B1)) iff $A1 \subseteq A2$ or equivalently, $B2 \subseteq B1$. We denote $\leq$-sign to express this relation and thus we have (A1, B1) $\leq$ (A2, B2): $\Leftrightarrow A1 \subseteq A2$ or $B2 \subseteq B1$. We say (A1, B1) is proper sub-concept of (A2, B2) if (A1, B1) $\neq$ (A2, B2) holds.

An example of formal context is shown in Table 1. Rows represent the objects with their unique object IDs while column represent the attributes of objects. Presence of an attribute in an object is shown by 'x' symbol in the context. Let object set $A_I = \{1, 2, 4\}$ and attribute set $B_I = \{c, d\}$, then (A_I, B_I) is a formal concept since $A_I^{\uparrow} = B_I$ and $B_I^{\downarrow} = A_I$. Let $A_J = \{1, 2\}$, then (A_J, B_I) is not a formal concept since $B_I^{\downarrow} \neq A_J$. Consider concepts Y = ({1, 2, 4}, {c, d}) and X = ({1, 4}, {c, d, f}), and we can say X is proper sub-concept of Y (or C2 < C1). This ordering can be expressed in the form of a lattice (see Fig. 1) where each node represents a concept derived from the context and it is connected to all related concepts. The concepts reachable from a particular concept in strictly upward direction in the lattice are super-concepts while the concepts reachable in strictly downward direction are called sub-concepts. The top concept in the lattice is computed using the null attribute set $\emptyset$ as $<\emptyset^{\downarrow}, \emptyset^{\downarrow\uparrow}>$ whereas the bottom concept is computed using the null object set $\emptyset$ as $<\emptyset^{\uparrow\downarrow}, \emptyset^{\uparrow}>$. Generally the top concept is equal to $<G, \emptyset>$ as no attribute is common to all objects in G while the bottom concept is equal to $<\emptyset, M>$ as no object contains all the attributes in M. The top and the bottom concepts are labeled with id C0 and C16 in the lattice.

The concept finding problem can also be viewed as a problem of discovering maximal rectangles of crosses 'x' in the context table. The transpose of a context table

Table 1. An example Formal Context, Objects 'G' in first column, Attributes 'M' in first row and attribute presence in an object is marked by 'x' mark.

	a	b	c	d	e	f	g
1			x	x	x	x	
2	x	x	x	x			x
3	x	x					
4	x			x	x		x
5	x			x		x	x

also contains the same number of maximal rectangles. Therefore if attributes are treated as objects and objects are treated as attributes, newly mined concepts will correspond to concepts from original context, but with interchanged extents-intent pair. So if the complexity of any concept mining algorithm depends un-evenly on context dimension, finding concepts on context transpose might reduce runtime. We utilize this property in our implementation.

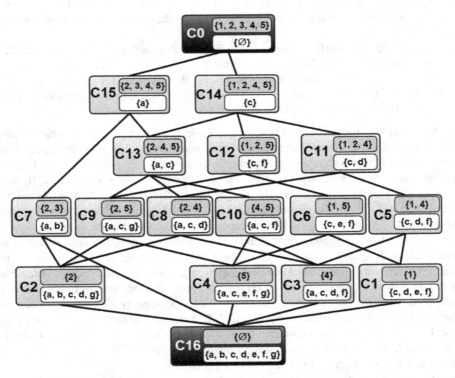

Fig. 1. Concept lattice corresponding to context in Table 1, each node representing concept with Id (left), Extent (top-right) and Intent (bottom-right)

3 Related Work

There are several stand-alone algorithms for concept mining [13–15]. As we are mainly interested in distributed mining algorithms, we compare our approach with two representative algorithms in this area, namely, Close-by-One [3] (referred as MR-CbO) and MR-Ganter [4]. Both of them are implemented using MapReduce paradigm. MR-CbO was the first attempt in parallelizing concept mining process by using several networked nodes to mine concepts in parallel. This algorithm mines concepts using a top-down approach. The top concept is evaluated in the driver code of MapReduce job. Then the iterations are launched with single key-value pair created from the top concept. In the Map phase of each iteration the mapper processes the input pair using intent of the concept and adds non-preexisting attributes to generate several concepts. These concepts are validated by the reducer using a canonicity test. The concepts which pass canonicity test in reduce phase are saved as valid concepts and are used in Map phase of next iteration for further concept generation. By using attribute ordering and canonicity test, the algorithm ensures that each concept is validated only once in a distributed setting. This allows it to run in continuous iterations without any synchronization with the driver. The only drawback with this algorithm is that it requires full context to be present on every node during the Map computation. This confines the algorithm to contexts which can fit in the memory of a single machine. However, as discussed earlier, several data-sets in practice have a large context.

The second algorithm MR-Ganter addresses the issue associated with large context storage. It allows context to be partitioned in several disjoint parts and stores them statically on different nodes. It takes advantage of the fact that concept intents are closed under intersection. Thus for an input intent and every non-preexisting attribute in it, the mappers generate new intermediate local intent(s) which are merged during reduce phase and checked for canonicity. However, this approach has some limitations. In this algorithm each intent can be generated multiple times within iteration as well as across different iterations. As only the new intents are required to be used as input for the next iteration, a repository needs to be maintained to keep track of al-ready generated intents and needs to be checked every time a concept is generated. MR-Ganter+, an enhanced version of MR-Ganter uses a distributed hash table to speedup this check. It is also able to mine concepts in fewer iterations. However, both MR-Ganter and MR-Ganter+ require the newly generated concepts to be broadcasted to all the mappers at the end of each iteration. As the number of concepts generated is substantial, this approach imposes huge network overhead. Further, both the above algorithms do not store the extent along with the intent, which if required needs re-computation.

Our approach neither requires scanning the context for concept generation nor does it require storing the entire context on a single node. Thus, we can process larger data sets simply by adding more machines.

4 Methodology

4.1 Data Format and Input

Conventional algorithms assume input context in tabular form with row-wise storage, i.e. object along with its attributes. But in practice, many data storage systems support append-only writes to avoid locking issues that arise from fine-grained up-dates to existing data objects. The incoming data in such cases is <object id, attribute id> pair. Thus, new objects and new attributes get added to the dataset over time. As big context tables are often very sparse, this representation (key-value pair) has immense storage benefits compared with the tabular representation. An object-attribute pair is added only for the existing attributes of the object whereas the tabular representation would have to store null values for every non-existing attribute in the table. We use the key-value representation in our system. In this paper, we restrict ourselves to mining formal concepts from a snapshot of the dataset taken at a particular time. Issues regarding the merging of formal concepts mined over different snapshots are beyond the scope of this paper.

4.2 Data Aggregation

Recall that finding concepts on the context table or its transpose yields the same result. Thus, we can aggregate data by objects or by attributes. As the total number of concepts is bounded by the number of different possible combinations of objects or attributes (whichever is lower), we aggregate on the dimension with lower count to reduce the search space for valid concepts. Spark has functions that can approximate the distinct number of objects/attributes within a specified timeout. We use that function to limit the maximum number of iterations required by the algorithm to mine all concepts. In the dataset corresponding to our example context, it can be found that the number of objects is less than the number of attributes. So we aggregate on the basis of object ID's. The aggregated key-value pairs are listed as candidate concepts of key size one (referred as CC_1) in Table 2.

4.3 Concept Finding Approach

The candidate concept set of key size 2 (CC_2, Table 3) is generated using CC_1 table as follows: we take all combinations of the keys from CC_1 to produce the candidate concept keys of CC_2; the candidate concept values are generated by intersecting the corresponding values of the keys in CC_1. Those keys in CC_2 which have their value-part as null are discarded from the candidate set. In general, candidate concept set of higher order e.g. CC_{N+1} is generated from candidate concept set CC_N by merging key-value pairs in CC_N where the keys differ only in a single element.

   If the value corresponding to any candidate concept in CC_1 is repeated in CC_2, then that candidate concept in CC_1 is not considered to be a valid concept. The rest of the candidate concepts from CC_1 (whose values are not regenerated in CC_2) are copied to Valid Concepts of key size 1 (referred as VC_1, Table 4). Thus, 4 out of the 5 candidate key-value pairs of size 1 are declared as valid concepts. Continuing in this manner, CC_2 is used to generate CC_3 (Table 5). Filtering out the candidate concepts in CC_2 whose values are regenerated in CC_3, we are left with 6 out of 10 pairs that are valid (VC_2 - Table 6). It may also be noted that CC_3 has only 7 elements out of the 10 possible combinations. The idea of generating 'N + 1'th order candidate set with reduced number of elements using filtered candidates from 'N'th order candidate set is borrowed from Chap. 6 in [11].

We now generalize the process of concept mining. Let CC_N be the set of candidate key-value pairs $<K_N, V>$ of key size 'N' and CC_{N+1} be the candidate set of pairs $<K_{N+1}, V>$ with key size 'N + 1'. Let $V_X = \{V| < K_{N+1}, V > \in CC_{N+1}\}$, be the set of values in CC_{N+1}. Then valid concept set of key size N (VC_N) is given by:

$$VC_N = \{ <K_N, V > \,|\, <K_N, V > \, \in CC_N \text{ and } V \notin V_X\} \tag{1}$$

4.4 Additional Important Insights

It may be noticed that key-value pairs in CC_1 (number of elements = 'N') are listed in lexicographic order of the keys. To generate elements in CC_2 (number of elements = $^NC_2$) each key in CC_1 is combined with all the keys that succeed in the order. So from N keys in CC_1, first key will be used to generate first $N - 1$ elements of CC_2, 2nd key will generate next $N - 2$ elements, and so on. In general, the K'th key in CC_1 is paired with the next 'N-K' elements to generate elements in CC_2 (highlighted in Tables 2 and 3). By enforcing this ordering on the keys, we ensure that the same combination is not regenerated. The value (Set) in each pair of CC_2 is evaluated by intersecting the value from parent key pairs in CC_1. In a distributed implementation, we could partition the computation such that the 'N-K' combinations of the K'th key reach a single node. This way of splitting will however cause uneven number of key-value pairs across nodes causing communication (shuffling) bottlenecks. To minimize the communication overhead, we reorder the keys in CC_1 in ascending (non-descending) order of the number of elements in the value. After reordering, the first key in CC_1 will have least number of elements in the value. The number of combinations of this key in CC_2 will be largest ('N − 1') but the number of elements in each one of them will be small (the cardinality of the intersection operation cannot be greater than the cardinality of the smallest set). Thus by reordering strategy, even when we have large number of keys reaching a node, the number of elements associated to them will be small. Thus, we can reduce the communication overhead.

We now illustrate the combination of two ordered keys of size N to generate a new concept key of size N + 1. Let us assume two ordered keys of size N, $P_N = \{I_1, I_2 \ldots I_{N-1}, A\}$ and $Q_N = \{I_1, I_2 \ldots I_{N-1}, B\}$ which have the first $n - 1$ elements common. We combine them to give a new ordered key of size 'N + 1' as:

$$K_{N+1} = \{I_1, I_2 \ldots I_{N-1}, A, B\} \text{ only if } A < B \tag{2}$$

In this way candidate keys are combined to create next order candidate keys. The effect can be observed in highlighted keys in Tables 5, 7 and 8.

Table 2. Candidate concepts of key-size = 1 (CC_1)

Key	Value
{1}	{c, d, e, f}
{2}	{a, b, c, d, g}
{3}	{a, b}
{4}	{a, c, d, f}
{5}	{a, c, e, f, g}

Table 3. Candidate concepts of key size = 2 (CC_2)

Key	Value
{1, 2}	{c, d}
{1, 3}	{∅}
{1, 4}	{c, d, f}
{1, 5}	{c, e, f}
{2, 3}	{a, b}
{2, 4}	{a, c, d}
{2, 5}	{a, c, g}
{3, 4}	{a}
{3, 5}	{a}
{4, 5}	{a, c, f}

Table 4. Valid concepts of key size = 1 (VC_1) using CC_1 and CC_2

Id	Extent	Intent
C1	{1}	{c, d, e, f}
C2	{2}	{a, b, c, d, g}
C3	{4}	{a, c, d, f}
C4	{5}	{a, c, e, f, g}

Table 5. Candidate concepts of key-size = 3 (CC_3)

Key	Value
{1, 2, 4}	{c, d}
{1, 2, 5}	{c}
{1, 4, 5}	{c, f}
{2, 3, 4}	{a}
{2, 3, 5}	{a}
{2, 4, 5}	{a, c}
{3, 4, 5}	{a}

Table 7. Candidate and valid concepts of key size = 4 (VC_4), since no element for CC_5

Id	Key / Extent	Value / Intent
C14	{1, 2, 4, 5}	{c}
C15	{2, 3, 4, 5}	{a}

Table 6. Valid concepts of key size = 2 (VC_2) using CC_2 and CC_3

Id	Extent	Intent
C5	{1, 4}	{c, d, f}
C6	{1, 5}	{c, e, f}
C7	{2, 3}	{a, b}
C8	{2, 4}	{a, c, d}
C9	{2, 5}	{a, c, g}
C10	{4, 5}	{a, c, f}

Table 8. Valid concepts of key size = 3 (VC_3) using CC_3 and CC_4

Id	Extent	Intent
C11	{1, 2, 4}	{c, d}
C12	{1, 4, 5}	{c, f}
C13	{2, 4, 5}	{a, c}

5 Implementation Using Spark

Apache Spark [5] is a popular open-source distributed data processing framework, which is optimized to best utilize main memory of network nodes and hence is faster than previous technologies. Spark defines its distributed storage abstraction as Resilient Distributed Datasets (RDDs) [6]. It provides two sets of operations – transformations and actions. Transformation allows coarse-grained manipulation of the data in RDD. These transformations are carried out when an action is specified. For more details, refer to Scala API documentation [7].

Data can be inputted from local file or any distributed file system to create a temporary RDD (say R1). This RDD contains object-attribute pairs. Recall our discussion from Sect. 4.2 that we need to aggregate on the dimension with lower count to reduce the search space. As the size of the dimensions is not known apriori, we approximate the count with the help of "map" followed by "countApproxDistinct" transformation. This gives us an approximate number of distinct objects and attributes in the dataset. We aggregate on the dimension with the lower count. For instance, if the number of objects is lower than the number of attributes, we aggregate attributes treating object as key using "combineByKey" transformation to create new RDD, (say R2). Thus object is paired with attributes <key=object Id, value={attribute Id, attribute Id …}>. If the attributes are less, then we aggregate objects based on attributes: <key=attribute Id, {value=object Id, object Id …}>. Next we order the keys within the chosen dimension according to the number of elements. We count the number of elements in the values of each key by using "countByKey" action. We re-label keys in ascending numeric value according to increasing number of elements in their values. This RDD corresponds to CC_1. At this point we no longer require R1 and R2 RDDs, so we remove them from memory.

We create CC_2 RDD using "cartesian" transformation of CC_1 with itself followed by "filter" transformation as specified in Eq. 2. Then using CC_1 and CC_2, we generate VC_1 using "reduceByKey" followed by "filter". As soon as VC_1 is generated, CC_1 is not required anymore and thus can be purged from memory. For the subsequent candidate set generation (e.g. CC_3), we use "map" on the previous candidate set (e.g. CC_2) followed by self-join (using "join" followed by "filter"). The data pipeline is shown in Fig. 2. The top and the bottom concepts are evaluated using reduce operations on CC_1.

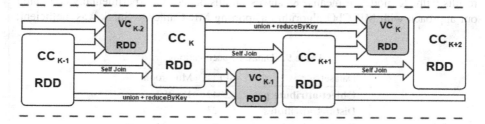

Fig. 2. Spark data pipeline for our implementation

We used Scala interactive shell for our experiments. Scala shell is a single threaded application and thus allows us to run a single job at a time on the cluster. However, Spark also supports running several jobs launched by different threads in parallel. If we use this Spark feature in our application then after generating CC_{K+1} from CC_K, we can immediately proceed to generate CC_{K+2} without waiting for the generation of VC_K. VC_K can be generated by a separate thread and thus execution gets speeded up. The new pipeline in this case will look similar to the one in Fig. 3.

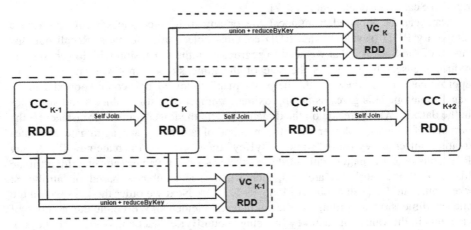

Fig. 3. A parallel (Multithreaded) pipeline for implementation

6 Evaluation and Results

For experiments we used two standard datasets from [8]. The multivalued attributes in data were translated to binary attributes. Then the binary attributed context(s) were converted into text file of randomly ordered object-attribute pairs (one per line) before giving them as input to our algorithm. The details about the converted datasets are shown in Table 9. We used 5 lab machines with core i5-2310 (2.9 GHz) processor, 4 GB Memory and running Ubuntu 12.04 LTS operating system. We ran Spark master on one node and used others as slaves to run Spark standalone cluster. Each slave was configured to use a single CPU core and 512 MB of memory. In figures, when we show results with 'K' nodes, it means 'K' slaves. In this paper, we experimentally compared our approach with MR-CbO algorithm as porting MR-Ganter to Spark was inefficient.

Table 9. Dataset Specifications

Dataset	SPECT	Mushroom
Object-attribute pairs	2042	186852
Distinct attributes	23	119
Distinct objects	267	8124
Concepts	21550	238710

For the smaller dataset (SPECT), MR-CbO performs much faster than our algorithm as the storage of such context takes very less space in memory and scanning small context is not computationally expensive (Figs. 4 and 5).

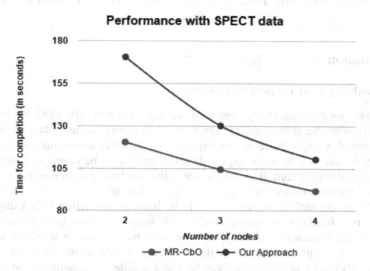

Fig. 4. Result comparison on SPECT dataset

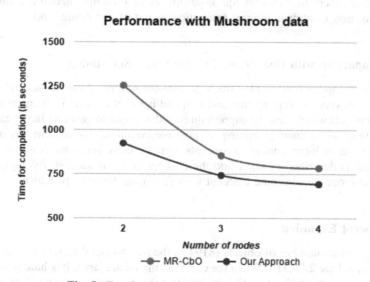

Fig. 5. Result comparison on Mushroom dataset

For the larger dataset (Mushroom), our algorithm performs faster than MR-CbO. Recall that MR-CbO stores the entire context on every node. As the dataset increases in size, the performance is limited by the memory on the machine. Storing large context with limited memory and scanning it several times to generate every new concept is computationally expensive. Thus, MR-CbO algorithm did not perform well for large data set.

7   Discussion

7.1   Scalability with Respect to Context

In this paper, we experimentally compared our approach with MR-CbO algorithm. As MR-CbO requires the entire context to be stored in memory, we used datasets that fit in the memory of a single node in our experiments. But our algorithm can scale with larger context size as it does not require the entire context to be stored on a single node at any step of the algorithm. It should be noted that the first step (generating CC_2) uses "cartesian" transformation followed by "filter" whereas the later steps use "map-join-filter" transformation sequence. We do so because generating CC_2 using "map-join-filter" transformation sequence would result in entire context to be generated on a single node as intermediate data. The "cartesian" transformation although not very efficient is a distributed operation, and we employ it only in the first step. We can improve performance of the other steps by using a different transformation sequence (like "map-aggregateByKey-flatMap") thereby avoiding "join" transformation for generating next level candidate concept set. Testing the performance of this optimization and others like custom Spark partitioner to minimize network shuffling of keys during new candidate concept generation is part of our future work.

7.2   Comparison with Distributed Frequent Item-Set Mining

Although our approach resembles frequent item-set mining, there are several notable differences between concept mining and frequent item-set mining. In frequent item-set mining, item-sets which pass the support threshold are used to generate larger candidate item-sets whereas in concept mining all possible combinations of item-sets are considered to generate larger candidate concepts. Further, these generated concepts have to be validated as described in Eq. 1 and the concept lattice is formed. By applying the threshold criteria, we can mine frequent item-sets from the concept lattice.

7.3   Concept Explosion

Even with a small number of objects (8194 in the Mushroom data-set), the number of concepts mined are 2,38,710. When the concepts mined are large, it is hard to visualize them. This raises several interesting questions regarding concept generation methodology - "should all concepts be generated? Can we rank concepts?" We are currently exploring methods to handle the concept explosion problem.

7.4   Mining Links Between Concepts

Currently, no distributed algorithm mines links between concepts. This would be useful in visualization. In our algorithm, the concepts of different sizes are present in different RDDs. Hence, a supplementary algorithm needs to be designed for mining links between concepts. Concept lattice could be represented using Spark's graph processing component namely "GraphX" or any other graph framework for visualization or further analytics.

8   Conclusion

In this paper, we presented an incremental approach to mine formal concepts from a context which is assumed to be present in the form of object-attribute pairs. We validated our approach by comparing the concepts generated with that in MR-CbO. Our approach is more scalable than the earlier approaches as it neither requires scanning the context for concept generation nor does it require storing the entire context on a single node. Thus, we can process larger data sets simply by adding more machines. Experimental results show that our algorithm outperforms the previously proposed algorithms as the data-set size grows. Thus, our algorithm is suitable for practical concept mining applications.

Acknowledgments. Authors would like to thank Dr. Sriram Kailasam, Assistant Professor at IIT Mandi for his help in improving the manuscript.

References

1. Ganter, B., Wille, R.: Formal Concept Analysis. Springer, Berlin (1999)
2. Wille, R.: Restructuring lattice theory: an approach based on hierarchies of concepts. In: Ferré, S., Rudolph, S. (eds.) ICFCA 2009. LNCS, vol. 5548, pp. 314–339. Springer, Heidelberg (2009)
3. Krajca, P., Vychodil, V.: Distributed algorithm for computing formal concepts using map-reduce framework. In: Adams, N.M., Robardet, C., Siebes, A., Boulicaut, J.-F. (eds.) IDA 2009. LNCS, vol. 5772, pp. 333–344. Springer, Heidelberg (2009)
4. Xu, B., de Fréin, R., Robson, E., Ó Foghlú, M.: Distributed formal concept analysis algorithms based on an iterative mapreduce framework. In: Domenach, F., Ignatov, D.I., Poelmans, J. (eds.) ICFCA 2012. LNCS, vol. 7278, pp. 292–308. Springer, Heidelberg (2012)
5. Zaharia, M., Chowdhury, M., Franklin, M.J., Shenker, S., Stoica, I.: Spark: cluster computing with working sets. In: Proceedings of the 2nd USENIX Conference on Hot Topics in Cloud Computing, pp. 10–10 (2010)
6. Zaharia, M., Chowdhury, M., Das, T., Dave, A., Ma, J., McCauley, M., Franklin, M., Shenker, S., Stoica, I.: Resilient distributed datasets: a fault-tolerant abstraction for in-memory cluster computing. In: Proceedings of the 9th USENIX Conference on Networked Systems Design and Implementation, pp. 2–2. USENIX Association (2012)

7. Spark programming guide. http://Spark.apache.org/docs/latest/programming-guide.html. Accessed 01 July 2015
8. UCI Machine Learning Repository: Data Sets. http://archive.ics.uci.edu/ml/datasets.html. Accessed: 01 July 2015
9. Pasquier, N., Bastide, Y., Taouil, R., Lakhal, L.: Efficient mining of association rules using closed itemset lattices. Inf. Syst. **24**, 25–46 (1999)
10. du Boucher-Ryan, P., Bridge, D.: Collaborative recommending using formal concept analysis. Knowl.-Based Syst. **19**(5), 309–315 (2006)
11. Rajaraman, A., Ullman, J.: Mining of Massive Datasets. Cambridge University Press, New York (2012)
12. Ying., W., Mingqing, X.: Diagnosis rule mining of airborne avionics using formal concept analysis. In: International Conference on Cyber-Enabled Distributed Computing and Knowledge Discovery (CyberC). IEEE (2013)
13. Ganter, B., Reuter, K.: Finding all closed sets: a general approach. Order **8**(3), 283–290 (1991)
14. van der Merwe, D., Obiedkov, S., Kourie, D.G.: AddIntent: a new incremental algorithm for constructing concept lattices. In: Eklund, P. (ed.) ICFCA 2004. LNCS (LNAI), vol. 2961, pp. 372–385. Springer, Heidelberg (2004)
15. Kuznetsov, S.O.: Learning of simple conceptual graphs from positive and negative examples. In: Żytkow, J.M., Rauch, J. (eds.) PKDD 1999. LNCS (LNAI), vol. 1704, pp. 384–391. Springer, Heidelberg (1999)

Khanan: Performance Comparison and Programming α-Miner Algorithm in Column-Oriented and Relational Database Query Languages

Astha Sachdev[1], Kunal Gupta[1], and Ashish Sureka[2]([✉])

[1] Indraprastha Institute of Information Technology, Delhi (IIITD), New Delhi, India
http://www.iiitd.ac.in/
[2] Software Analytics Research Lab (SARL), New Delhi, India
ashish@iiitd.ac.in
http://www.software-analytics.in/

Abstract. Process-Aware Information Systems (PAIS) support business processes and generate large amounts of event logs from the execution of business processes. An event log is represented as a tuple of CaseID, Timestamp, Activity and Actor. Process Mining is a new and emerging field that aims at analyzing the event logs to discover, enhance and improve business processes and check conformance between run time and design time business processes. The large volume of event logs generated are stored in the databases. Relational databases perform well for a certain class of applications. However, there is a certain class of applications for which relational databases are not able to scale well. To address the challenges of scalability, NoSQL database systems emerged. Discovering a process model (workflow) from event logs is one of the most challenging and important Process Mining tasks. The α-miner algorithm is one of the first and most widely used Process Discovery techniques. Our objective is to investigate which of the databases (Relational or NoSQL) performs better for a Process Discovery application under Process Mining. We implement the α-miner algorithm on relational (row-oriented) and NoSQL (column-oriented) databases in database query languages so that our application is tightly coupled to the database. We conduct a performance benchmarking and comparison of the α-miner algorithm on row-oriented database and NoSQL column-oriented database. We present the comparison on various aspects like time taken to load large datasets, disk usage, stepwise execution time and compression technique.

Keywords: Apache Cassandra · α-miner algorithm · Column-oriented database · MySQL · Process Mining · Performance comparison · Row oriented database

1 Research Motivation and Aim

A PAIS is an IT system that manages and supports business processes. A PAIS generates data from the execution of business processes. The data generated

© Springer International Publishing Switzerland 2015
N. Kumar and V. Bhatnagar (Eds.): BDA 2015, LNCS 9498, pp. 165–180, 2015.
DOI: 10.1007/978-3-319-27057-9_12

by a PAIS like Enterprise Resource Planing (ERP) and Customer Relationship Management (CRM) [11] is in the form of event logs (represented as a tuple of <CaseID, Timestamp, Activity, Actor>). In an event log, a particular CaseID, that is a process instance, has a set of activities associated with it, ordered by timestamp. Process Mining is a new and emerging field which consist of analyzing event logs generated from the execution of business process. The insights obtained from event logs helps the organizations to improve their business processes. There are three major techniques within Process Mining *viz.* Process Discovery, Process Conformance and Process Enhancement [14]. The classification of Process Mining techniques is based on whether there is a priori model and how the a priori model is used, if present. In this paper we focus on Process Discovery aspect of Process Mining. In Process Discovery, there is no a priori model. Process Discovery aims to construct a process model, which is a computationally intensive task, from the information present in event logs. One of the most fundamental algorithm under Process Discovery is the α-miner algorithm [13] which is used to generate a process model from event logs.

Before the year 2000, majority of the organizations used traditional relational database management systems (RDBMS) to store the data. Most of the traditional relational databases focus on Online Transaction Processing (OLTP) applications [10] but are not able to perform Online Analytical Processing (OLAP) applications efficiently. Row-oriented databases are not well suited for analytical functions (like Dense_Rank, Sum, Count, Rank, Top, First, Last and Average) but work fine when we need to retrieve the entire row or to insert a new record. Recent years have seen the introduction of a number of NoSQL column-oriented database systems [12]. These database systems have shown to perform more than an order of magnitude better than the traditional relational database systems on analytical workloads [3]. NoSQL column-oriented databases are well suited for analytical queries but result in poor performance for insertion of individual records or retrieving all the fields of a row. Another problem with traditional relational databases is impedance matching [5]. When representation of data in memory and that in database is different, then it is known as impedance matching. This is because in-memory data structures use lists, dictionaries, nested lists while traditional databases store data only in the form of tables and rows. Thus, we need to translate data objects present in the memory to tables and rows and vice-versa. Performing the translation is complex and costly. NoSQL databases on the other hand are schema-less. Records can be inserted at run time without defining any rigid schema. Hence, NoSQL databases do not face the problem of impedance matching.

There is a certain class of applications, like facebook messaging application, for which row-oriented databases are not able to scale. To handle such class of applications, NoSQL database systems were introduced. Process Discovery is a very important application of Process Mining. Our objective is to investigate an approach to implement a Process Discovery α-miner algorithm on a row-oriented database and a NoSQL column-oriented database and to benchmark the performance of the algorithm on both the row-oriented and column-oriented databases. A database query language is one of the most standard way to interact with the database. Structured Query Language (SQL) has grown over the past few years and has become a fairly complex language. SQL takes care of the various aspects like storage management, concurrent access, memory leaks and fault tolerance and also gives the flexibility of tuning the database [1]. A lot of research has been done in implementing data mining algorithms in database query languages. Previous work suggests that tight coupling of the data mining algorithms to the database systems improves the performance of the algorithms significantly [8]. We aim to implement α-miner algorithm in the specific database query languages so that our Process Discovery application is tightly coupled to the database.

There are various NoSQL column-oriented databases [12] but for our current work, we will focus on Apache Cassandra[1] (NoSQL column-oriented database) and MySQL[2] (row-oriented database).

The research aim of the work presented in this paper is the following:

1. To investigate an approach to implement α-miner algorithm in Structured Query Language (SQL). The underlying row-oriented database for implementation is MySQL using InnoDB[3] engine.
2. To investigate an approach to implement α-miner algorithm in Cassandra Query Language (CQL) on column-oriented database Cassandra.
3. To conduct a series of experiments on a publicly available real world dataset to compare the performance of α-miner algorithm on both the databases. The experiments consider multiple aspects such as α-miner stepwise execution time, bulk loading across various datasets, write intensive time and read intensive time and disk space of tables.

2   Related Work and Novel Contributions

In this Section, we present a literature review of papers closely related to the work presented in this paper and list the novel contributions of our work in context to existing work. We divide related work into following three lines of research:

2.1   Implementation of Mining Algorithms in Row-Oriented Databases

Ordonez et al. present a method to implement k-means clustering algorithm in SQL. They cluster in large datasets in RDBMS [1]. Their work concentrates on defining suitable tables, indexing them and writing suitable queries for clustering purposes. Ordonez et al. presents an efficient SQL implementation of the EM algorithm to perform clustering in very large databases [2]. Sattler et al.

---

[1] http://cassandra.apache.org/.

[2] http://www.mysql.com/.

[3] http://dev.mysql.com/doc/refman/5.5/en/innodb-storage-engine.html.

present a study of applying data mining primitives on decision tree classifier [8]. Their framework provides a tight coupling of data mining and database systems and links the essential data mining primitives that supports several classes of algorithms to database systems.

2.2 Implementation of Mining Algorithms in Column-Oriented Databases

Rana et al. conducted experiments on the utilization of column oriented databases like MonetDB with oracle 11 g which is a row oriented data store for execution time analysis of Association Rule Mining algorithm [4]. Suresh L et al. implemented k-means clustering algorithm on column store databases [9].

2.3 Performance Comparison of Mining Algorithms in Column-Oriented and Graph Databases

Gupta et al. conduct a performance comparison and programming alpha-miner algorithm in relational database query language and NoSQL column-oriented using Apache Phoenix [6]. Joishi et al. [7] presents a performance comparison and implementation of process mining algorithms (organizational perspective) in graph-oriented and relational database query languages.

In context to existing work, the study presented in this paper makes the following novel contributions:

1. While there has been work done on implementing data mining algorithms in row-oriented databases, we are the first to implement Process Mining α-miner algorithm in row-oriented database MySQL using Structured Query Language(SQL).
2. While data mining algorithms have been implemented in column-oriented databases, we are the first to implement Process Mining α-miner algorithm in column-oriented database Cassandra using Cassandra Query Language(CQL).
3. We present a performance benchmarking and comparison of α-miner algorithm on both row-oriented database MySQL and column-oriented database Cassandra.

3 α-Miner Algorithm

The α-miner algorithm is a Process Discovery algorithm used in Process Mining [13]. It was first put forward by van der Aalst, Weijter and Maruster. Input for the α-miner algorithm is an event log and output is a process model. The α-miner algorithm consists of scanning the event logs for discovering causality between the activities present in the event log.

The stepwise description of the α-miner algorithm can be given as:

1. Compute Total Events which represents the set of distinct activities present in the event log.
2. Computes Initial Events which represents the set of all the initial activities of corresponding trace.
3. Compute Final Events which represents the set of distinct activities which appear at the end of some trace in the event log.
4. Compute the relationships between all the activities in Total Events. This computation is presented in the form of a footprint matrix and is called pre-processing in α-miner algorithm. Using the footprint matrix we compute pairs of sets of activities such that all activities in the same set are not connected to each other while every activity in first set has causality relationship to every other activity in the second set.
5. Keep only the maximal pairs of sets generated in the fourth step, eliminating the non-maximal ones.
6. Add the input place which is the source place and the output place which is the sink place in addition to all the places obtained in the fifth step.
7. Present all the places including the input and output places and all the input and output transitions from the places.

4   Implementation of α-Miner Algorithm in SQL on Row-Oriented Database (MySQL)

We present a few segments of our implementation due to limited space in the paper. The entire code and implementation can be downloaded from our website[4]. Before implementing α-miner algorithm, we do pre-processing in JAVA to create the following two tables viz. causality table (consists of two columns eventA and eventB) and NotConnected table (consists of two columns eventA and eventB).

1. We create a table eventlog using create table[5] keyword consisting of 3 columns (CaseID, Timestamp and Activity) each of which are varchar datatype except Timestamp which is of timestamp datatype. The primary key is a composite primary key consisting of CaseID and Timestamp.
2. We load the data into table eventlog using LOAD DATA INFILE[6] command.
3. For Step 1, we create a table totalEvent that contains a single column (event) which is of varchar datatype. To populate the table we select distinct activities from the table eventlog and insert into table totalEvent.
4. For Step 2, we create a table initialEvent that contains a single column (initial) which is of varchar datatype. To populate the table
   (a) We first select minimum value of Timestamp from table eventlog by grouping CaseID.

---

[4] http://bit.ly/1C3JgIx.
[5] http://dev.mysql.com/doc/refman/5.1/en/create-table.html.
[6] http://dev.mysql.com/doc/refman/5.1/en/load-data.html.

(b) Then we select distinct activities from table eventlog for every distinct value of CaseID where Timestamp is the minimum Timestamp.

5. For Step 3, we create a table finalEvent that contains a single column (final) which is of varchar datatype. To populate table
   (a) We first select maximum Timestamp from table eventlog by grouping CaseID.
   (b) Then we select distinct activities from table eventlog for every distinct value of CaseID where Timestamp is the maximum Timestamp.

6. For Step 4, we create five tables *viz.* SafeEventA, SafeEventB, EventA, EventB and XL. All the five tables contain two columns (setA and setB) which are of varchar datatype.
   (a) In table causality we use group_concat[7] to combine the values of column eventB for corresponding value of column eventA and insert the results in table EventA.
   (b) In table causality we use group_concat to combine the values of column eventA for corresponding value of column eventB and insert the results in table EventB.
   (c) To populate tables SafeEventA and SafeEventB-
       (i) Select setA and setB from tables EventA and EventB
       (ii) For every value of setB in table EventA, if value is present in table notconnected, insert the corresponding value of setA and setB in table SafeEventA. Repeat the same step for populating table SafeEventB.
   (d) To populate table XL, we insert all the rows from the three tables SafeEventA, SafeEventB and causality.

7. For Step 5, we create three tables *viz.* eventASafe, eventBSafe and YL. All the three tables contain two columns (setA and setB) which are of varchar datatype.
   (a) We create a stored procedure to split the values of column setB of table SafeEventA on comma separator. Insert the results in safeA table.
   (b) We create a stored procedure to split the values of column setA of table SafeEventB on comma separator. Insert the results in safeB table.
   (c) To populate table eventASafe, insert all the rows from table safeA.
   (d) To populate table eventBSafe, insert all the rows from table safeB.
   (e) To populate table YL, insert all the rows from tables SafeEventA, SafeEventB and causality excluding all rows in tables eventAsafe and eventSafeB.

8. For Step 6, we create two tables *viz.* terminalPlace that contains a single column (event) which is of varchar datatype and PL which also contains a single column (Place) which is of varchar datatype.
   (a) To populate table terminalPlace, insert 'i' and 'o' in the table. 'i' and 'o' represent the source and sink places respectively.

---

[7] http://dev.mysql.com/doc/refman/5.0/en/group-by-functions.html#function_group-concat.

  (b) To populate table PL, we use concat_ws [8] to combine the values of column setA and column setB of table YL using & separator and insert the results in table PL. Furthermore, we insert all the rows of table terminalPlace into table PL.

9. For Step 7, we create 3 tables *viz.* Place1 and Place2 which consist of two columns (id and value) which are of varchar datatype and FL which consists of two columns (firstplace and secondplace) which are of varchar datatype.

  (a) To populate table Place1, we use concat_ws to combine the values of column setA and column setB of table YL using & separator. Insert the results in column setB of table Place1. Insert all the values of column setA of table YL into column setA of table Place1.

  (b) To populate table Place2, we use concat_ws to combine the values of column setA and column setB of table YL using & separator. Insert the results in column setA of table Place2. Insert all the values of column setB of table YL in column setB of table Place2.

  (c) We create a stored procedure to split column setB of table Place1 on comma separator. In stored procedure we create table temp_place2 to insert the results.

  (d) We create a stored procedure to split column setA of a table Place2 on comma separator. In stored procedure we create table temp_place2 to insert the results.

  (e) To populate a table FL, insert all the rows from tables temp_place1 and temp_place2. Insert the results of cross join of two tables *viz.* terminalPlace and intialEvent and of table finalEvent and table terminalPlace.

5 Implementation of α-Miner Algorithm on NoSQL Column-Oriented Database Cassandra

Before implementing α-miner algorithm, we do pre-processing in JAVA to create the following two tables *viz.* causality table (consists of two columns eventA and eventB) and NotConnected table (consists of two columns eventA and eventB).

The data in Cassandra is modelled as a wide column family, where CaseID is the partition key and Timestamp is the clustering key. Timestamp represents the cell names and Activity represents the cell values. Since Timestamp is the clustering key, all the Activities are stored in ascending order of Timestamp values for a particular partition key, that is CaseID.

1. Create keyspace.
   We create a keyspace called eventdataset. In Cassandra, keyspace is the container for the data we need to store and process.
2. Create and populate table eventlog.
   We create a table eventlog with CaseID as the partition key and Timestamp as the clustering key and load the dataset into the table eventlog using COPY command.

---

[8] http://dev.mysql.com/doc/refman/5.0/en/string-functions.html#function_concat-ws.

3. Create and populate table totalEvents.
   The Create command creates the table totalEvents with tevents(that represents activities in the eventlog) as the primary key for storing the total distinct activities in the eventlog. We use the COPY command two times to obtain the set of distinct activities. The first COPY command loads all the activities of the eventlog into 'totalEvents.csv' file. The second COPY command copies the activities stored in 'totalEvents.csv' file to the table totalEvents.
4. Create and populate table for storing all the initial activities.
   The table startevents is used to store all the initial activities i.e., all those activities that appear in the start of some trace. We create the table initial with the rows being ordered in the decreasing order of Timestamp and load the data from 'eventlog.csv' into it. The columns CaseID, Timestamp and Activity of table initial are copied to the file 'inital.csv'. Therefore, the file 'initial.csv' will contain the rows in decreasing order of timestamp. Then we load the data from file 'initial.csv' into table starteve. The row with the earliest value of timestamp corresponding to a CaseID will sustain in the table. Finally, we create the table startevents with ievents(that represent activities in the eventlog) as the primary key and copy the column sevents, which represents activities in the eventlog into the file 'startEve.csv' and load this file into the table startevents giving all the distinct initial activities in the eventlog.
5. Create and populate table finalEvents.
   The table finalEvents is used to store all the ending activities i.e., all those activities that appear in the last of some trace. The query can be explained as: We create the table final and load the data from 'eventlog.csv' into it. Since only CaseID is the primary key in the table final, it will contain only rows with the highest value of Timestamp corresponding to a CaseID. The column Activity of table final is copied to file 'finalEve.csv'. Finally, we create the table finalEvents with fevents(that represent activities in the eventlog) as the primary key. We load the data from file 'finalEve.csv' into the table finalEvents.
6. Perform preprocessing to create the footprint matrix.
   We create a table trace with CaseID as the primary key and list of events corresponding to each CaseID.
   (a) We iterate over the table eventlog and store the list of activities corresponding to each CaseID in an arraylist traceList.
   (b) We insert the value of traceList corresponding to each CaseID in table trace.
   (c) We create the table called preprocesstable with ACTIVITY as the primary key and columns as the number of activities in the event log. We initialize all the values in the preprocesstable as NOT CONNECTED.
   (d) We scan the table trace and update the corresponding entries in the table preprocesstable.

```
UPDATE preprocesstable SET activityA='RELATION' WHERE
    activity='activityB';
```

7. Create and populate Table SetsReachabeTo and SetsReachableFrom. We create table SetsReachableTo with 3 columns - Place which is the primary key, activityin which represents the set of input activities and activityout which represents the set of the output activities. Similarly, we create table SetsReachableFrom with 3 columns - Place, activityout, activityin. For each activity in the totalActivities table, we read from the preprocesstable its relation to every other activity. If the relation is CAUSALITY, then we insert it into table setsreachablefrom. Similarly, we populate table setsreachableto. Finally we merge the two tables using COPY command.

8. Create and Populate Table YW.
   We create a table YW with Place as the primary key and columns-activityin storing the input activities and column activityout storing the output activities. We iterate over the table XW and check if a particular place is a subset of other place. If Place X is a subset of Place Y, we insert Place Y in table YW.

9. Create Places.
   We alter the table YW by adding a column called placeName. For each input and output activity in table YW, we concatenate the activity values and insert into the corresponding value of column placeName. Then, we insert the input place i.e. the source place represented as 'iL' and the output place i.e. the sink place represented as 'oL'.

10. Insert the set of initial and final events.
    (a) We create two hashsets initialActivity and finalActivity.
    (b) We read from the table initial obtained in Step 2 and add the activities to hashset initialActivity. Similarly, we obtain the hashset finalActivity.
    (c) Finally, we insert both the hashsets into table YW for corresponding input and output places.

6 Experimental Dataset

We use Business Process Intelligence 2013(BPI 2013)[9] dataset to conduct our experiments. The log contains events from an incident and problem management system called VINST. The event log is provided by Volvo IT Belgium. The data is related to the process of serving requests in an IT department. The process describes how a problem is handled in the IT services operated by Volvo IT. The dataset is provided in CSV format. We use the VINST cases incidents CSV file dataset, which contains 65533 records. We use the following fields:

1. Problem Number: It represents the unique ticket number for a problem. It is represented as CaseID in our data model.
2. Problem Change Time: It represents the time when the status of the problem changes. It is represented as Timestamp in our data model.
3. Problem Substatus: It represents the current state of the problem. It is represented as Activity in our data model.

---

[9] http://www.win.tue.nl/bpi/2013/challenge.

7   Benchmarking and Performance Comparison

Our benchmarking system consists of Intel Core i3 2.20 GHz processor, 4 GB Random Access Memory (RAM), 245 GB Hard Disk Drive (HDD), Operating System (OS) is Windows 2008 LTS. The experiments were conducted on MySQL 5.6 (row-oriented database) and Cassandra 2.0.1 (NoSQL column-oriented database). We conduct series of experiments on a single machine.

The α-miner algorithm interacts with the database. The underlying data model for implementing α-miner algorithm consists of 3 columns (CaseID, Timestamp and Activity) each of which are of varchar datatype except Timestamp which is of timestamp datatype. We use the same data model while performing bulk loading of datasets through the database loader. We take each reading five times for all the experiments and the average of each reading is reported in the paper.

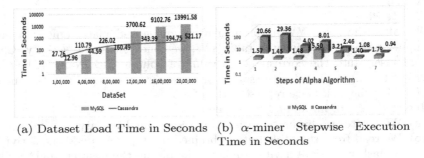

(a) Dataset Load Time in Seconds   (b) α-miner Stepwise Execution Time in Seconds

Fig. 1. Dataset load time and α-miner stepwise execution time

Our first experiment consists of investigating the time taken to perform bulk loading in both the databases across various dataset sizes. Figure 1(a) shows that the time taken to load data in MySQL is initially lower as compared to Cassandra. However, as the dataset size increases beyond a certain point, the time taken to load data in MySQL increases as compared to Cassandra. On an average the time taken to perform bulk loading in Cassandra across various dataset sizes is 16 times lower than that of MySQL. We believe the reason for the increase in load time in MySQL when the dataset size increases can be the difference between how bulk loading is performed in both the databases. Bulk loading in MySQL is done using LOAD DATA INFILE command which is designed for mass loading of records in a single operation as it overcomes the overhead of parsing and flushing batch of inserts stored in a buffer to MySQL server. LOAD DATA INFILE command also creates an index and checks uniqueness while inserting records in a table. Bulk loading in Cassandra is done using COPY command which expects the number of columns in CSV file to be the same as the number of columns in the table metadata. When the size of the dataset increases then in case of MySQL most of the time is spent in checking uniqueness and creating indexes.

There is no such overhead in Cassandra. Hence, the time taken to load the data in MySQL increases when the dataset size increases.

α-miner algorithm is a seven step algorithm (Refer to Section 3). Few steps are read intensive (Steps 1–3) while few steps are write intensive (Steps 4–7). We perform an experiment to compute the α-miner algorithm execution time of each step in both MySQL and Cassandra to examine which database performs better for each step. In MySQL default size of innodb_buffer_pool_size is 8 MB that is used to cache data and indexes of its tables. The larger we set this value, the lesser is the disk I/O needed to access the data in tables. Figure 1(b) reveals that the stepwise time taken in MySQL and Cassandra varies differently for each of the steps. We conjecture the reason for the difference in time taken can be the difference in the internal architecture of MYSQL and Cassandra and the number of reads and writes performed at each step. For the first three steps, the time taken in Cassandra is 12 times more as compared to MySQL. The reason for this is that we copy the data to and from CSV files in order to obtain the total, initial and final activities. We create a number of tables and load the data a number of times to get the set of activities. This overhead of reading from CSV files and writing to CSV files is not there in MySQL. The fourth step involves reading from the tables created in the first three steps, the causality table and the eventlog table to create the table XL. In MySQL, in order to read the data from a table we need to scan the B-Tree index to find the location of block where data is stored. In case of Cassandra data is read from the memtable. If values are not in memtable they are read from Sorted String Tables (SSTables). All entries of a row are present across multiple SSTables. Thus, the read operation in Cassandra involves reading from the Memtable and multiple SSTables. Hence, read performance of MySQL is better as compared to Cassandra. The fifth step includes more number of insert operations as compared to read operations. In MySQL, in order to write data, the entire B-Tree index needs to be scanned to locate the block where we need to write data. Cassandra follows log structure merge tree index. In case of Cassandra, values are written in an append only mode. The writes in Cassandra are sequential. There are no in place updates. Hence, Cassandra gives better write performance as compared to MySQL. Similarly for Step 6, there are more number of insert operations and hence, Cassandra gives a better performance for step 6. Step 7 involves the execution of stored procedures and a lot of data is read from the database, processed and inserted into the FL table. However, in Cassandra, Step 7 involves inserting only the set of initial and final activities and adding the input and output place names to the YL table. Since, the number of insert operations performed are more as compared to the select operations, the overall time taken in MySQL is more as compared to Cassandra.

We conduct an experiment to compare which of the database performs better for read and write operations in both MySQL and Cassandra. As can be seen from Fig. 2(a), the total time taken in MySQL to read data is 3.7 times lower than the time taken to read data in Cassandra. According to us, the reason for Cassandra giving better read performance can be the difference in the data

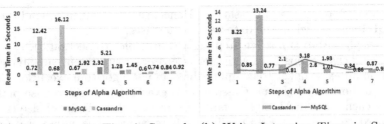

(a) Read Intensive Time in Seconds   (b) Write Intensive Time in Seconds

Fig. 2. Read and write intensive time

structure used by both the databases. In MySQL, only B-Tree index needs to be scanned to find the location of block where the data is stored. In case of Cassandra data is read as described below-

1. To find the data, Cassandra client first scans the memtable.
2. When the data is not found in the memtable, Cassandra scans all the SSTables as all the fields of a particular record can be present across multiple SSTables.

Figure 2(b) shows that the write performance of Cassandra is better as compared to MySQL except for the first three steps as the first three steps have the overhead of copying to and from CSV files. For the remaining steps Cassandra performs writes 1.37 times faster than MySQL. We believe the reason for Cassandra giving better write performance for the remaining steps can be the difference in the way writes are performed in both the databases. In MySQL, the B-Tree index needs to be scanned to find the location of block where the data needs to be written. Almost all the leaf blocks of B-Tree are stored on the disk. Hence, at least one I/O operation is required to retrieve the target block in memory. Figure 2(b) illustrates that Step 5 and Step 7 of α-miner algorithm in MySQL are more write intensive than the other steps. We believe the reason can be the generation of maximal sets and places by stored procedures in MySQL. A large number of insert operations are executed in the stored procedure to generate the maximal sets. In Cassandra we perform the same steps, that is all the analytical processing using Java because CQL does not support advanced features of SQL. Writes in Cassandra are performed in an append only mode. There is no overwrite in place. All update operations append the new data which gets merged with the older data in the background. Thus, writes in Cassandra are more optimized as compared to MySQL.

We perform an experiment to investigate which database can efficiently store the results of each step of α-miner algorithm using minimum disk space. We include only the data length (excluding the size of the index table) in the disk space of a table. Figure 3(a) reveals that Cassandra on an average uses disk space 4.06 times lower than that of MySQL for tables created at each step of the algorithm. The cumulative disk space for storing all the tables in MySQL

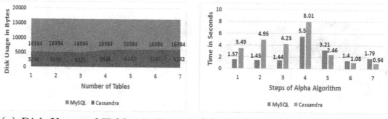

(a) Disk Usage of Tables in Bytes

(b) α-miner Stepwise Execution Time in Java

Fig. 3. Disk usage of tables in bytes and α-miner stepwise execution time in Java

is 162388 bytes while for Cassandra the space is 39742 bytes. We believe the underlying reason for MySQL occupying more space is the difference in the way memory is allocated to tables in both the databases. In MySQL, the operating system allocates fixed size blocks of size 16 KB for the data to be stored in a table. Number of blocks assigned to a table is equal to the dataset size divided by the block size. In MySQL, if a particular set of blocks or block has been allocated for a table then that particular set of blocks or block can be used only by that table. Either the table completely utilizes the space provided to it or the space in the last block is not utilized. Storing tables of size less than 16 KB leads to under-utilization of space and the remaining space cannot be utilized by other tables. Cassandra stores the key-value pairs in an in memory data structure called memtable. Memtables are flushed to the disk when the size of the data increases beyond a certain threshold value. The data is then written to the disk in data files called SSTables which is a file of key-value string pairs and is equal to the size of the data flushed from the memtable. Hence, the disk space at each step is more efficiently utilized in Cassandra as compared to MySQL.

The step wise execution time of α-miner algorithm for the first three steps in Cassandra is very high as compared to MySQL. The reason is the overhead of copying data to and from CSV files to get the desired results. In order to avoid this overhead, we instead of using the COPY command use only Select and Insert statements with some Java processing. We create a table trace that stores CaseID as the primary key and list of activities ordered by timestamp. We extract the first activity from the list corresponding to each CaseID and insert it in the table storing initial activities. We extract the last activity from the list corresponding to each CaseID and insert it in the table storing the final activities. Similarly we insert all the activities in the list and insert the values in the table storing all the activities. As can be seen from Fig. 3(b), the stepwise execution time in Cassandra reduces by 4.26 times as compared to the time taken using COPY command. Thus, the performance of Select and Insert statements with Java processing gives a much better performance as compared to the COPY command.

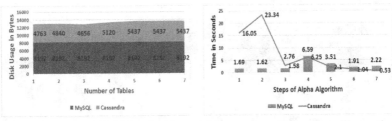

(a) Disk Usage of Tables in Bytes   (b) α-miner Stepwise Execution
with Compression   Time with Compression

Fig. 4. Disk usage of tables in bytes and α-miner stepwise execution time with compression

Disk space can be efficiently utilized by using the compression technique. We conduct an experiment to compute the disk space occupied by tables at each step of the α-miner algorithm with compression enabled. Figure 4(a) illustrates that when we compare the disk space occupied by each table without compression and with compression the compression ratio (Actual size of table/Compressed size of table) is better in MySQL as compared to Cassandra. The maximum and minimum compression ratio in MySQL is 2. Similarly, the maximum compression ratio in Cassandra is 1.15 and minimum compression ratio is 1.05. We believe the reason for MySQL having a better compression ratio as compared to Cassandra is the difference in the compression techniques used by both the databases. MySQL uses zlib compression technique which provides a better compression ratio but not a good decompression speed while Cassandra uses LZ4 compression technique which does not provide a very good compression ratio but provides very fast decompression speed.

We conduct an experiment to examine the time taken by each step of the α-miner algorithm with compression technique. Figure 4(b) reveals that the stepwise performance improves for each step in Cassandra while it degrades for each step in MySQL. We believe the reason for performance degradation when compression is enabled can be the difference in the way compression is performed in both the databases. MySQL uses blocks of sizes 1 KB, 2 KB, 4 KB, 8 KB and 16 KB. The default block size after compression in MySQL is 8 KB. Thus, if a block size after compression is 5 KB, then the block will be first uncompressed, then split into two blocks and finally recompressed into blocks of size 1 KB and 4 KB. Cassandra does not have a fixed block constraint after compressing a block. Also, with compression Cassandra can quickly find the location of rows in the SSTables. SSTables in Cassandra are immutable and hence recompression is not required for processing write operations. We observe that the total time taken in executing α-miner algorithm by Cassandra without compression is 2.02 times lower than time taken with compression. Similarly, the total time taken in MySQL with compression is 1.11 times lower than time taken without compression.

8 Conclusion

In this paper, we present an implementation of α-miner algorithm in MySQL and Cassandra using the database specific query language (SQL and CQL). Furthermore, we present the performance comparison of α-miner algorithm in MySQL and Cassandra. The α-miner implementation in MySQL is a one tier application which uses only standard SQL queries and advanced stored procedures. Similarly, implementation in Cassandra is done using CQL and Java. We conclude that when the size of the dataset increases, the time taken by Cassandra on an average is 16 times faster than MySQL. Based on experimental results, we conclude that Cassandra outperforms MySQL in loading real time large datasets data (event logs).

The total time taken to read the data while execution of α-miner algorithm is 3.70 times lower in MySQL as compared to Cassandra. Similarly, for writing the data, time taken by Cassandra is 1.37 times lower as compared to MySQL. Cassandra outperforms MySQL in terms of the disk usage of tables. The disk space occupied by tables in Cassandra is 4.06 times lower as compared to MySQL. Thus, we conclude that Cassandra is more efficient than MySQL in terms of storing data and performing query. When compression is enabled, performance of Cassanadra improves by 0.22 % while that of MySQL degrades by 0.19 %.

References

1. Carlos, O.: Programming the k-means clustering algorithm in SQL. In: ACM SIGKDD International Conference on Knowledge Discovery and Data Mining, pp. 823–828 (2004)
2. Ordonez, C., Cereghini, P.: SQLEM: fast clustering in SQL using the EM Algorithm. In: International Conference on Management of Data, pp. 559–570 (2000)
3. Abadi, D.J., Madden, S.R., Hachem, N.: Column-stores vs. row-stores: how different are they really? In: SIGMOID (2008)
4. Rana, D.P., Mistry, N.J., Raghuwanshi, M.M.: Association rule mining analyzation using column oriented database. Int. J. Adv. Comput. Res. 3(3), 88–93 (2013)
5. Finn, M.A.: Fighting impedance mismatch at the database level. White paper (2001)
6. Gupta, K., Sachdev, A., Sureka, A.: Pragamana: performance comparison and programming alpha-miner algorithm in relational database query language and NoSQL column-oriented using apache phoenix. In: Proceedings of the Eighth International C* Conference on Computer Science & Software Engineering, C3S2E 2015, pp. 113–118 (2008)
7. Joishi, J., Sureka, A.: Vishleshan: performance comparison and programming process mining algorithms in graph-oriented and relational database query languages. In: Proceedings of the 19th International Database Engineering and Applications Symposium, IDEAS 2015, pp. 192–197 (2014)
8. Sattler, K.-U., Dunemann, O.: SQL database primitives for decision tree classifiers. In: Conference on Information and Knowledge Management, pp. 379–386 (2001)
9. Suresh, L., Simha, J., Velur, R.: Implementing k-means algorithm using row store and column store databases-a case study. Int. J. Recent Trends Eng. 4(2) (2009)

10. Plattner, H.: A common database approach for OLTP and OLAP using an in-memory column database. In: ACM SIGMOD International Conference on Management of Data (2009)
11. Russell, N.C.: Foundation of process-aware information systems. Dissertation (2007)
12. Sharma, V., Dave, M.: SQL and NoSQL database. Int. J. Adv. Res. Comput. Sci. Softw. Eng. **2**(8), 20–27 (2012)
13. Weerapong, S., Porouhan, P., Premchaiswadi, W.: Process mining using α-algorithm as a tool. IEEE (2012)
14. Aalst, W.V.D.: Process mining: overview and opportunities. ACM Trans. Manage. Inf. Syst. **3**(2), 1–17 (2012)

A New Proposed Feature Subset Selection Algorithm Based on Maximization of Gain Ratio

Arpita Nagpal[✉] and Deepti Gaur

Computer Science Department, Northcap University, Gurgaon, India
{arpitanagpal,deeptigaur}@ncuindia.edu

Abstract. Feature subset selection is one of the techniques to extract the highly relevant subset of original features from a dataset. In this paper, we have proposed a new algorithm to filter the features from the dataset using a greedy stepwise forward selection technique. The Proposed algorithm uses gain ratio as the greedy evaluation measure. It utilizes multiple feature correlation technique to remove the redundant features from the data set. Experiments that are carried out to evaluate the Proposed algorithm are based on number of features, runtime and classification accuracy of three classifiers namely Naïve Bayes, the Tree based C4.5 and Instant Based IB1. The results have been compared with other two feature selection algorithms, i.e. Fast Correlation-Based Filter Solution (FCBS) and Fast clustering based feature selection algorithm (FAST) over the datasets of different dimensions and domain. A unified metric, which combines all three parameters (number of features, runtime, classification accuracy) together, has also been taken to compare the algorithms. The result shows that our Proposed algorithm has a significant improvement than other feature selection algorithms for large dimensional data while working on a data set of image domain.

Keywords: Classification · Feature selection · Filter method · Mutual information

1 Introduction

Nowadays, the data is increasing at tremendous speed in terms of volume and number of features. The major difficulty is called as 'the curse of dimensionality' [20]. The learning algorithms are greatly affected by the dimensionality of the data. The task of dimension reduction is the process of reducing the number of features or variables of an object under consideration.

Dimension reduction and feature selections are two techniques which can reduce the attributes of data for classification tasks. But still there lies some difference in both the techniques. Dimensionality reduction is creating new attributes as a combination of the old attributes like in PCA (Principal Component Analysis) whereas in feature selection some attributes whose information overlap with other attributes called redundant attributes are removed from the dataset. PCA involves feature transformation and obtains a set of transformed features rather than a subset of the original features [17]. Dimension

© Springer International Publishing Switzerland 2015
N. Kumar and V. Bhatnagar (Eds.): BDA 2015, LNCS 9498, pp. 181–197, 2015.
DOI: 10.1007/978-3-319-27057-9_13

reduction of the Big Data (i.e. Voluminous data) can help in the easy processing of data for some decision-making. Generally, there are four types of feature selection techniques filter, wrapper, embedded and hybrid technique. The filter approach to feature selection is to remove the features based on the general characteristics of the training data without involving any learning algorithm [4, 6]. The wrapper method involves a classification algorithm to determine the efficiency of the subset generated. The embedded methods are specific to the learning algorithm and during its training phase feature selection algorithms are applied. Hybrid approach which has been recently been proposed for high dimensional data is a combination of both filter and wrapper method [1, 2], [4], [5].

Janecek et al. [6] have proven by experimental results that among the feature selection methods, wrappers tend to produce the smallest feature subsets with very comprehensive classification accuracy, in many cases the best overall dimension reduction methods. But the wrapper method is computationally expensive as it needs the learning algorithm to evaluate the selected features performance and find the final selected set. When there is a small set of features wrapper can be applied, but when the number of features becomes very large, filter model is usually chosen due to its computational accuracy and efficiency [4]. In high dimensional dataset, feature selection becomes more efficient than a dimension reduction technique of PCA.

This work is based on feature selection using a filter approach. A new algorithm which can efficiently remove both irrelevant and redundant features for Big Data has been developed. Here, we have experimentally shown its performance by taking some of the high dimensional data sets. Our method calculates Gain Ratio between each feature and the class attributes. The feature having highest gain ratio value becomes the first node of the list. Second highest gain ratio value feature is now considered. It's gain ratio is calculated with the first feature and if it satisfies the condition then it is added to the list otherwise ignored. This method is based on the multiple feature correlation technique in which next feature's correlation is checked with the correlation of all the features present in the list. If the feature not present in the list satisfies the condition, then it is added to the list otherwise it is denied and not involved in further computations. Final list depict the set of selected features. Multiple feature correlation technique reduces the number of computations and produces a subset of independent feature free from overlap of information contained in them. The Proposed algorithm is tested on 9 datasets from different domains (image, microarray and text data). Our method has been compared with two filter feature selection algorithms: Fast-Correlation based Filter (FCBS) [4] and FAST [7] and it shows that the Proposed algorithm outperforms them in terms of classification accuracy, runtime and number of features selected in most data sets.

The rest of the paper has been organized as follows: in Sect. 2, related work will be explained. In Sect. 3, we describe the theoretical background. Section 4 discusses the complete algorithm with an example. Section 5 gives the result and comparisons with other algorithm based on dimension of data sets and domain. Finally, in Sect. 6 we draw conclusions based on the experimental results.

2 Related Work

Feature selection aims to find the subset of features from the original set of features by removing irrelevant and redundant features. Within the filter model of feature selection there have been many algorithms proposed such as Relief [11], Relief-F [12], FOCUS, FOCUS-2[13], Correlation based Feature Selection (CFS) [8], FCBS[4], FAST[7]. Relief [11] and Correlation based Feature Selection (CFS) [8] methods remove only the irrelevant features. The algorithms proposed later remove both irrelevant and redundant features.

Liu and Yu [10], has given that the general process of feature selection is divided into four processes: subset generation, subset evaluation, stopping criterion and subset validation.

Each of the algorithms described in literature uses one of the subset generation techniques either complete search, sequential search or random search, all of either in forward, backward or bidirectional directions [3, 10]. After generating a subset, this subset needs to be evaluated. Form data set with 'n' features 2n subsets can be generated. A search algorithm is often employed to find the optimal feature subsets. To find which the optimal subset is, each algorithm has an evaluation technique based on different heuristics. Generally, the statistics used as evaluation measures are distance based measures, Information gain [4], correlation coefficient [9], consistency measures [3]. The process terminates when it reaches a stopping criterion.

CFS (Correlation-based Feature Selection), one of the feature selection method uses forward greedy feature selection method. It is based on the hypothesis that a good feature subset is the one that contains features highly correlated to the class, yet uncorrelated to each other [8].

Fast-Correlation based Filter (FCBS) algorithm given by Yu and Liu [4] removes both irrelevant and redundant features by the use symmetric uncertainty as an evaluation measure. It uses the concept of correlation based on information theory of mutual information and entropy to calculate the uncertainty of a random variable. It removes features by performing a pairwise correlation.

Recently, an algorithm named FAST has been developed by Song et al. (2013) which uses symmetric uncertainty as an evaluation measure to remove both irrelevant and redundant features. It generates a Minimum Spanning Tree (MST) by calculating the correlation of each feature with every other feature. Then it partitions the MST in forest with each tree representing a cluster, represented features are then selected from each cluster. These representative features form a final subset of features.

Quite different from FAST algorithm, our Proposed algorithm uses Gain Ratio as an evaluation measure to remove irrelevant and redundant features. It does not calculate the correlation of each feature with every other feature instead, it calculates correlation with only those present in the feature subset formed. The problem becomes NP-hard if data are high dimensional and we keep on finding correlation of each feature with every other feature in the dataset. Unlike, FCBF it does not perform pairwise correlation, instead it performs a correlation with all present in the feature subset. It is a greedy forward selection method and adds features in forward direction.

3   Theoretical Background

Entropy is a measure of uncertainty of a random variable. If X is a discrete random variable with alphabet x and probability mass function $p(x) = PR \{X = x\}$. The probability mass function is denoted by $p(x)$. The entropy $H(X)$ of a discrete random variable X is defined by:

$$H(X) = -\sum\nolimits_x p(x) \log_2 p(x) \tag{1}$$

Information gain is a measure of the amount of information that one random variable contains about another random variable. The information gain $I(X; Y)$ give the relation between two variables. Information gain or Mutual Information [16] is given by

$$I(X; Y) = H(Y) - H(Y|X) = H(X) - H(X|Y)$$
$$= H(Y) + H(X) - H(X, Y) \tag{2}$$

Where $H(X)$, $H(Y)$ is the individual entropies of two random variables X and Y. Entropy of X is based on the individual probabilities of variables in X. It gives the diversification in values.

Our algorithm is based on the concept of information theory. It is based on the assumption that if there are two different random variables, then larger the value of information gain between them, stronger the relationship they share. Theorem 1 as given in [14].

Theorem 1: *For any discrete random variable Y and Z $I(Y;Z) \geq 0$. Moreover, $I(Y; Z) = 0$ if and only if Y and Z are independent.*

Let D be a full feature set, $fi \in D$ be one of the feature. C is the target class attribute. The definitions can be defined as follows:

Definition 1 (Relevance): *A feature fi is relevant to the class C if and only if $GR(fi,C) \geq \theta$ i.e. the gain ratio value between a feature and class attribute should be greater than a predefined threshold θ.*

Definition 2 (Redundancy): *Let D be a full set of features in the dataset, Two features fi and fj are redundant peers if and only if $GR(fi,fj) > GR(fi,C) \cap GR(fi,fj) > GR(fj,C)$. Otherwise they are not redundant.*

Redundant features are those that contain much of the common information. Definition 2 indicates that a feature is redundant to other feature in the dataset, if the correlation between them is greater than the correlation of feature with the Class C. Here, Information gain (I) is used to measure the correlation between the two features. The drawback of information gain is that it is biased towards the feature with all different values. It prefers to select the attribute having large number of different values in its instances. For example, consider an attribute student_ID in the students' record data that has all different values in it. Therefore, the information gained on this attribute will be maximal. To overcome this drawback, we use an extension of information gain known as gain ratio, which overcomes this bias. It normalizes information gain using a "split info" value defined as:

$$\text{SplitInfoB}(D) = -\sum_{i=1}^{u} \frac{|D_i|}{|D|} \times \log_2\left(\frac{|D_i|}{|D|}\right) \tag{3}$$

The data set D is split into u portions of attribute B. $|D_i|$ is total number of tuples in the ith portion and $|D|$ is the number of attributes in complete dataset. Splitinfo gives the information generated after partitioning whereas information gain, measures the information with respect to classification that is obtained based on the same partitioning. The gain ratio is defined as

$$\text{Gain Ratio}(B) = \text{Gain}(B)/\text{SplitInfo}(B) \tag{4}$$

Definition 3 (maxGR): It is the largest value of Gain ratio(GR) found after calculating the gain ratio of the new feature fi (fi ∈ D) with all the features already present in the tree.

Suppose at any step (i-1), some features are already present in tree U. To add a new feature f_i ($f_i \in D\backslash U_{i-1}$) to the tree find GR ($f_i$; f_j) for each feature $f_j \in U$. The largest value of GR (f_i; f_j) is the maxGR value.

Definition 4 (Relevantf): It gives us the relation between the feature fi (fi ∈ D) and the class C. The relevance between the feature and the class is found on the basis of the value of the Gain ratio value between them. It is denoted by GR (f, c).

Definition 5 (Redundantf): A feature is added as the tree node if, fi ∈ D and maxGR(X; Y) < GR(Y,C). This means that both features (X,Y) are not correlated with each other.

Our algorithm is based on the assumption that stronger the relation between two variables, larger the value of gain ratio they will have. A feature becomes redundant if its relation is stronger with any of the feature already present in the feature subset than its relation with its class attribute.

4 Algorithm and Analysis

The Proposed algorithm depicted in Figs. 1 and 2 is based on the methodology of gain ratio as described before. Input to the algorithm is all the features given in the data set $D = \{f_1, f_2, \ldots\ldots f_m\}$ and Class C. The first task is to remove the irrelevant features. Relevantf gives the value of $GR(f_i, C)$. If this value is greater than the predefined threshold, then those features are kept as relevant ones, others are ignored.

The next step is to remove redundant features. To do this, first arrange the list of all relevant features (D′) found along with their Gain ratio value (G′) in descending order. The first feature in the D′ list will be the feature having the highest value of gain ratio with the class. According to our assumption made the first feature in D′ is most relevant and has to be kept.

Input: D(f₁,f₂,......f_m, C), the given dataset
        θ   // Relevant Threshold
Output: F   //final feature subset
Begin:
// Irrelevant feature removal
 1.   For each feature, i=1 to m do
 2.   Relevantf= GR(f$_i$,C)
 3.   If Relevantf > θ
 4.   Append f$_i$ to Snewlist
 5.   End;
 6.   End

//Redundant Feature removal from the elements in Snewlist
which has 'k' relevant features

 7.   D'=Arrange Snewlist in Descending order.
 8.   G'=Arrange GR(f,C) in descending order.
 9.   ΔT.firstnode ← get first element from G'
10.   Y ← second element from G'
11.   L ← 1
12.   F=sub (ΔT,Y,L,G')
13.   End;

Fig. 1. Algorithm

To find correlation in polynomial time, we arrange it in descending order and find correlation of new feature with every feature in tree U ignoring redundant features found.

This step starts with an empty list named T. First add the first feature from D' and keeps on adding non redundant features into it. Check the first feature with every other feature in terms of the redundancy, according to Definition 5. The features found redundant with the first feature is ignored and their redundancy is never again checked with any other feature.

Suppose at any step (i-1), some features are already present in Tree U. To add a new feature f$_i$ (f$_i$ ∈ D\U$_{i-1}$) to the list first it finds GR (U$_{s-1}$; f$_i$). The following criterion is used:

$$f_{(i)} = \text{argmax } GR(U_{s-1}; f_i)$$

This means that from the feature in the list which has the largest value of GR with f$_i$ is picked.

This approach maximizes the gain ratio between feature subset found and the class attribute. If maxGR with all features in U at step i-1 is less than GR of new feature and class C then a new feature gets added to the list. If this condition is not satisfied, then the feature has lost the opportunity to be added in the list and hence ignored. Figure 1 gives a method to remove the irrelevant features. The remaining features are then arranged in descending order. Pass the first node to list T, the first element from D'.

Algorithm: sub(ΔT,Y,L,G')

    Input:(ΔT,Value of Gain ratio's G',

                Next element Y, Current depth L, number of relevant features k)

    Output: Final tree, F

    Begin:

1.   F=ΔT.Lth Node;
2.   For every element X $\in$ F {
3.   Calculate GR(X;Y)
4.   Extract maxGR(X;Y) as defined in Definition 3
5.   }
6.   If(max GR(X;Y)<GR(Y,C)) {
7.   Extract Y from G'
8.   Add to ΔT.Lth Node
9.   }
10.   If(L $\leq$ k) {
11.   Y=get next element from G';
12.   L $\leftarrow$ L+1;
13.   sub (ΔT,Y,L,G')}**End;**

Fig. 2. The subroutine of the algorithm

Then T is passed to the subroutine sub given in Fig. 2. Figure 2 keeps on adding the new features to T according to maxGR explained in Definition 3. If maxGR(X;Y) > GR (Y,C) then the algorithm will ignore the feature and move to the next feature. Suppose the number of features found after removing irrelevant features is k. The searching process terminates when all the 'k' features in the dataset have been examined.

To clarify the search procedure, we explain the algorithm through an example. Let the set of features in the dataset is D = {a,b,c,d,e,f} and the class attribute is C. 'm' is the number of features in the dataset. Here, m = 6. Suppose after going through steps 1 to 5 in Fig. 1 all feature's Relevantf value except feature f satisfies the predetermined threshold and gets added in the Snewlist. Snewlist becomes {a,b,c,d,e}. k i.e. the number of features in Snewlist becomes 5. To further process Snewlist, it is arranged in descending order in G'{a, d, b, e, c} according to their gain ratio value with the class. Figure 3 depicts the search procedure to add the new feature to the empty data structure T. First the list T is empty $\Delta T = \{\}$. At level 1, the first node 'a', from G' is taken and added to the list. Second value from G' i.e. d is taken. Calculate GR (a, d) and compare it with GR (d, class C) according to step 6 of Fig. 2. 'd' satisfies the condition so list adds 'd' to itself.. Pick the third element from G' which is 'b'. Calculate GR (a, b) and GR (d, b). Pick the maximum GR value from them and compare it with GR (b, class). According to steps 6 to 8 of Fig. 2, it does not satisfy the condition, so it is not added to the list and it never used again in further comparisons. The next element from the list is 'e'. Repeat the same steps with e as done with last element 'b'. Here, we found that e satisfies the condition so it is added to the T. The last element is 'c' Calculate GR (a, c), GR (d, c) and GR (e, c). Take out the maximum value of GR out of these three values and Compare it with GR (c, Class). It is observed that c does not satisfy the condition

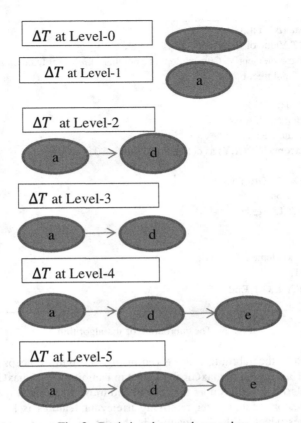

Fig. 3. Depicting the search procedure

so it is filtered out. Finally ΔT at level-5 contains the feature subset after removing both irrelevant and redundant features.

5   Empirical Study

5.1   Datasets

In our experiment we have employed 11 datasets which are from different domains, text, image, Microarray. The number of features varies from 36 to 10, 000 features. The data sets used in the experiments are taken from the UCI machine learning repository [18], tunedit.org/repo/Data/Text and featureselection.asu.edu [21]. Microarray datasets of Colon_1 [22] actually contained 22883 features, but a preprocessing strategy [23] has reduced the features to 8826. Leukemia [24] is one of the cancer classification data which comes under microarray domain has also been pre-processed. The features with a value less than 20 and more than 16000 were removed. The summary of a data set is given in Table 1.

Table 1. Summary of data sets

Data set	Number of instances	Number of features	Number of classes	Domain
WarpAR10P	130	2400	10	Image, face
Chess	3196	36	2	Text
WarpPIE10p	210	2420	10	Image, Face
Arcene	100	10000	2	Image
Coil2000	134	86	2	Text
Email word subject	64	242	2	Text
tox-171	100	5749	3	Microarray
Pix10P	100	10000	10	Image,face
orlaws10p	100	10304	10	Image, face
Colon_I	37	8826	2	Microarray
Leukemia	72	7128	3	Microarray

5.2 Experimental Results and Comparisons

To verify the experimental results three parameters percentage of selected features, runtime and Classification accuracy has been calculated. Two feature selection algorithms FCBF and FAST have been compared with the Proposed algorithm on these three parameters. In the performed experiments, the relevant threshold, θ is the GR((ain Ratio) value of the $\llcorner m/\log m \lrcorner_{th}$ ranked feature for all the datasets. This threshold is as a suggestion given by Yu and Liu [4]. By applying, 10-fold cross validation classification accuracies of three different classifiers (Naïve Bayes, C4.5, and IB1) on all the datasets accurate results could be achieved.

The Proposed algorithm has also been compared with FCBF and FAST on the basis of multi-criteria Metric EARR (Extended Adjusted Ratio of Ratios) proposed by Wang [15]. Under one unified metric, the classification accuracy with a runtime and number of features selected are integrated. This unified metric EARR evaluates the performance by taking the ratio of the metric values. Let $D = \{D_1, D_2, \ldots., D_n\}$ be a set of n data sets, and $A = \{A_1, A_2, \ldots. A_n)$ be a set of M FSS algorithms. Then, the $EARR$ of A_i to A_j over D_k be defined as:

$$EARR_{A_i,A_j}^{D_k} = \frac{acc_i^k / acc_j^k}{1 + \propto . \log\left(t_i^k / t_j^k\right) + \beta . \log(n_i^k / n_j^k)} \quad (1 \leq i \neq j \leq M, 1 \leq k < N \quad (5)$$

$\propto$ and β are user defined parameters, which tells us how much importance should be given to the runtime and number of features selected respectively. acc_i^k is the accuracy of ith algorithm of 'k' th dataset. t_i^k and n_i^k are the runtime and number of selected features of dataset 'k' on ith algorithm respectively.

This will allow the user to tell how much the runtime and feature selected should dominate accuracy. When comparing multiple feature selection algorithms, it takes the arithmetic mean of the $EARR_{A_i,A_j}^{D_k}$ of A_i to another algorithm A_j on D. It is defined as:

$$EARR_{A_i}^{D_k} = \frac{1}{M-1} \sum\nolimits_{j=1\&j\neq i}^{M} EARR_{A_i,A_j}^{D_k} \qquad (6)$$

The larger the value of EARR, better is the corresponding algorithm on a given data set D [15].

5.3 Dimension Wise Comparison of Feature Selection Algorithms

Tables 2 and 3 depict the comparison of low dimensional data set and large dimensional data set respectively, of three feature selection algorithm on the basis of three parameters (percentage of feature selected, runtime and accuracy of three different classifiers). According to our assumption low dimension datasets consisting of less than 200 features and high dimensional data sets are datasets with features greater than 200 or more. Accuracy on all three classification algorithm on all the data sets is conducted in Weka [19].

We observe from Tables 2 and 3 that the Proposed algorithm is performing better in terms of percentage of the selected features and runtime for large dimensional data rather than for low dimensional data. The Proposed algorithm is securing first position for all the evaluation metrics for Arcene data, PIX10P,ORL10P set which have around 10, 000 features. So, we can say that this technique works well on large dimensional data sets.

5.4 Domain Wise Comparison of Feature Selection Algorithms

Data sets used in the experiments belongs to three types of Domain Text, Image and Microarray. Tables 4, 5, 6, 7, 8 gives the average values obtained domain wise for three performance metrics (Percentage of selected features, Runtime and Classification accuracy). If we observe the percentage of the selected features and runtime in Tables 4 and 5, data sets in image domain are showing a comparable performance. In case of text dataset, there is an improvement in some cases. Table 4 elaborates averages of the three feature selection algorithm on each data set domain wise.

Table 4 shows that the Proposed algorithm selects fewer features than FCBF and FAST in all three domains text, Image and Microarray. Further Comparisons depicts that:

1. For text datasets, Proposed algorithm selects 5.89 percent of the features. FCBF and FAST have a margin of 1.28 percent between them.
2. For image datasets, Proposed algorithm ranks 1 by selecting 0.334 percent of features with a margin of 0.15 from FCBF and 5.25 from FAST.
3. For Microarray datasets, Proposed algorithm selects 1.25 and 6.7 lesser percentages of features than FCBF and FAST respectively.

Table 2. Comparison of feature selection algorithm for low- dimensional data sets

Data set	Feature selection algorithm	Percentage of selected features	Runtime (s)	Accuracy by Naïve Bayes	Accuracy by C4.5	Accuracy byIB1
Chess	FCBF	16.6	25.36	92.5	94.08	92.05
	FAST	5.5	164.42	75.4	75.4	70.3
	Proposed	11.11	56.24	67.08	69.8	63.7
Coil2000	FCBF	3.48	0.190	92.5	95.5	94.77
	FAST	2.3	1.093	94.04	94.02	93.04
	Proposed	2.32	0.32	94.06	95.52	94.77

Table 3. Comparison of feature selection algorithm for large – dimensional data sets

Data set	Feature selection algorithm	Percentage of selected features	Runtime (s)	Accuracy by Naïve Bayes	Accuracy by C4.5	Accuracy by IB1
ORL10P	FCBF	0.39	0.53	48	44	45
	FAST	0.39	69.21	49	50	59
	Proposed	0.39	0.36	62	63	58
WarpAR10P	FCBF	0.041	7.15	16.15	16.92	17.69
	FAST	0.19	1476	15.03	18.69	15.33
	Proposed	0.041	8.35	33.84	33.07	26.15
Warp PIE10p	FCBF	0.041	11.19	32.95	34.28	35.23
	FAST	0.133	7411	33.75	36.60	34.92
	Proposed	0.041	0.78	32.8	34.28	35.2
Arcene	FCBF	0.01	23.143	58	54	61
	FAST	0.01	5164	57	55	59
	Proposed	0.03	94.8	64	64	58
PIX10P	FCBF	1.953	0.482	90	98	97
	FAST	27.34	60.3	89.07	98.07	97
	Proposed	1.17	0.78	90	98.08	97
TOX-171	FCBF	0.39	0.0040	40	37	46
	FAST	0.39	0.0025	40	37	44
	Proposed	0.39	0.44	40	40	47
Email-word subject	FCBF	8.26	0.157	67.18	67.18	57.8
	FAST	24.38	8.23	67	66.08	59.9
	Proposed	4.54	0.046	67.18	67.18	60.9
Colon_1	FCBF	0.05	4.72	32.43	89.18	81.08
	FAST	0.30	8.66	72.5	88.5	80.8
	Proposed	0.02	2.79	83.78	75.65	81.08
Leukemia	FCBF	0.02	42.64	52.77	52.77	56.94
	FAST	0.07	69.21	77.16	52.77	55
	Proposed	0.01	28.46	52.77	52.77	56.94

Table 4. Comparison based on percentage of selected features

Dataset	Domain	Proposed	FCBF	FAST
Chess	Text	11.11	16.6	5.5
Coil2000	Text	2.32	3.48	2.3
Email word	Text	4.25	8.26	24.38
Average (Text)		5.89	9.44	10.72
WarpAR10P	Image	0.041	0.041	0.19
Warp PIE10p	Image	0.041	0.041	0.133
Arcene	Image	0.03	0.01	0.01
PIX10P	Image	1.17	1.953	27.34
ORL10P	Image	0.39	0.39	0.39
Average (Image)		0.3344	0.487	5.61
Tox-171	Microarray	4.54	8.26	24.38
Leukemia	Microarray	0.01	0.02	0.07
Colon_I	Microarray	0.02	0.05	0.30
Average (Microarray)		1.52	2.77	8.25

Table 5. Comparison based on runtime

Dataset	Domain	Proposed	FCBF	FAST
Chess	Text	56.24	25.6	164.42
Coil2000	Text	0.32	0.190	1.093
Email word	Text	0.046	0.157	8.23
Average (Text)		18.868	8.649	57.91
WarpAR10P	Image	8.35	7.15	1476
Warp PIE10p	Image	0.78	11.19	7411
Arcene	Image	94.8	11.19	7411
PIX10P	Image	0.78	0.482	60.3
ORL10P	Image	0.36	0.53	69.21
Average (Image)		21.008	6.1084	3285.5
Tox-171	Microarray	0.44	0.0040	0.0025
Leukemia	Microarray	28.46	42.64	69.21
Colon_I	Microarray	2.79	4.724	8.66
Aveage (Microarray)		10.56	15.788	25.95

If we observe the runtime, the Proposed algorithm is showing a significant improvement compared to FAST and FCBF algorithm in all the domains. Table 5 depicts the average runtime of all three algorithms domain wise.

For text data set, the Proposed algorithm is 39.05 times faster at runtime than FAST. For Image data set, it is 3,264.49 times faster than the FAST algorithm. In case of microarray data, the runtime of Proposed algorithm has decreased by 5.22 and 15.39 as compared to FCBF and FAST respectively.

Tables 6, 7, 8 depicts the 10-fold cross validation classification accuracies of three classifiers on 11 data sets domain wise.

Table 6. Average accuracy domain wise for Naïve Bayes classifier

Dataset	Domain	Proposed	FCBF	FAST
Chess	Text	67.08	92.5	75.4
Coil2000	Text	94.02	92.5	94.04
Email word	Text	67.18	67.18	67
Average (Text)		76.09	84.06	78.81
WarpAR10P	Image	33.84	16.5	15.03
Warp PIE10p	Image	32.8	32.95	33.75
Arcene	Image	64	58	57
PIX10P	Image	90	90	89.07
ORL10P	Image	62	48	49
Average (Image)		56.52	49.09	48.77
Tox-171	Microarray	40	40	40
Leukemia	Microarray	52.77	52.77	77.16
Colon_1	Microarray	83.78	32.43	72.5
Average (Microarray)		58.85	41.73	63.22

Table 7. Average accuracy domain wise for C4.5 classifier

Dataset	Domain	Proposed	FCBF	FAST
Chess	Text	69.8	95.5	94.02
Coil2000	Text	95.52	95.5	94.02
Email word	Text	67.18	67.18	66.08
Average (Text)		77.5	86.06	84.70
WarpAR10P	Image	33.07	16.92	18.69
Warp PIE10p	Image	32.8	32.95	33.75
Arcene	Image	64	54	55
PIX10P	Image	98.08	98	98.07
ORL10P	Image	**63**	**44**	**50**
Average (Image)		58.19	49.17	51.102
Tox-171	Microarray	40	37	37
Leukemia	Microarray	52.77	52.77	52.77
Colon_I	Microarray	75.65	89.18	88.5
Average (Microarray)		56.14	59.65	59.42

We observe that Naïve Bayes classification accuracy after applying feature selection algorithm has a positive improvement in all the domains. It is noted that:

1. Under Image dataset domain FCBF, FAST is 86.8 percent and 86.2 percent better in accuracy than Proposed algorithm.
2. For Arcene dataset, i.e. a large dimensional dataset the Naïve Bayes classification accuracy of Proposed algorithm has been increased by 6, 7 times by FCBF and FAST respectively.

Table 8. Average accuracy domain wise for IB1 classifier

Dataset	Domain	Proposed	FCBF	FAST
Chess	Text	63.7	92.05	70.3
Coil2000	Text	94.77	94.77	93.04
Email word	Text	60.9	57.8	59.9
Average (Text)		75.35	81.54	74.41
WarpAR10P	Image	26.15	17.69	15.33
Warp PIE10p	Image	35.2	35.2	34.92
Arcene	Image	58	61	59
PIX10P	Image	97	97	97
ORL10P	Image	58	45	59
Average (Image)		54.87	51.178	53.05
Tox-171	Microarray	47	46	44
Leukemia	Microarray	56.94	56.94	55
Colon_I	Microarray	81.08	81.08	80.8
Average (Microarray)		61.67	61.34	59.93

3. For WarpAR10p, datasets i.e. a large dimensional dataset the Naïve Bayes classification accuracy of Proposed algorithm has been increased by 17.34 and 18.81 times for FCBF and FAST respectively.
4. The Proposed algorithm has increased the classification accuracy of the Naïve Bayes classifier by 0.9 times than that of FAST and is performing almost the same in case of FCBF for WarpPie10p dataset.
5. For microarray dataset Colon_1 Naïve Bayes accuracy of Proposed algorithm has increased by 38.7 percent and 86.5 percent from FCBF and FAST respectively.

For C4.5 classifier, we observe from Table 7 that:

1. For Image dataset, FCBF and FAST have 9.02, 7.08 lesser accuracy value than the Proposed algorithm.
2. For Arcene dataset, one of a large dimensional data set in image domain the classification accuracy of Proposed algorithm has been increased by 10, 9 times by FCBF and FAST respectively.
3. For WarpAR10p datasets i.e. a large dimensional image datasets the classification accuracy of Proposed algorithm has been increased by 16.15 and 14.38 times for FCBF and FAST respectively.
4. For WarpPIE10p dataset Proposed algorithm is performing almost in a similar way as FCBF and FAST.
5. In case of microarray datasets Tox-171 the accuracy of Proposed algorithm has increased 3 times from FAST and FCBF. In case of Colon_1 it has increased 13.53 times and 12.85 times for FCBF and FAST respectively.

We observed the classification accuracies for IB1 classifier in Table 8 and noted that:

1. For Image dataset FCBF and FAST have a difference of 3.69 and 1.82 respectively, than Proposed algorithm.

2. For Arcene dataset, i.e. a large dimensional dataset the classification accuracy of Proposed algorithm has been decreased by 3, 1 margin by FCBF and FAST respectively.
3. For WarpAR10p datasets one of a large dimensional datasets the classification accuracy of Proposed algorithm has been increased by 8.46 and 10.82 value for FCBF and FAST respectively.
4. For WarpPie10p dataset Proposed algorithm is performing almost in a similar way as FCBF and FAST.
5. For microarray data, Proposed algorithm has increased the classification accuracy for Tox-171 and Colon_l dataset by 5.4 percent and 1.4 percent by FAST algorithm.

In order to further explore, which feature selection algorithm is performing better, a unified, multi-criteria metric EARR (Wang et al. 2013) has been used. We have taken number of features selected, runtime and Naïve Bayes classification accuracies values from Tables 4, 5, 6 respectively. Using Eq. 5, we calculate the EARR values of Proposed algorithm with FCBF and FAST on all datasets. Table 9 depicts the different EARR values found between two different algorithms.

According to Wang et al., the value of EARR A_i, A_j is greater than (or equal to, or smaller than) that of EARR A_i, A_j indicates that A_i is better than (or equal to, or worse than) A_j.

The Proposed algorithm when compared with FCBF on Image dataset, the EARR (Proposed, FCBF) value is 1.15 which is greater than EARR (FCBF, Proposed) in value of 0.868 at $\alpha = \beta = 0.001$. When comparing Proposed algorithm with FAST on image data set gives a value of EARR (Proposed, FAST) as 1.16 and EARR (FAST, Proposed) as 0.85. Here also we can say that Proposed is better than FAST.

The EARR value of text dataset at $\alpha = \beta = 0.001$, when compared with FCBF is EARR (Proposed, FCBF) is 0.905 and EARR (FCBF, Proposed) is1.115. Comparing Proposed algorithm with FAST algorithm gives a value of EARR (Proposed, FAST) as 0.965 and EARR (FAST, Proposed) as 1.035.Here we found that FCBF and FAST are better than Proposed.

For Microarray dataset, EARR value (Proposed, FCBF) is a 1.411 and EARR value (FCBF, Proposed) is 0.708. This implies that Proposed algorithm is better than FCBF. In case of FAST algorithm, EARR (Proposed, FAST) is 0.931 and EARR (FAST, Proposed) is 1.072 indicates FAST is better than Proposed.

So, from Table 9 it can be observed that the value of EARR Proposed algorithm is better in case of an image dataset when compared with both FCBF and FAST. The Proposed algorithm is also better than FCBF in case of microarray data. However, for text datasets FCBF and FAST are better than the Proposed algorithm.

Table 9. EARR values calculated to compare two algorithms

	Image			Text			Microarray		
	Proposed	FCBF	FAST	Proposed	FCBF	FAST	Proposed	FCBF	FAST
Proposed		0.8688	0.85		1.115	1.035		0.708	1.072
FCBF	1.15		0.990	0.9051		0.936	1.4116		1.512
FAST	1.16	1.0133		0.965	1.129		0.9319	0.660	

6 Conclusion

In this paper, a new feature selection technique which can work well on high dimensional data has been introduced. To reach this goal a correlation based filter approach using gain ratio is implemented to find the optimal and complete feature subset. The Proposed algorithm can eliminate both irrelevant and redundant features. By extensive experiments and calculations, we have shown that it works well for large dimensions (thousands of features) data set for classification.

The performance of the Proposed algorithm has been compared with two of the existing feature selection algorithms FCBF and FAST on the different data sets. Datasets belong to three domain, text, image and microarray data. We found that the proposed method ranks 1 for image data set and microarray dataset in case of three classifiers naïve Bayes, C4.5 and IB1. Comparing the Proposed algorithm on a unified metric, also led us to decide that the Proposed algorithm is better for the image dataset than FCBF and FAST. FCBF and FAST are good alternatives for text dataset and micro array data sets.

Our further work will be to extend this method for much higher dimensionality (more than ten thousand features). We will try to explore the different methodology which can improve text data.

References

1. Kohavi, R., John, G.H.: Wrapper for feature subset selection. Artif. Intell. **97**, 273–324 (1997)
2. Das, S.: Filter, wrapper and a boosting-based hybrid for feature selection. In: Proceedings of Eighteenth International Conference on Machine Learning, pp. 74–81 (2001)
3. Dash, M., Liu, H., Motoda, H.: Consistency based feature selection. In: Terano, T., Liu, H., Chen, A.L.P. (eds.) PAKDD 2000. LNCS, vol. 1805, pp. 98–109. Springer, Heidelberg (2000)
4. Yu, L., Liu, H.: Feature selection for high-dimensional data: a fast correlation-based filter solution. In: Proceedings of the Twentieth International Conference on Machine Learning (ICML-2003), Washington DC (2003)
5. Huang, J., Cai, Y., Xu, X.: A filter approach to feature selection based on mutual information. In: 5th IEEE international Conference (2006)
6. Andreas, G.K. Janecek, A., Gansterer, W.N., Demel, M.A., Ecker, G.F.: On the relationship between feature selection and classification accuracy. In: JMLR: Workshop and Conference Proceedings, vol. 4, pp. 90–105 (2008)
7. Song, Q., Ni, J., Wang, G.: A fast clustering based feature subset selection algorithm for high dimensional data. IEEE Trans. Knowl. Data Eng. **25**(1), 1–14 (2013)
8. Hall M.A.: Correlation-based feature selection for discrete and numeric class machine learning. In: Proceedings of 17th International Conference on Machine Learning, pp. 359–366 (2000)
9. Hall, M.A.: Correlation based feature selection for machine learning. Thesis, Department of Computer Science, University of Waikato, Hamilton, New Zealand (1999)
10. Liu, H., Yu, L.: Toward integrating feature selection algorithms for classification and clustering. IEEE Trans. Knowl. Data Eng. **17**(4), 491–502 (2005)

11. Kira, K., Rendell, L.A.: The feature selection problem: traditional methods and a new algorithm. In: Proceedings of 10th National Conference Artificial Intelligence, pp. 129–134 (1992)
12. Kononenko, I.: Estimating attributes: analysis and extensions of RELIEF. In: Proceedings of European Conference Machine Learning, pp. 171–182 (1994)
13. Almuallim H., Dietterich T.G.,: Algorithms for Identifying Relevant Features, Proc. Ninth Canadian Conf. Artificial Intelligence, pp. 38–45 (1992)
14. Cover, T.M., Thomas, J.A.: Elements of Information Theory. Wiley, New York (1991)
15. Wang, G., Song, Q., Sun, H., Zhang, X., Xu, B., Zhou, Y.: A feature subset selection algorithm automatic recommendation method. J. Artif. Intell. Res. **47**, 1–34 (2013)
16. Gray, R.M.: Entropy and Information Theory. Springer, New York (1991)
17. Mitra, P., Murthy, C.A., Pal, S.K.: Unsupervised feature selection using feature similarity. IEEE Trans. Pattern Anal. Mach. Intell. **24**, 301–302 (2002)
18. Blake, C., Merz: UCI repository of machine learning databases. http://www.ics.uci.edu
19. Witten, I.H., Frank, E., Hall, M.A., Mining, D.: Practical Machine Learning Tools and Techniques, 3rd edn. Morgan Kaufmann, Burlington (2011)
20. Powell, W.B.: Approximate Dynamic Programming: Solving the Curses of Dimensionality, 1st edn. Wiley-Interscience, New York (2007)
21. Zhao, Z., Morstatter, F., Sharma, S., Alelyani, S., Anand, A., Liu, H.: Advancing feature selection research. Technical report, Arizona State University (2011)
22. Laiho, P., Kokko, A., Vanharanta, S., Salovaara, R., Sammalkorpi, H., Jarvinen, H., Mecklin, J.P., Karttunen, T.J., Tuppurainen, K., Davalos, V., Schwartz, S., Arango, D., Makinen, M.J., Aaltonen, L.A.: Serrated carcinomas form a subclass of colorectal cancer with distinct molecular basis. Oncogene **26**(2), 312–320 (2007)
23. Ramaswamy, S., Tamayo, P., Rifkin, R., Mukherjee, S., Yeang, C.H., Angelo, M., Ladd, C., Reich, M., Latulippe, E., Mesirov, J.P., Gerald, W., Loda, M., Lander, E.S., Golub, T.R.: Multiclass cancer diagnosis using tumor gene expression signatures. Proc. Nat. Acad Sci. USA **98**(26), 15149–15154 (2001)
24. Golub, T.R., Slonim, D.R., Tamayo, P., Huard, C., Gaasenbeek, M., Mesirov, J.P., Coller, H., Loh, M.L., Downing, J.R., Caligiuri, M.A., Bloomfield, C.D., Lander, E.S.: Molecular classification of cancer: class discovery and class prediction by gene expression monitoring. Science **286**, 531–537 (1999)

Big Data in Medicine

Genomics 3.0: Big-Data in Precision Medicine

Asoke K. Talukder$^{(\boxtimes)}$

InterpretOmics India Pvt. Ltd., Bangalore, India
asoke.talukder@interpretomics.co
http://interpretomics.co/

Abstract. The Human genome project transformed biology and pharmacology into a computational, mathematical, and big-data science. In this paper we dissect the science and technology of big-data translational genomics and precision medicine - we present various components of this complex *Genomics 3.0* science. We also identify diverse idiosyncrasies of big-data with respect to application of computer algorithms and mathematics in genomics. We discuss the 7Vs of big-data in biology; we discuss genomic data and its relevance with respect to formal database systems. Genomics big-data analysis is a combination of *top-down, bottom-up, and middle-out* approaches with all the constituent parts integrated into a single system through complex meta-analysis. Finally, we present two big-data platforms *iOMICS* and *DiscoverX*. iOMICS platform is deployed at Google cloud for translational genomics; whereas, DiscoverX is deployed at Amazon Web Services for precision medicine.

Keywords: Genomics 3.0 · Big-data genomics · Precision medicine · Top-down bottom-up and middle-out · Patient stratification · iOMICS · DiscoverX · 7Vs of big-data · Systems biology · Exploratory data analysis

1 Introduction

The approach in biology has been mostly empirical, that relied on intuitions from observations and experiments. Empirical evidence is also at the foundation of *evidence-based medicine* (EBM) or *evidence-based practice* (EBP). EBP is defined as integrating individual clinical expertise with the best available external clinical evidence from systematic research [1]. For centuries, clinicians examined the external appearance (*phenotype*) of a disease to build these intuitions and followed them to treat a symptom. However, experimental facts remain blind without a mechanistic approach that defines the laws or principles behind these observations [2]. In 21st Century however, following the sequencing of Human genome [3] and the integration of *electronic health records*, EBP will be termed as *big-data* driven *precision medicine*. We are now moving towards a model of a cell [4] and even a complete human [5] in a computer; and then towards designing the line of treatment customized for an individual that will be effective without any side-effect.

© Springer International Publishing Switzerland 2015
N. Kumar and V. Bhatnagar (Eds.): BDA 2015, LNCS 9498, pp. 201–215, 2015.
DOI: 10.1007/978-3-319-27057-9_14

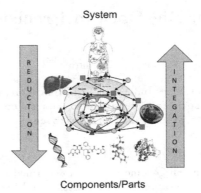

Fig. 1. Reduction versus Integration

We have been looking at a disease only from its phenotypic variations that can also be termed as its *morphological manifestation*, occasionally combined with pathological data like blood, X-Ray etcetera. To understand the disease biology, biologists, researchers, and clinicians always used the reduction methods where a disease or a biology problem is broken into manageable constituent parts (Fig. 1); and, then studied. In the process of reduction, the system view is lost and it is difficult to understand the holistic cause of the disease and impact of a drug at a system level. Adding to this, if there were multiple drugs in use, the drug-drug interactions in the patient's body were completely unknown. These resulted in side-effects and toxicity of the drugs. To ensure right therapeutics, the entire system needs to be understood through the process of integrative systems biology - from the parts to the whole (Fig. 1).

According to the National Institute of Health (NIH), USA, precision medicine is an approach for disease management (treatment and prevention) that takes into account individual variability in genes, environment, and lifestyle for each patient. The schematic of precision medicine that will need diverse data is shown in Fig. 2. This will combine patient's *genotype*, patient's *phenotype*, the environmental data, along with the background *population* data. While advances in precision medicine have been made for some cancer treatments, the practice is not currently common for most other diseases. To accelerate the pace, President Obama unveiled the precision medicine initiative (PMI) - the use of precision medicine in every day clinical practice [6].

It is known that the same drug works differently in different bodies. Therefore, as part of precision medicine, the patient is required to be *stratified* based on his genetic makeup and the *mechanism of action* (MoA) of the drug. Looking at the individual's genetic structure, the right drug with right dose will be administered so that the drug works with highest efficacy and without any side-effects. Precision medicine of the future will be a refinement of evidence based medicine, amalgamated with *Genomics 3.0*, so that the outcome of a treatment will be measurable. It will be empirical and mechanistic, with an understanding of various macromolecules that are part of the biological system and their

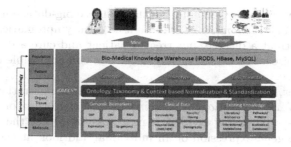

Fig. 2. Data driven 21st century quantitative medicine

interactions. A biological system is multi-scale, from a molecule (micrometer) to a population (kilometer). The quantification of these parts, their functions, and their interactions will build the theoretical basis with the help of genomics, mathematical sciences, computational sciences, and network sciences.

This article is about Genomics 3.0 – the process to integrate big-data in the journey towards the goal of precision medicine and next generation genomic research. We present the 7Vs of biological big-data; we also present the relevance of formal-databases in genomics. We discuss the data-sciences driven top-down, graph-theory driven bottom-up, and middle-out approaches of systems biology to create the mechanistic model. We also discuss a critical piece of *big-data genomics - patient stratification* where we stratify the patients based on their characteristics. Finally, in this paper we take two case studies of *cloud computing* based *multi-scale multi-omics big-data* platforms viz., *iOMICS* for translational research and *DiscoverX* for precision medicine deployed at Google Cloud and Amazon Web Services respectively.

2   Genomics 3.0

Genetics is derived from the word gene whereas genomics is derived from the word genome (DNA). A gene is only a small part of the genome. Therefore, genetics can be interpreted as a study of a gene or a part of the genome; whereas, genomics is the study of the whole genome or the DNA (all chromosomes). Genetic data analysis is mostly *hypothesis driven*; whereas, genomic data analysis is always exploratory and *hypothesis creating*.

NGS data introduced a component of data-driven mechanistic science into evidence-based medicine - bringing in computer scientists and mathematicians to help a clinician. *Genomics 1.0*, started with the Human genome project, was the genomics used by academics and researchers to understand the disease dynamics and the genotype phenotypic association of a living system. Genomics then graduated to *Genomics 2.0* when it entered the clinic and pharmaceutical companies through *translational genomics*. *Genomics 2.0* is used today as a tool for diagnosis of non-communicable and genetic diseases. Clinicians use *Genomics 2.0* to not just treat symptoms; but, to treat the disease. Holistic precision medicine will be driven by Genomics 3.0 that will use big-data genomic analytics of the 21st Century. *Genomics 3.0* will be used for asymptomatic disease onset. It will not just treat a disease, but treat a patient and cure a disease – be it a cardiovascular disease or cancer or any other non-communicable environmental or genetic disease.

In November, 2013, the US Food and Drug Administration (FDA) had approved the *Next Generation Sequencing* (NGS) platforms for in vitro diagnostic (IVD) uses [7]. Using NGS it is now possible to get the whole-genome or genome-wide gene expression of an individual and look at the patient from inside - from the molecular perspective or the genetic structure of an individual. Targeted NGS data of 100 genes with an average gene-size of 10,000 nucleotides and 300x depth of sequencing will generate 1 Giga Byte (GB) of data. An exome (only the protein coding region of DNA) with 300x will generate 80 GB data; and the DNA of a human will generate 3.2 Tera Bytes (TB) of data. This is a giant leap towards *Genomics 3.0.*

3 Dimensions of Big-data

Gartner defined big-data in 2001 through the three dimensional space of 3Vs. These three Vs are *Volume, Velocity, and Variety.* Volume is defined in terms of the physical volume of the data that need to be online, like giga-byte (10^9), tera-byte (10^{12}), peta-byte (10^{15}) or exa-byte (10^{18}) or even beyond. For example, dbNSFP is a database developed for functional prediction and annotation of all potential non-synonymous single-nucleotide variants (nsSNVs) in the human genome [8]; the size of the latest version (v 2.5) dbNSFP is 52 GB. Velocity is about the data-retrieval time or the time taken to service a request. Velocity is also measured through the rate of change of the data volume. Variety relates to heterogeneous types of data like text, structured, unstructured, video, audio etcetera. Some authors added one more V for *Veracity* - it is another dimension to measure data reliability - the ability of an organization to trust the data and be able to confidently use it to make crucial decisions.

Unlike business or www big-data, life-sciences big-data has three additional dimensions or three additional Vs. These dimensions are *Vexing, Variability,* and *Value.* Vexing covers the effectiveness of the algorithm. The algorithm needs to be designed to ensure that data processing time is close to linear and the algorithm does not have any bias; irrespective of the volume of the data, the algorithm is able to process the data in reasonable time. The other dimension is Variability. Variability is the scale of data. Data in biology is multi-scale, ranging from sub-atomic ions at picometers, macro-molecules, cells, tissues and finally to a population [9] at thousands of kilometers. Finally the last dimension is Value - the final actionable insight or the functional knowledge. The same mutation in a gene may have a different effect depending on the population or the environmental factors. Many of these considerations will have direct implications on life or the environment. Removal of confounding factors with the discovery of independent variables and the causal attributes is the key in value; this value will finally be consumed as the knowledge or actionable insight.

4   Genomic Big-data

Genomic data can be grouped into two major categories:

1. Patient data or data generated from one subject (n = 1)
2. Background databases (or cohort data) from a population (n = N).

4.1   Patient Data

This is the high-throughput data generated from the patients bio-specimen. This data can be in giga-bytes. This data will be used for precision medicine or translational research. For a large cohort, it can even be in tera-bytes or peta-bytes. The expression data that is generated by microarray experiments are generally smaller is size compared to the NGS data.

4.2   Background Databases

There are many background data required to arrive at some meaningful biological insights. These start from reference genomes to many interactome data. All these files are regularly updated and available for download or online access. The latest human reference genome as of June 2015 is GRCh38.p3 (Genome Reference Consortium human version 38 patch level 3); it has a data volume of 3.2 GB. When you generate human DNA data - be it whole-genome, exome, or a targeted sequence, the data will be aligned with this version of the human genome. Other frequently used databases are GWASdb2 (Genome Wide Association Study database), dbSNP (Single Nucleotide Polymorphism database), ClinVar (Genomic variation database related to phenotypic/clinical importance), wwPDB (World Wide Protein Database), additional databases from *NCBI* (National Center for Biotechnology Information), databases from *EMBL* (European Bioinformatics Institute) etcetera.

There are two types of databases available in the biomedical domain. These are downloadable databases and online databases. Most of the downloadable biomedical databases are TAB delimited. However, there are many other databases that have complex structures. Some of these databases are stored as formal databases and some are even complex graph databases. Some of these databases cannot be downloaded, but can be accessed online. Many of these databases even include a functional layer on top of the database. This functional part does some functions and returns the final data. These are generally accessed through *web APIs* (Application Programming Interface).

Along with the genome, there is other information like genes, exons, introns, intergenic regions, known disease causing variations etc. Also, there are many other databases that include gene functions, drugs, diseases and associations between them. For details you can refer to the list of biological databases in Wikipedia [10]. Also, an important resource for finding biological databases is a special yearly issue of the journal Nucleic Acids Research (NAR). The 2015 Nucleic Acids Research Database Issue and molecular biology database collection are available at [11].

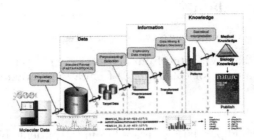

Fig. 3. Steps in exploratory data analysis in genomics

5   Exploratory Data Analysis

Biological information needs to be mined from big genomic data. This is achieved by using *exploratory data analysis* (EDA). EDA was introduced by John Tukey. Most of the data used in industry segments from telecom to financial, have a structure - because they are defined by people like us. Also, the pattern of such data are always known. For example we know how to compute the interest of 1000 Rupees at the end of the year with 3 % interest. However, the data of a living organism are created by nature and our understanding of them is never complete; therefore, the processing must be exploratory. In EDA however we do not rely upon any assumptions about the data and what kind of model the data follows, with the more direct approach of allowing the data itself to reveal its underlying structure and model [12]. EDA is an approach/philosophy to,

1. maximize insight into a data set
2. uncover underlying structure
3. extract important variables
4. detect outliers and anomalies
5. test underlying assumptions
6. develop parsimonious models
7. determine optimal factor settings

EDA is not a collection of techniques; it is instead a philosophy as to how we dissect a dataset. The exploratory analysis can be either *parametric* or *non-parametric*. The schematic of exploratory data analysis is shown in Fig. 3. EDA is also known as data mining where you mine the data to discover a consistent pattern. EDA or data mining is used to discover unknown knowledge from the data.

6   Big-data to Information

This is the first step to discover a pattern from the biological data. The bio-specimen will be used to generate *high-throughput data* from blood, tissue (biopsy), bacteria, or some other bio-specimens. Macromolecules like *DNA, miRNA, mRNA, proteins, metabolites* etc. are extracted from the bio-specimen through complex chemistry experiments. Experiments such as NGS, microarray, mass spectrometry provides genome sequence (exome, target and whole genome data), gene expression, protein expression and metabolite data. These data volumes range from hundreds of mega-bytes (MB) to TB (Tera Bytes).

The data to information part of *big-data genomics* is a *top-down* technique where we use statistical techniques. Following many experiments, and processing tera-bytes of genomic data, we now know what statistical distribution and model will fit in this step for a particular type of data. This makes this part of the analysis *parametric*, though there could be cases for *nonparametric* as well. Majority of the Open Source software written by academicians and research labs fall in this category.

This *top-down exploratory data analysis* undergoes different stages of processing as shown in Fig. 3. This involves *preprocessing, exploratory analysis* to find some patterns statistically. In this step, we evaluate whether the concluded pattern may occur by chance (probability within the confidence interval) or due to the specific nature of the case. We compute the *Type-I* (false positive) and *Type-II* (false negative) errors statistically and finally accept the solution that has minimum Type-I and Type-II errors. Type-I error is quantitatively expressed through p-value; whereas, Type-II error is represented through q-value or FDR (False Discovery Rate).

Finally we generate an n by p matrix of n genes and p patients. In this matrix a column is a vector of about 20,000 values (for 20,000 genes) for some individuals. In genetics, n >> p, where the number of observations p is much smaller than the number of independent variables n.

7 Information to Knowledge

In this phase we do bottom-up analysis or what is commonly known as functional analysis. This step is completely exploratory and most often non-parametric. This phase is also known as functional genomics. In this phase we use the knowledge of various macromolecules produced by *genomic, transcriptomic, metabolomic, phenomic* etc. experiments and already available in background *big-data databases*. We normally use the association fallacy (guilt by association) to arrive at a function of an object from other known objects.

This phase of analysis relates to network sciences with various interaction networks. Some of the common interaction networks are, gene-gene interaction network *BioGrid* [13], protein-protein interaction network *IntAct* [14], DNA-protein interaction network *TransFac* [15] and metabolic networks *ReconX* [16]. Also, there are other comprehensive databases like *GO* [17], *KEGG* [18], *PANTHER* [19], *DAVID* [20] etc. that contains multiple interaction networks and pathways.

8 Integrative Systems Biology

Biological systems are highly complex networks of *interlinked macromolecules*. In this step we try to understand the whole - at the system level (Fig. 1). *Systems biology* is sometime referred to as the middle-out paradigm, where many knowledge-bodies are combined to obtain a holistic system-level view. This requires meta-analysis of multi-scale multi-omics data from different sources. For example we may like to study the impact of mutations on proteins in cancer at a population level. In this case, we will need the DNA data to analyze and discover the mutations. We also require the gene expression data for the same set of patients to quantify protein production for genes which have these mutations. We then combine the mutation data with expression analysis results to arrive at a conclusion about the impact of the mutations on gene expression. The *meta-analysis* of the data will depend on the level of structural and functional complexity of the data. It may be noted that these analysis are self-similar, no particular scale has privileged relevance for systems biology. Starting from a cell to the whole body, similar algorithms will be applicable, because they are systems at different levels and scales. Systems biology will be used to model an organ, a cell or even a part of a cell.

Most of these studies will be in the form of clinical research, where a patient population is observed for an extended period of time for their clinical and phenotypic characteristics. Such studies can be either retrospective or prospective. For example, for a *retrospective cancer* study you will look at the patient data at a hospital and then select a population best suited for the study. Then, take the respective patients' tumors from the tumor bank to generate data. If some patients died you know their survival and drug usage patterns. Advantage of such studies are that the study period is less and a very focused population can be selected. Also, in such studies the end results are known. In *prospective studies* however, the study starts with the recruitment of patients and continues for long time in the future. All clinical trial studies are prospective in nature.

At the systems biology stage, the association between genotype and phenotype is established. *Genotype* is the cause (or perturbation) and *phenotype* is the external manifestation of this genotype. For any type of management, it is absolutely necessary to have a cause-effect equation established. Once the cause-effect is understood, we can tune various health and therapeutics parameters for the best possible precision medicine.

9 Patient Stratification

In *precision medicine*, patient stratification is a critical step. Patient stratification is also critical in *clinical trials*. In patient stratification, you stratify the patient (or the patient subpopulation) based on clinical, phenotype, or the genotype traits. In a *familial study*, stratification is necessary based on ethnicity or sex. *Stratification* will be done with genomic data and clinical data like progression free survivability. Clinical data will include *re-hospitalization* as well. This will be based on certain types of biomarkers. Patients will be stratified based on high or low expression of genes compared to healthy. Also, stratification can play an important role in identifying responders and non-responders to medications, avoiding adverse events, and optimizing drug dose.

There is a table provided by *FDA* at the FDA web site http://www.fda.gov/drugs/scienceresearch/researchareas/pharmacogenetics/ucm083378.htm   that lists *FDA-approved* drugs with pharmacogenomic information and their labeling. This table includes specific actions to be taken based on the genomic information of the patient. These genetic markers are germline or somatic mutations, functional deficiencies, expression changes, and chromosomal abnormalities. Some selected protein biomarkers that are used to select patients for treatment are also included in this page.

For cancer, *NCI* (National Cancer Institute) has made the clinical data of 8,689,771 cancer patients available. These data have been collected from 1973 to 2012 and are very useful for prognosis calculations. These data are available at the *SEER* (Surveillance, Epidemiology, and End Results Program) site [21]. The NCI SEER dataset contains both categorical and numerical data. The broad category of patients' SEER data types include (i) *clinical* or *phenotypic* and (ii) *demographics* details. Clinical or phenotypic data contains information such as cancer type, subtype, diagnosis, treatment type, cancer stage (TNM staging), survival state and survival period in months etc. Demographics contains information such as age, sex, race and ethnicity etc. One of the main application of the NCI SEER dataset is patient stratification through cancer survivability analysis. Prognosis is the key attribute which helps to understand the likely outcome of cancer for a patient. The statistical models like Kaplan Meier and Cox-regression model are used for the prognosis calculation and individual patient stratification like high or low risk groups.

10   Characteristics and Life of Genomic Big-data

Genomic data have some unique characteristics - they are mostly categorical without a collating sequence. Unlike a person's name (text) or bank balance (real number), a set of gene names cannot be sorted meaningfully either alphabetically, numerically, or even functionally. Given two gene names it cannot be said which gene comes first. For example, *KRAS, TP53, BRCA1, BRCA2* are bi-modal and function as both oncogenes (causing tumor formation) and tumor suppressor (stopping tumor growth) genes. In some context these genes help in cancer progression; under certain conditions they stop cancer. This makes normalizing genomics data complex.

The top-down part of the data analytics that we talked about earlier, is generally *single-write single-read*. Once the information is obtained, the data loses its life. The data generated by NGS will be a file in *FASTQ* format with the nucleotides and quality information. After NGS FASTQ data are aligned with a *reference genome*, *SAM* (Sequence Alignment Map) or *BAM* (Binary Sequence Alignment Map) file [22] will be generated. Once the BAM file is generated, most of the software will use this BAM file, making the raw FASTQ file redundant.

This is unlike any other data (financial, telecom, or any other industry data) lifecycle - where data is read over and over again (single write multiple reads). When you read a data over and over again, it needs to be stored in such a fashion that it can be retrieved fast - this is why we normalize the data to bring in a structure and use a database. However, as the raw NGS data is never used again, it need not be stored in any database. Though, *Integrated Rule-Oriented data System* (iRODS) [23] is now being used to store such raw files in the cloud so that many people can use them without copying them to the local machine.

Once the raw BAM file is processed, it is necessary to perform downstream analysis and derive knowledge out of the data using EDA. This data will be required to be processed multiple times to minimize Type-I errors and select the most optimal result. Sometime the result set is too large, then we increase the precision or specificity and use a smaller set of data with a higher threshold and rerun the data. This phase of the analysis is therefore *single-write multiple-read*. An in-memory database like *HANA* [24] will improve the performance at this level.

It can be debated whether you need a *commercial database system* like *Oracle* or *Teradata* for genomic big-data either at a clinic level or for a research institute. A formal database is useful when there are multiple-read, multiple-write, deletion of existing data, or insertion of new data. Single-read data need not be online; however, data that need multiple-write and insert/deletes need a formal structure for better performance. Relational databases will be used for patient data in precision medicine; however, controlled-vocabulary or ontology based graph databases are most useful as background databases. We mentioned that genomic data are categorical; the sequence and meaning of an object in such an environment depends only on the context. This is where *graph database* plays a significant role. In such databases genes will be nodes with edges being the context, function, or relation. In a metabolic database, metabolites will be the nodes with reactions being edges. The graph may be undirected, directed, or even weighted. One of the most frequently used databases for *functional genomics* is GO (Gene Ontology), which is a graph database. There are other medical databases built around graphs.

Formal relational databases like MySQL are used in iOMICS (Fig. 4) to store genomic metadata that are accessed quite often. Also, they are used to generate reports and trace objects. All these metadata will need multiple-read, multiple-write, and multiple-inserts. In addition, the final result from most of the sub-systems of a genomic analysis will be a *biomarker*. This biomarker could be a gene, mutation, small molecule, metabolite, or even chromosome. Example of a mutation biomarker is the *BRCA1* mutation Rs80357713 believed to be causal for breast cancer. All these biomarkers will be multiple-write multiple-read. A formal database will also be necessary to store user information (like user name, credentials etc.) or information related to samples, specimens, patients or information that are necessary for *LIMS* (Laboratory Information Management System).

Medical records of a patient are multiple-write multiple-read. These comprise of patients' clinical, pathological, and genomic data. Such records are updated, inserted, deleted quite often. Therefore, they will need formal databases like Oracle or any other relational database. This type of data has a definite structure and is written, read, updated, inserted, and deleted multiple times. At the level of integration of an *EMR* (Electronic Medical Record) or *EHR* (Electronic Health Record), with the patient's genomic data, there will be a seamless integration between *Variability and Variety*.

11   Mark-up Languages to Represent Biological Data

Most of the Biological databases are TAB delimited text files. To allow fast access of such TAB delimited text files, *TABIX* API is developed [25] that can index a TAB delimited file and can access records in the text file through the index, as if it is stored in a database. Many interactome files are in TAB delimited adjacency list format. Many of them even use markup languages like *SBML* [26], *CellML* [27], *FieldML* [28] etc.

12   The Big-data Genomics Platform iOMICS

iOMICS is a big-data multi-scale multi-omics analytics platform [29] that includes all the empirical mechanistic top-down and bottom-up analytics systems as described above. The high level architecture of the iOMICS system is shown in Fig. 4. iOMICS is a cloud ready system that can be commissioned either as a private or a public cloud. The public cloud version of iOMICS is available at Google cloud (http://iomics-research.interpretomics.co/). A private cloud version of iOMICS is used by a research group like at the University of Copenhagen for animal health, breeding and productivity.

iOMICS is build around *RESTful* architecture. The iOMICS engine includes, Play framework for the UI (User Interface) development and rendering. An exploratory data analysis paradigm demands extensive data visualization.

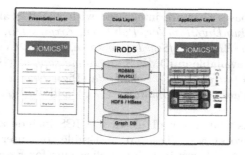

Fig. 4. iOMICS Architecture

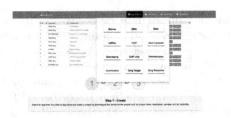

Fig. 5. The iOMICS App store

Keeping the complex visualization in mind, *D3* is used for dynamic graphics. Other technologies used are *HTML5, CSS, JQuery, and D3JS.*

iOMICS offers parallelization and *job scheduling.* Sun grid engine is used to manage the jobs initiated by the user to optimize compute resources. Polyglot programming (Python, R, C, C++, SQL, Perl, Shell etc.) is used to analyze and interpret big-data and to derive biological insights. Cytoscape and JQuery plugins are used for on-the-fly filtering and interactive graph representations and reporting. Standard Google cloud storage is used to store user specific input data and results. Google compute persistent storage is used for intermediate and faster read/write operations. iOMICS supports widely used reference genomes with flexibility to add more reference genomes.

As part of *PaaS* (Platform as a Service), *MPI* is used for parallel processing. *Hadoop HBase* is used in iOMICS for storing the user input data and the results. In the database layer, iOMICS includes iRODS, and MySQL. *IRODS* is used for single-write genomic data storage; whereas MySQL is used for multiple-write multiple-read metadata management. MySQL is also at the core for the management of user, security, and accounting.

iOMICS applications will be run on *on-demand pre-built compute* instances based on data set and user choice. Below are widely used instance types

- N1-Standard-4 - 4 cpu 15 GB ram
- N1-Standard-8 - 8 cpu 30 GB ram
- N1-Standard-16 - 16 cpu 60 GB ram
- N1-Standard-32 - 32 cpu 120 GB ram

Biological databases that are integrated with iOMICS are *1000 Genomes, dbSNP, dbNSFP, HumDiv/HumVar, PolyPhen, coxpressDB, ClinVar, Uniprot, Ensemble, GO.db, miRBase, RefSeq, Interactome, OMIM, COSMIC and SnpEff.* Reference genomes available in iOMICS are *Homo sapiens* (Human), *Mus musculas* (Mouse), *Bos taurus* (Cow), *Sus scrofa* (Pig), *Ovis aries* (Sheep), *Equus caballus* (Horse), *Canis lupus familiaris* (Dog) and *Arabidopsis* (Arabidopsis thaliana).

The applications that are available in iOMICS include all types of biological data analysis workflows. These are accessible to a user through the App Store (Fig. 5). The App Store includes applications for Exome analysis; DNA and de novo and reference assembly; RNA NGS, microarray gene expression

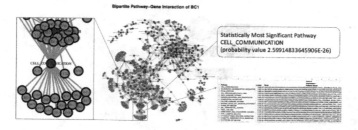

Fig. 6. The interaction between genes and pathways (bipartite graph) for a breast cancer patient (ERR166303) with the implicated pathway and its genesets

analysis with ab-initio gene modeling; discovery of known and novel genes, target identification of micro-RNAs; conservational study with phylogenetically related species; Chromatin immunoprecipitation analysis for histone modification, transcription factor, RNA-DNA hybrid and DNA replication analysis; gene expression, comparative genomics, co-expression and case/control study; DNA methylation analysis, patient stratification, drug target discovery, drug response analysis, quantitative trait loci analysis (QTL); population genetics; Chem-Seq analysis. Some of these applications refer to online databases through Web API; databases that are integrated are KEGG, GO, NCBI etc.

13 Live Genome Research Case

A use-case of big-data analytics platform *iOMICS* is already reported [30]. This use-case is about the reanalysis of a *breast cancer cohort* dataset comprising of 11 non-BRCA1/BRCA2 familial breast cancer patients that was originally published in 2013 [31]. The same data was rerun using exome workflow of iOMICS followed by extensive graph theoretic analysis of the data. The big-data paradigm described in this article was able to unleash critical actionable information that the original research work failed to discover [31]. The results are available at the iOMICS site at http://www.iomics.in/research/XomAnnotate. Figure 6 shows a bipartite graph of a cancer patient from this dataset with id ERR166303. Figure 6 shows the *Pathway-gene bipartite graph* with red nodes representing pathways and green nodes representing the genes. For this patient, the CELL_COMMUNICATION pathway was identified as the most significant with a *p-value* of $2.6e^{-26}$. The table (spreadsheet) with other pathways and their crossover points are also shown in Fig. 6.

14 Live Genomics and Precision Medicine Case

We present here another big-data application, DiscoverX, (Fig. 7) developed by InterpretOmics for precision medicine and used for clinical genetic tests in India for cancer, metabolic, pediatric, neurological, and other known hereditary diseases. *DiscoverX* is a comprehensive clinical genetics software for identification

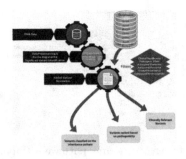

Fig. 7. The DiscoverX flowchart

and annotation of variants from DNA data. It consumes deep sequencing data, to identify causal germline and somatic mutations from whole genome, whole exome or targeted DNA sequences. This ambidextrous system identifies *high precision clinically relevant variants* with *high sensitivity/high specificity* and annotates them simultaneously identifying known as well as novel genetic mutations. The software annotates the variants from major databases like ClinVar, dbSNP, dbNSFP, COSMIC, SnpEff etc. Filtering modules such as autosomal dominant, autosomal recessive, compound heterozygote, X-linked etc. make disease associated variant prioritization accurate and easy. Sensitivity and specificity of variant detection coupled with HL7 compliant reporting assists in informed decision making which helps in management of disease and treatment.

The precision medicine system *DiscoverX* developed by *InterpretOmics* that runs on Amazon cloud with 32 core 64 GB RAM with 6 patient samples in parallel takes about 3 hours. The patient samples are around 1 GB for 300x depth with 96 GB of background databases. The patient samples are targeted sequences for 318 neurological, 91 pediatric, 55 oncology and 123 metabolic disorders (inclusive of subtypes). DiscoverX has been exclusively developed for Applied Genetics Diagnostics India Pvt. Ltd. (www.appgendx.com), a wholly owned subsidiary of Singapore Life Sciences Pvt. Ltd.

References

1. Sackett, D.L., Rosenberg, W.M., Gray, J., Haynes, R.B., Richardson, W.S.: Evidence based medicine: what it is and what it isn't. Br. Med. J. (BMJ) **312**(7023), 71 (1996)
2. Di Ventura, B., Lemerle, C., Michalodimitrakis, K., Serrano, L.: From in vivo to in silico biology and back. Nature **443**(7111), 527–533 (2006)
3. Venter, J.C., Adams, M.D., Myers, E.W., Li, P.W., Mural, R.J., Sutton, G.G., Smith, H.O., Yandell, M., Evans, C.A., Holt, R.A., et al.: The sequence of the human genome. Science **291**(5507), 1304–1351 (2001)
4. Karr, J.R., Sanghvi, J.C., Macklin, D.N., Gutschow, M.V., Jacobs, J.M., Bolival, B., Assad-Garcia, N., Glass, J.I., Covert, M.W.: A whole-cell computational model predicts phenotype from genotype. Cell **150**(2), 389–401 (2012)

5. Kohl, P., Noble, D.: Systems biology and the virtual physiological human. Mol. Syst. Biol. **5**(1), 292 (2009)
6. Precision medicine initiatives. http://www.nih.gov/precisionmedicine/
7. Collins, F.S., Hamburg, M.A.: First FDA authorization for next-generation sequencer. N. Engl. J. Med. **369**(25), 2369–2371 (2013)
8. Liu, X., Jian, X., Boerwinkle, E.: dbNSFP v2.0: a database of human non-synonymous SNVs and their functional predictions and annotations. Hum. Mutat. **34**(9), E2393–E2402 (2013)
9. Steinhauser, M.O.: Computational Multiscale Modeling of Fluids and Solids. Springer, New York (2008)
10. List of biological databases. https://en.wikipedia.org/wiki/List_of_biological_databases
11. Galperin, M.Y., Rigden, D.J., Fernández-Suárez, X.M.: The 2015 nucleic acids research database issue and molecular biology database collection. Nucleic Acids Res. **43**(D1), D1–D5 (2015)
12. Engineering statistics handbook: Exploratory data analysis. http://www.itl.nist.gov/div898/handbook/eda/eda.htm
13. Biogrid. http://thebiogrid.org/
14. Intact molecular interaction database. https://www.ebi.ac.uk/intact/
15. Transfac. http://www.gene-regulation.com/pub/databases.html
16. Reconx. http://humanmetabolism.org/
17. Geneontology. http://geneontology.org/
18. Kyoto encyclopedia of genes and genomes. http://www.genome.jp/kegg/
19. Panther. http://www.pantherdb.org/pathway/
20. David. http://david.abcc.ncifcrf.gov/
21. Surveillance, epidemiology, and end results program. http://seer.cancer.gov/data/
22. The sam/bam format specification working group, sequence alignment/map format specification (2015). https://samtools.github.io/hts-specs/SAMv1.pdf
23. Integrated rule-oriented data system irods. http://irods.org/
24. Hana. http://hana.sap.com/
25. Li, H.: Tabix: fast retrieval of sequence features from generic tab-delimited files. Bioinformatics **27**(5), 718–719 (2011)
26. Sbml. http://sbml.org/Basic_Introduction_to_SBML
27. Cellml. https://www.cellml.org/about
28. Fieldml. http://physiomeproject.org/software/fieldml/about
29. iomics. http://iomics.in
30. Talukder, A.K., Ravishankar, S., Sasmal, K., Gandham, S., Prabhukumar, J., Achutharao, P.H., Barh, D., Blasi, F.: Xomannotate: analysis of heterogeneous and complex exome-a step towards translational medicine. PLoS ONE **10**, e0123569 (2015)
31. Gracia-Aznarez, F.J., Fernandez, V., Pita, G., Peterlongo, P., Dominguez, O., de la Hoya, M., Duran, M., Osorio, A., Moreno, L., Gonzalez-Neira, A., et al.: Whole exome sequencing suggests much of non-BRCA1/BRCA2 familial breast cancer is due to moderate and low penetrance susceptibility alleles. PloS one **8**(2), e55681 (2013)

CuraEx - Clinical Expert System Using Big-Data for Precision Medicine

Mohamood Adhil, Santhosh Gandham, Asoke K. Talukder (✉),
Mahima Agarwal, and Prahalad Achutharao

InterpretOmics India Pvt. Ltd., Bangalore, India
{mohamood.adhil,santhosh.gandham,asoke.talukder,
mahima.agarwal,prahalad}@interpretomics.co
http://interpretomics.co/

Abstract. Cancer is a complex non-communicable disease with many types and subtypes, where the same treatment does not work for all cancers. Moreover cancer drugs have tremendous side effects. Deciding a suitable line of treatment for cancer, demands complex analytics of diverse distributed numeric and categorical data. Suitable therapy depends on factors like tumor size, lymph node infection, metastasis, genetic patterns of the tumor and patient's clinical history. We present CuraEx, a Clinical Expert System (CES) that uses clinical and genomic marker of the patient combined with a knowledge-base created from distributed, dissimilar, diverse big-data. This system computes cancer staging based on constraints defined by the American Joint Committee on Cancer (AJCC). It predicts prognosis using a cancer registry compiled between 1997 to 2012 in the US. Semi-structured data mining on disease association data is used to determine the most appropriate approved drug for the cancer type. Additionally, suitable clinical trial information will be retrieved based on the patient's geographicals location and phenotype. We then integrate the genomic marker and clinical data of the patient which paves the way for precision medicine. Molecular information or genomics biomarkers of the patient helps in treatment selection, increases the likelihood of therapeutic efficacy and minimize the drug toxicity. Our clinical expert system is availabe at http://www.curaex.org/ for public use.

Keywords: Clinical expert system (CES) · Computational models · Cancer staging · Prognosis · Cancer therapeutics · American joint committee on cancer (AJCC) · Precision medicine

1 Introduction

Cancer is a complex disease which is caused by environmental factors and inherited genetics. It has many types and subtypes. In cancer, most of the research and efforts are focused on improving patient's survival [1]. The cancer treatment lifecycle is divided into three stages; viz. (i) Diagnosis - cancer type, histological grade and stage of the disease are assessed. Also, whether the cancer is

© Springer International Publishing Switzerland 2015
N. Kumar and V. Bhatnagar (Eds.): BDA 2015, LNCS 9498, pp. 216–227, 2015.
DOI: 10.1007/978-3-319-27057-9_15

restricted to the primary (original) site or it has metastasised or spread to other parts of the body is determined, (ii) Prognosis - during this step the survivability and likely outcome of therapeutic intervention is assessed. This depends on the molecular, clinical, and pathological state of the patient. This also depends on the therapeutic burden, and (iii) Therapeutics - this step is concerned with the treatment of disease which includes medicine, doses, frequency, and cost of the treatment etc.

Cancer drugs are mostly pathway inhibitors and potentially can have serious side effects. Moreover, cancer drugs are very expensive. It is therefore imperative that proper diagnosis and correct assessment of the state is done. Staging is an important process in cancer diagnosis, as it helps the oncologist to find the amount of cancer cells present in the body and also where it is located. It is crucial step while planning treatment and also helpful to predict the prognosis or survival of the patient using previous history or incidence records. The prognosis helps to predict the treatment outcome. It helps to choose the best line of treatment with least side effects based on the patient's tumour profile done using molecular (gene expression or mutation) or clinical (stage, histological grade, age, weight, ethinicity and gender etc.) markers. Prognosis can also be used to obtain the optimum cost-effective outcome. Using these approaches, we can minimize the trade off between drug benefits, and cost and side effects of the treatment.

One of the ways to reduce the disease burden and improve the quality of treatment is by using a clinical expert system (CES). CES plays a major role in helping with the treatment decision and in turn increasing the therapeutic outcome [2]. There are many hurdles to be crossed before developing such a clinical expert system. They are, (i) mining the right data for the knowledge base where majority of the data are categorical, (ii) interpretation of the unstructured pathological information, (iii) interpretation of all possible clinical phenotypes, (iv) identifying features that explain the heterogeneity of patient's, (v) redundancy, and (vi) choosing the right mathematical and statistical models [3,4]. The inference through expert system will help to achieve improved outcome in terms of patient's survival and reduced cost due to precise treatments. Such an expert system should have an ideal knowledge base, analytical engine and communication portal. Based on the user input, the system uses the knowledge base to infer and communicate the output to the user in a short time. In this paper, we introduce a clinical expert system CuraEx, which we have developed that takes the patient specific information i.e., both clinical and genetic information and helps in diagnostics and patient stratification by providing cancer staging, prognosis and therapeutics.

The rest of the paper is organized as follows. Section 2 is an overview of CuraEx with architecture. Section 3 describes types of cancers available and the information needed to calculate staging of a cancer patient. Section 4 gives details about CuraEx and how it helps oncologist's in decision making. In Sect. 5, we talk about the knowledge bases used in CuraEx and Sect. 6 describes software stack used to develop CuraEx.

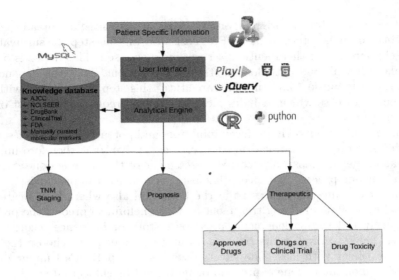

Fig. 1. Architecture of CuraEx

2   CuraEx Overview

CuraEx is derived from the Latin word "cura" which means "care" or "concern" [5]. The CuraEx system helps the physician or oncologist to compute the clinical/pathological stage of cancer as recommended by AJCC (American Joint Committee of Cancer) in their 7th Edition of the Cancer Staging Manual [6]. The staging classifies the extent of disease (EOD) in the cancer patient's. The staging can be performed at two levels (i) clinical and (ii) pathologic staging. In clinical staging the extent of the disease is determined before the treatment whereas in pathologic staging the extent of the disease is determined after the surgery. The system can be used to infer disease and the patient specific prognosis using the NCI SEER dataset as the background knowledge base [7]. The prognosis is used to identify the likely outcome of cancer for an individual, based on the survival of population having similar clinical and genetic features [8,9]. CuraEx is also used to identify suitable drugs (approved and on clinical trials) based on the clinical and genetic information of the patient. This clinical expert system requires user input such as T (Tumour), N (Node), M (Metastasis), demographic information and genetic markers of the patient. Using these informations, the system calculates the stage of cancer, prognosis (disease and patient specific) and suggests a suitable drug for the individual patient. The architecture of CuraEX is shown in the Fig. 1. Each category in the architecture is explained in detail with an example in the following section.

3   Patient Specific Information

Patient specific information such as cancer type, TNM information (T - size of the tumour, N - Number of lymph nodes involved and M - presence or absence

Patient Details

Patient id *		Treatment Type	Chemotherapy ▼
Age *		Date of Diagnosis	
Gender *	Male ▼	Drug Prescribed	Yes ▼
Race *	White ▼	Duration of Drug Prescribed (Months)	
Tumor Size (cm)		Name of Drug Prescribed	
Laterality	Right ▼	Histological grade	Grade1 ▼

* marked are mandatory

Select methods which you would like to perform: ☑ Staging ☑ Prognosis ☑ Therapeutics

Breast cancer Clinical Staging Form

Primary Tumor(T)

☐	TX	Primary tumor cannot be assessed
☐	T0	No evidence of primary tumor
☐	Tis	Carcinoma in situ
☐	Tis(DCIS)	Ductal carcinoma in situ
☐	Tis(LCIS)	Lobular carcinoma in situ
☐	Tis(Paget's)	Paget's disease of the nipple is NOT associated with invasive carcinoma and/or carcinoma in situ (DCIS and/or LCIS) in the underlying breast parenchyma. Carcinomas in the breast parenchyma associated with Paget's disease are categorized based on the size and characteristics of the parenchymal disease, although the presence of Paget's disease should still be noted
☐	T1	Tumor ≤ 20 mm in greatest dimension
☐	T1mi	Tumor ≤ 1 mm in greatest dimension
☐	T1a	Tumor > 1 mm but ≤ 5 mm in greatest dimension
☐	T1b	Tumor > 5 mm but ≤ 10 mm in greatest dimension
☐	T1c	Tumor >10 mm but ≤ 20 mm in greatest dimension
☑	T2	Tumor > 20 mm but ≤ 50 mm in greatest dimension
☐	T3	Tumor > 50 mm in greatest dimension
☐	T4	Tumor of any size with direct extension to the chest wall and/or to the skin (ulceration or skin nodules)*
☐	T4a	Extension to the chest wall, not including only pectoralis muscle adherence/invasion
☐	T4b	Ulceration and/or ipsilateral satellite nodules and/or edema (including peau d'orange) of the skin which do not meet the criteria for inflammatory carcinoma
☐	T4c	Both T4a and T4b
☐	T4d	Inflammatory carcinoma

Lymph nodes(N)

☐	NX	Regional lymph nodes cannot be assessed
☐	N0	No regional lymph node metastasis
☐	N1	Metastases to movable ipsilateral level I, II axillary lymph node(s)
☑	N2	Metastases in ipsilateral level I, II axillary lymph nodes that are clinically fixed or matted; or in clinically detected* ipsilateral internal mammary nodes in the absence of clinically evident axillary lymph node metastases
☐	N2a	Metastases in ipsilateral axillary lymph nodes fixed to one another (matted) or to other structures
☐	N2b	Metastases only in clinically detected*** ipsilateral internal mammary nodes and in the absence of clinically evident axillary lymph node metastases
☐	N3	Metastases in ipsilateral infraclavicular (level III axillary) lymph node(s) with or without level I, II axillary lymph node involvement; or in clinically detected* ipsilateral internal mammary lymph node(s) with clinically evident level I, II axillary lymph node metastases; or metastases in ipsilateral supraclavicular lymph node(s) with or without axillary or internal mammary lymph node involvement
☐	N3a	Metastases in ipsilateral infraclavicular lymph node(s)
☐	N3b	Metastases in ipsilateral internal mammary lymph node(s) and axillary lymph node(s)
☐	N3c	Metastases in ipsilateral supraclavicular lymph node(s)

Metastasis(M)

☑	M0	No clinical or radiographic evidence of distant metastases (no pathologic M0; use clinical M to complete stage group)
☐	cM0(+)	No clinical or radiographic evidence of distant metastases, but deposits of molecularly or microscopically detected tumor cells in circulating blood, bone marrow or other non-regional nodal tissue that are no larger than 0.2 mm in a patient without symptoms or signs of metastases
☐	M1	Distant detectable metastases as determined by classic clinical and radiographic means and/or histologically proven larger than 0.2 mm

Submit

Fig. 2. Patient details form along with breast cancer TNM form based on AJCC guideline in CuraEx

Table 1. Most prevalent cancer types and subtypes available in the current version of the CuraEx

Cancer types	Sub-types
Head and neck	(i) Lip and oral cavity
	(ii) Pharynx (iii) Larynx (iv) Nasal cavity and paranasal sinuses
	(v) Thyroid
Digestive system	(i) Stomach (ii) Colon and rectum (iii) Liver
	(iv) Exocrine and endocrine pancreas
Thorax	(i) Lung
Breast	(i) Breast
Gynecological	(i) Cervix uteri (ii) Ovary and primary peritoneal carcinoma
Genitourinary	(i) Prostate (ii) Kidney (iii) Urinary bladder

of distant metastasis), demographics, genetic marker and other information such as age, race, gender, tumour size, laterality, treatment type, date of diagnosis, drugs prescribed, duration of the drug, histological grade, biomarker and genetic variants are taken as inputs from the user. Using the given patient specific information, CuraEx performs cancer staging, patient prognosis and prepares therapeutic reports. The TNM values are required from the user for cancer staging calculation. Figure 2 shows the patient details form and breast cancer staging form based on the AJCC guideline. Most common cancer types are made available on the current version of the system as shown in Table 1.

4   Analytical Engine

4.1   Cancer Staging

Staging is the process, used during diagnosis which helps the oncologist to better understand the patient's disease condition. Staging is performed using rule based technique where the stage of a cancer subtype is calculated based on the different combination of TNM values [10]. The cancer stage and TNM mapping information for each cancer subtype is normalized and stored in relational data model. TNM staging algorithm is unique for every anatomic site or sub-type where the tumour can possibly originate. An example of breast cancer stage for specific TNM values from CuraEx is shown in Fig. 3.

4.2   Prognosis

Prognosis is the key factor to understand the likely course and outcome of a cancer. The prognosis of the patient is studied by survival analysis using previous cancer registry data set from NCI SEER collected over 1997 to 2012 [11,12]. This data set contains over 8 million records of various cancer patient's and each record has more than 100 fields. The format of NCI SEER is, SAS (data type)

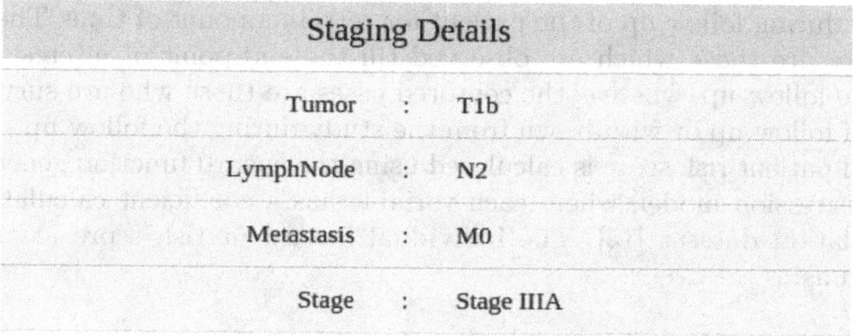

Staging Details		
Tumor	:	T1b
LymphNode	:	N2
Metastasis	:	M0
Stage	:	Stage IIIA

Fig. 3. Staging report for breast cancer with T1b, N2 and M0

Table 2. Example of coded categorical (DERIVED AJCC-6 M) and numerical (SURVIVAL MONTHS) variable

Variable	Data type	Codes	Value
DERIVED AJCC-6 M	Categorical	99	MX
		00	M0
		10	M1
		11	M1a
		12	M1b
		13	M1c
		19	M1 NOS
		88	NOT APPLICABLE
SURVIVAL MONTHS	Numerical	000-9998	000-9998 months
		9999	Unknown

and stored in ASCII text. The SAS data set contains two files, one file contains the encrypted data values which are organized as a table of observation, where row contains the patient's information and column contains the variables. The other file contains the mapping or descriptor information such as the type and length of the variables. The variables in the data are of both categorical and numerical type. For illustration, an example of (i) coded categorical variable and (ii) coded numerical variable are shown in Table 2. During pre-processing, all these codes are taken into account with right statistical corrections.

The prognosis analysis in CuraEx is an evidence based technique to predict the outcome of cancer and the probability of patient survivability. Cox-regression model, which is a semi-parametric model, is used to study the effects of several covariates (i.e., age, sex, stage, grade, ethnicity and receptor information like ER/PR/HER2 types for breast cancer) on survival. This model is used to estimate the influence of multiple covariates on the survival distribution including censored cases [13]. To perform the cox-regression, two variables are required for survival distribution, which is survival of the patients (Number of years the patient has survived) and event state (uncensored and censored) which is measured during follow up of the patient for certain amount of time. The uncensored cases are those which are observed till the end-point of interest (death) during the follow up, whereas the censored cases are those who are survived till the end of follow up or withdrawn from the study during the follow up [14]. The individual patient risk score is calculated using the hazard function generated by the cox-regression model, where each variable has a coefficient calculated from the population dataset [15]. The individual hazard or risk score at time t is calculated as:

$$h(t) = h_0(t) * exp(coef_{age} * age + coef_{sex} * sex + coef_{stage} * stage + coef_{grade} * grade + coef_{race} * race) \quad (1)$$

The $h_0(t)$ is the baseline or underlying hazard function and $coef_{(variables)}$ is regression coefficient calculated from the population dataset.

The Kaplan-Meier estimator is used to estimate the survival curve, using the NCI SEER population data, which calculates the proportion surviving at each point under similar circumstances. The result of estimation using Kaplan-Meier includes a life table and survival curve. Life table gives information about the proportion surviving at each interval. The survival curve shows the pattern of survival rates over time [16]. Two types of cause specific survival analysis are performed in CuraEx (i) disease - specific survival curve which is based on the cancer type and stage, (ii) patient - specific survival curve which is based on cancer type, stage, grade, age and race of the patient [17]. Figures 4 and 5 illustrates disease and patient specific survival curve for breast cancer patients. Y-axis represents proportion of the population that has survived (0–100 %) and x-axis represents the survival time of the population (1–15 years). The SEER dataset is filtered based on the cancer subtype of the patient before carrying out the survival analysis.

4.3 Therapeutics

Following the staging and survivability analysis, CuraEx reports the most suitable drug based on the patient disease, clinical and genomic marker. This is based on the FDA approved drugs and the drugs that are currently studied on clinical trial. All these information helps the doctor in treating the patient and find the right therapeutic solution. Drugbank [18], clinicaltrial.gov [19] and FDA [20] databases are used at this stage as a knowledge base along with manually curated database at InterpretOmics by Ph.D quality scientists and biologists from bibliomics data which contains information about the impact of genetic variation on drug response for specific disease type from which the right treatment related information can be extracted. This helps to classify patients between responders and non-responders to medication. Manually curated database is periodically updated. These data are normalized, indexed and stored in the form of relational model to perform accurate and faster analytics. Several drug attributes such as taxonomy, pharmacological, drug target and properties etc. are represented in the form of a table with the filtering options on each field which

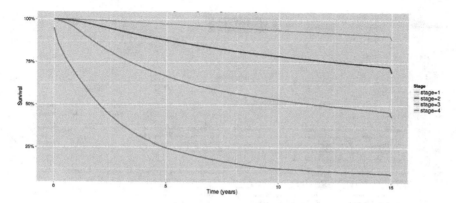

Fig. 4. Disease specific survival curve for breast cancer based on the cancer stage. Each curve represents a cancer stage. There are 232,985 individuals with breast cancer type, in which stage1, stage 2, stage3 and stage 4 have 112314, 90910, 20470 and 9291 individuals

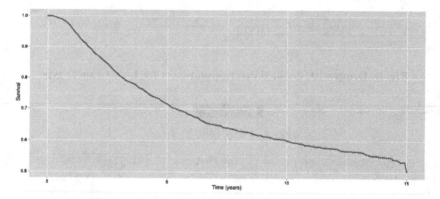

Fig. 5. Patient specific survival for breast cancer based on the patient age, sex, grade and stage. There are 2,613 individuals with breast cancer of age group 45–49, female, stage3, and histological grade 3

helps the doctor to narrow down the data set. For example doctor can check for the FDA approved small molecule drugs and biotech drugs, based on the type of the cancer. Along with drug features, pharmacogenomics information is also reported, where the response to drugs and prognosis varies significantly based on the genetic mutations of the patient. Also by using the patients molecular and clinical information, a suitable drug can be identified which is more likely to be successful than traditional approach. Figures 6 and 7 illustrates few of the available drugs and drugs in clinical trial for breast cancer type from CuraEx.

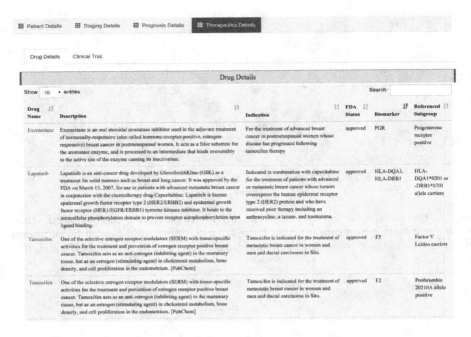

Fig. 6. Drugs with detailed description report for breast cancer type

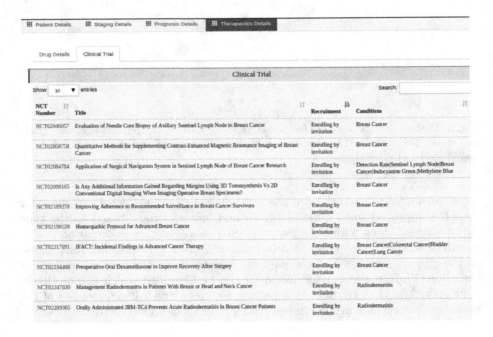

Fig. 7. Clinical trial report for breast cancer type

5 Knowledge Database

In summary at present, six background knowledge bases are used such as AJCC (rule based), NCI SEER (Evidence based), Drugbank, clinicaltrial.gov, FDA and Manually curated database (drug associated genomic marker). These data are stored in the relational database and used by the analytical engine to retrieve the patient specific information.

6 Software Stack and Data Management

Keeping future enhancements in mind, a highly scalable and inter-operable software architecture is used to develop CuraEx. Play framework is a high-scalable and fast web application framework that is used to develop the front-end interactive application [21]. The background knowledge base, which is used to perform analytics are normalized, indexed and stored in MySQL relational databases. The databases is updated once in three months. For powerful statistical computing and graphic tool, R is used to perform analytics and generate visuals.

7 Conclusion

The CuraEx system which we have developed, using the advanced software techniques and validated knowledge base can be used by the physician or oncologist in assisting the decision making during diagnosis as well as therapeutics. The major advantage of this system is that it uses clinical and molecular information of the patient to perform patient stratification which helps in selection of the most suitable line of treatment. This will lead to increase in the survival period of the patient compared to the general treatment strategies. At present, capturing the genetic information of the patient is made easy by high throughput genomics techniques. Identifying molecular markers and genetic variants are made possible from population study using big genomics data [22]. For example, data from the 1000 genome project, in which the volume is approximately 500 TB, help us to understand the genetic variants better in the population. Using the results from the population studies, genetic testing is designed using high throughput genomic techniques which is helpful to capture the patients genomic marker status. The genomic marker and genetic variant information along with the drug responses are made available in CuraEx which helps to perform precision medicine.

In future, the CuraEx will focus on developing an automatic staging system from free-text pathology report which uses natural language processing and machine learning techniques to predict TNM values and to determine the cancer stage [23]. In CuraEx, the staging is based on the five main cancer types, but in future it will include other types of cancers as well. Currently, the prognosis in CuraEx is based on the overall survival; soon, other type of prognosis such as disease free, progression free and recurrence free survival will be considered based on the availability of the dataset [24].

References

1. MacDermid, E., Hooton, G., MacDonald, M., McKay, G., Grose, D., Mohammed, N., Porteous, C.: Improving patient survival with the colorectal cancer multidisciplinary team. Colorectal Dis. **11**(3), 291–295 (2009)
2. Hernández, K.R.D., Lasserre, A.A.A., Gómez, R.P., Guzmán, J.A.P., Sánchez, B.E.G.: Development of an expert system as a diagnostic support of cervical cancer in atypical glandular cells, based on fuzzy logics and image interpretation. Comput. Math. Methods Med. **2013**, 387–796 (2013)
3. Edwards, G.A.: Expert systems for clinical pathology reporting. Clin. Biochem. Rev. **29**(Suppl 1), S105 (2008)
4. Zhang, Y., Fong, S., Fiaidhi, J., Mohammed, S.: Real-time clinical decision support system with data stream mining. BioMed Research International 2012 (2012)
5. Reich, W.T.: Encyclopedia of Bioethics: Revised Edition. Macmillan Library Reference, New York (1995)
6. Edge, S.B., Byrd, D.R., Compton, C.C., Fritz, A.G., Greene, F.L., Trotti, A. (eds.): AJCC Cancer Staging Handbook: From the AJCC Cancer Staging Manual. Springer, New York (2010)
7. Surveillance, epidemiology, and end results (seer) program. www.seer.cancer.gov
8. Maltoni, M., Caraceni, A., Brunelli, C., Broeckaert, B., Christakis, N., Eychmueller, S., Glare, P., Nabal, M., Vigano, A., Larkin, P., et al.: Prognostic factors in advanced cancer patients: evidence-based clinical recommendationsa study by the steering committee of the european association for palliative care. J. Clin. Oncol. **23**(25), 6240–6248 (2005)
9. Hou, G., Zhang, S., Zhang, X., Wang, P., Hao, X., Zhang, J.: Clinical pathological characteristics and prognostic analysis of 1,013 breast cancer patients with diabetes. Breast Cancer Res. Treat. **137**(3), 807–816 (2013)
10. National comprehensive cancer network, cancer staging guide. http://www.nccn.org/patients/resources/diagnosis/staging.aspx
11. Thein, M.S., Ershler, W.B., Jemal, A., Yates, J.W., Baer, M.R.: Outcome of older patients with acute myeloid leukemia. Cancer **119**(15), 2720–2727 (2013)
12. Wang, S.J., Fuller, C.D., Emery, R., Thomas Jr., C.R.: Conditional survival in rectal cancer: a seer database analysis. Gastrointest. Cancer Res. GCR **1**(3), 84 (2007)
13. Zwiener, I., Blettner, M., Hommel, G.: Survival analysis: part 15 of a series on evaluation of scientific publications. Deutsches Ärzteblatt Int. **108**(10), 163 (2011)
14. What is a cox model? http://www.medicine.ox.ac.uk/bandolier/painres/download/whatis/cox_model.pdf
15. Fox, J.: Cox proportional-hazards regression for survival data. An R and S-PLUS companion to applied regression, pp. 1–18. Sage Publications, Thousand Oaks (2002)
16. Goel, M.K., Khanna, P., Kishore, J.: Understanding survival analysis: kaplan-meier estimate. Int. J. Ayurveda Res. **1**(4), 274 (2010)
17. Gschwend, J.E., Dahm, P., Fair, W.R.: Disease specific survival as endpoint of outcome for bladder cancer patients following radical cystectomy. Eur. Urol. **41**(4), 440–448 (2002)
18. Law, V., Knox, C., Djoumbou, Y., Jewison, T., Guo, A.C., Liu, Y., Maciejewski, A., Arndt, D., Wilson, M., Neveu, V., et al.: Drugbank 4.0: shedding new light on drug metabolism. Nucleic Acids Res. **42**(D1), D1091–D1097 (2014)

19. clinicaltrials.gov, a service of the US national institutes of health. https://clinicaltrials.gov/
20. FDA pharmacogenomics. http://www.fda.gov/drugs/scienceresearch/researchareas/pharmacogenetics/ucm083378.htm
21. Play framework. https://www.playframework.com/
22. Stephens, Z.D., Lee, S.Y., Faghri, F., Campbell, R.H., Zhai, C., Efron, M.J., Iyer, R., Schatz, M.C., Sinha, S., Robinson, G.E.: Big data: astronomical or genomical? PLoS Biol **13**(7), e1002195 (2015)
23. Moore, D., McCowan, I., Nguyen, A., Courage, M.J., et al.: Trial evaluation of automatic lung cancer staging from pathology reports (2007). https://qccat.health.qld.gov.au/documents/moore-06-medinfo-preprint-abs.pdf
24. Dong, X.D., Tyler, D., Johnson, J.L., DeMatos, P., Seigler, H.F.: Analysis of prognosis and disease progression after local recurrence of melanoma. Cancer **88**(5), 1063–1071 (2000)

Multi-omics Multi-scale Big Data Analytics for Cancer Genomics

Mahima Agarwal, Mohamood Adhil, and Asoke K. Talukder[✉]

InterpretOmics, Bangalore, India
{mahima.agarwal,mohamood.adhil,asoke.talukder}@interpretomics.co
http://interpretomics.co

Abstract. Cancer research is emerging as a complex orchestration of genomics, data-sciences, and network-sciences. For improving cancer diagnosis and treatment strategies, data across multiple scales, from molecules like DNA, RNA, metabolites, to the population, need to be integrated. This requires handling of large volumes of high complexity "Omics" data, requiring powerful computational algorithms and mathematical tools. Here we present an integrative analytics approach for cancer genomics. This approach takes the multi-scale biological interactions as key considerations for model development. We demonstrate the use of this approach on a publicly available lung cancer dataset collected for 109 individuals from an 18 years long clinical study. From this data, we discovered novel disease markers and drug targets that were validated using peer-reviewed literature. These results demonstrate the power of big data analytics for deriving disease actionable insight.

Keywords: Integrative analysis · Network analysis · Multi-scale · Multi-omics · Patient stratification · Drug target · Precision medicine · Big data · Lung cancer

1   Introduction

For centuries, diseases have been studied and treated based on their external manifestations. Following the Human genome project, with an improved understanding of the genes and their interactions, the focus of cancer research has shifted to the genetic mechanisms which lead to disease development. The human genome consists of the DNA present within the cell nucleus, and is made up of over six billion nucleotides. These nucleotides code for molecules which make the different cells function properly. Any change in the six billion nucleotides is therefore capable of altering the functioning of cells. Such changes sometimes result in production of proteins with altered functions, or altered levels of proteins in the cells. This can result in loss of the homeostatic balance and uncontrolled growth of the cells. Such cells damage the surrounding tissue, resulting in tumor formation, leading to cancer. Research is now focused on understanding the root cause of the disease, which lies in the alterations in the genome (DNA) or gene

© Springer International Publishing Switzerland 2015
N. Kumar and V. Bhatnagar (Eds.): BDA 2015, LNCS 9498, pp. 228–243, 2015.
DOI: 10.1007/978-3-319-27057-9_16

expression. In the traditional empirical or reductionist approach, the problems are reduced to a single scale and studied in isolation. But, the connectivity and interdependence between the multiple levels of organization in a living system bestow upon it the unique properties which make it function as a whole [26]. Therefore the reductionist approach ignores many of the key features and complexity of the living system [27]. A more integrated, holistic approach is required for studying cancers.

Cancers are more responsive to treatment in early stages, compared to more advanced stages. This makes it essential to identify appropriate markers for diagnosis of cancer, as early as possible. When a patient is stratified and diagnosed correctly, appropriate treatment can start. However, cancers display a high level of variability between patients. Therefore, the same treatment/drugs may not be suitable for two patients. Precision medicine is based on this concept of individual patient variability [12]. This means that drugs should be highly focused for specific patient profiles right from development to treatment. This will reduce not only the treatment burden on patients, but also improve the efficacy of drugs, and trial success. This is of even more relevance since cancer drugs are expensive and can have severe side-effects. This type of patient variability based drug development and treatment approach, along with timely, high confidence diagnosis, requires an in-depth understanding of cancer. Unraveling these complex features requires an integrated system level approach instead of a reductionist approach [17]. This requires the integration of muti-scale "Omics" information, and is made tractable through big data analytics.

The development of high throughput technologies have made a lot of multi-scale "Omics" data available. These data capture DNA, RNA, protein, and metabolite level information in the form of genomics, transcriptomics, proteomics, phenomics, and metabolomics data, among others [24]. There has been large reduction in the cost and time involved in the generation of these data. It is estimated that over the next 10 years, Omics data will be at par, if not surpass data generated from sources such as astronomy, YouTube, and Twitter in terms of acquisition, storage, distribution and analysis [37]. The way the different forms of biological data are collected and represented makes high variety and variability inherent characteristics of these data. This makes integration across multiple datasets a challenge [36]. In addition, biological problems are usually NP-hard, and are therefore computationally intensive to solve [25]. These problems are further complicated by the high dimensionality of biological data, where the number of features (variables) for which observations are recorded is more than the number of samples by a few orders of magnitude. Therefore, the extraction of actionable biological and clinical insight from these data is riddled with some of the main challenges associated with the analysis of big data.

In this paper we show how big data analytics can help in understanding cancer genomics. We describe an integrative analysis framework which uses datasciences and network-sciences techniques for model creation from multi-scale, multi-omics data. This framework, shown in Fig. 1, is useful for discovering actionable insights in cancer. This framework consists of 4 stages. In the first

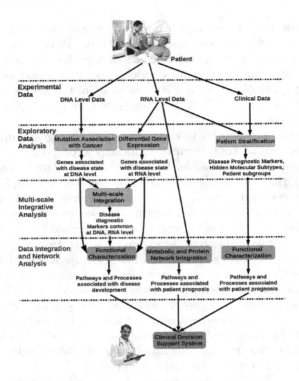

Fig. 1. Framework for integrative data analysis

stage, exploratory data analysis techniques are used for hypothesis creation from the experimental data, which includes DNA and RNA data. Traditional techniques are used to extract information from the individual datasets, to obtain disease biomarkers for diagnosis and prediction of patient survival/response. Next, the results from the exploratory data analysis are combined and filtered, within an appropriate biological context, in the multi-scale integrative analysis. This is a step towards developing a mechanistic model for the disease. Finally, the results from the exploratory data analysis and multi-scale integration steps are combined with information from existing knowledge-bases to obtain a functional understanding of the disease along with high quality biomarkers, and potential drug targets.

To demonstrate this integrative cancer genomics model, we have used a publicly available lung cancer (lung squamous cell carcinoma or SCC) clinical dataset, collected over 18 years [9] as an example. The data for this case study were downloaded from the Array Express database under accession id E-MTAB-1727 (www.ebi.ac.uk/arrayexpress). All analysis were run using the iOMICS platform that has been built by us and deployed in the Google cloud. This is accessible at http://iomics-clinical.interpretomics.co. This paper is organized into 5 main sections. A description of the input data, including experimental data and external knowledge-bases is provided in Sect. 2. Section 3 gives the key aims of the analysis. Section 4 describes the exploratory data analyses step of the analysis framework on the experimental data. Section 5 describes the multi-omics integrative step using results from exploratory data analysis. Finally, the integration of external knowledge-bases and application of network theory to derive actionable insights and biomarkers is described in Sect. 6.

2 Available Data

We have used multi-omics, multi-scale data for a group of lung cancer patients and healthy individuals to illustrate our analytics framework. These data were collected by the original authors [9] and made publicly available. They include DNA, RNA, and clinical data for 93 cancer patients and 16 healthy individuals. Together these make up the experimental datasets. Apart from the experimental datasets, various reference knowledge-bases are available, which have been used in the analytic framework. A description of all these available data is given, followed by a description of the key questions which can be answered using these multiple datasets.

2.1 DNA Level Data

The available DNA level data consist of information regarding DNA sequence alterations for 67 lung cancer patients [9]. This data was not available for the remaining 26 cancer patients and the 16 healthy individuals. For each of the over 300,000 DNA sequence sites captured, the genotype data provide the state of the DNA sequence (alleles) for both copies of DNA (one from each parent). These data were captured from genotyping experiments.

2.2 RNA Level Data

DNA sequence alterations can cause disease by altering the production of proteins in the cells. The first step in the translation of DNA sequence to proteins is the production of mRNA. mRNA levels in the cells are therefore a measure of the expression of DNA to proteins. mRNA levels were captured in the lung cancer study [9] and made available in the form of intensity measures from microarray experiments, for all 109 individuals (93 lung cancer patients and 16 healthy individuals). These intensity values need to first be normalized across samples and converted to expression measures before they can be used for analysis.

2.3 Clinical Data

Clinical data was recorded for all 93 lung cancer patients and 16 healthy individuals by the original authors [9]. These data contained patient information such as age at diagnosis, sex, disease stage, treatments received and other features related to disease risk and condition. A summary of the main sample characteristics for the 93 lung cancer patients from this dataset is given in Table 1.

Table 1. Sample characteristics

Gender	Male	89
	Female	4
Age at Diagnosis	Median	64
Histology	Well differentiated SCC	36
	Poorly differentiated SCC	15
	Mixed basaloid	18
	Pure basaloid	24
Stage	Stage I	55
	Stage II	19
	Stage III	17
	Stage IV	2

This information provides disease characteristics and can therefore be used to scale the molecular level (DNA, RNA) information, described earlier, with the disease state.

Survival Information. Survival information was also recorded for the 93 lung cancer patients. This information includes information regarding how long the patients survived during the study period. This includes both overall patient survival and survival without disease recurrence. While overall survival was recorded for all 93 patients, recurrence free survival was recorded for 87 cancer patients. One characteristic of survival information of this kind is that it is censored. This means that data is not available for those patients that survived beyond the duration of the clinical study, as well as for those that withdrew from the study. Therefore appropriate modeling algorithms, capable of handling censored data, are required in order to combine the survival data with other types of data from the patients (clinical, DNA, and RNA).

2.4 Background Databases

Vast quantities of biological knowledge, has been collected through biological experiments and is available in the public domain. This knowledge, in the form of reference databases can be used to extend the results of the experimental data, and provide them a functional context. This step is essential to obtain a mechanistic understanding of disease development, and for identifying drug targets. Three types of biological databases, namely functional characterization databases, metabolic databases, and protein interaction databases have been used in the analysis framework to complement the experimental data.

Functional Characterization Databases. Functional characterization databases contain information curated from research studies regarding the various biological properties of the protein products of genes. These include properties such as biological function, cellular localization and the high level pathways and processes. These functional properties provide biological relevance to lists of gene names, leading to the development of an explanation for why and how they are involved in the disease. We have used two such functional characterization databases for our analysis. These are the Gene Ontology database (GO) [5] and KEGG [20].

Metabolic Databases. Metabolic databases contain information regarding the multitude of biochemical reactions taking place in the living system. This information ranges from the small molecules (metabolites) being formed or destroyed, along with the involvement of genes in these processes. These biochemical (metabolic) reactions are responsible for the interaction of a living system with its environment, as well as the various processes taking place within the system. The collection of all these biochemical reactions in humans is called human metabolism. While information regarding human metabolism is growing, models of human metabolism exist which contain the current knowledge of metabolism. Recon X [39] is one such model, which contains information regarding metabolic reactions, their reactants, products, stoichiometry and associated genes, and is available in standard SBML format [18]. We have used Recon X with 7439 reactions and 2626 metabolites in our framework.

Protein Interaction Databases. At a level higher than metabolism, the functional characteristics of a living system arise from the interactions between proteins. Proteins transfer signals within and between cells, and lead to mediation of metabolic reactions based on these signals. The interactions between different proteins are captured in protein interaction databases. This information is represented as interaction networks with proteins forming the nodes, and edges representing the interactions between them. The protein-protein interactions can be directional or undirected, depending on the type of interaction. Our analytics framework uses the protein interaction database available from IntAct [31].

3   Key Aims

Based on the available experimental data, we have explored three main lines of analysis. The basaloid subtype of lung cancer is particularly aggressive and shows poor prognosis for the patients [9]. So, in the first, we aimed to identify the molecular differences between two cancer subtypes based on histology, the basaloid and SCC subtypes (Table 1), along with an understanding of how these molecular differences functionally result in differences in the two cancer subtypes. For the second line of analysis, we aimed to identify the molecular states associated with poor patient survival. In the third line of analysis, we compared the healthy individuals with the cancer patients using their molecular information, to identify therapeutic targets which can be used in drug development.

We show how the different datasets and steps in the analysis framework come together to answer the questions posed by these three lines of analysis.

4   Exploratory Data Analysis

The first step of the analysis framework is exploratory data analysis. This involves the analysis of individual experimental data sets, using traditional approaches, for hypothesis creation. The various analyses which can be performed depend on the type of experimental data available, and questions to answer. All the DNA, RNA, and clinical data were used to lay the foundation for the remaining analysis steps.

4.1   Mutation Association with Cancer State

For the first line of our analysis, we used the DNA level data to identify DNA sequence states which can differentiate the two cancer subtypes, namely the basaloid and the SCC. For each of the DNA sequence sites in the data, we first calculated the frequency of observing the least common sequence state for each cancer subtype. Based on these, odds were calculated for each disease subtype for observing the least common state $(p/(1-p))$. Then a ratio of these odds, called the odds ratio was taken for each site. Significant deviation of the odds ratio from one for a site signified that that particular site was associated with one or the other disease subtype. This association testing analysis was run using PLINK [32]. In order to identify meaningful results, we used high stringency cut-offs for the odds ratio and significance p-value (p-value $\leqslant$ 0.001, odds ratio $\geqslant$ 3). From this analysis, we were able to identify 735 disease subtype associated sites. Figure 2 shows the locations of these 735 sites along the chromosomes. This plot was generated using the quantsmooth R/Bioconductor package [30].

4.2   Differential Gene Expression

Cancer subtype differences can also manifest at the gene expression level, captured by the RNA data. We analyzed the RNA level data to study the differences between the two disease subtypes (basaloid and SCC) by identifying differentially

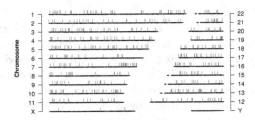

Fig. 2. Karyotype plot showing location of identified point mutations (red lines) along the chromosomes (Color figure online).

expressed genes. We used the R package LIMMA [34] for analyzing the expression level differences between the two disease subtypes. This algorithm is able to make statistical inferences even with a small number of samples [34]. It uses a linear model to model the expression values across samples, as a function of the disease subtypes. A separate model is fitted for each gene. This is followed by an empirical Bayes step across genes to identify the p-value and FDR (False Discovery Rate) adjusted p-value [34]. The log fold change between the disease subtypes is also estimated as the base 2 logarithm ratio of expression in the two states. Finally, we identified the differentially expressed genes which showed absolute log fold change > 0.6 with differential expression p-value < 0.0001. These cut-offs are variable and affect the stringency of the results. From this analysis, we identified 106 differentially expressed genes between the basaloid and SCC subtypes. Figure 3 shows the mRNA expression levels and hierarchical clustering of the 93 lung cancer patients for the identified differentially expressed genes. A clear separation in the expression values can be seen for the two subtypes.

For our third line of analysis, we needed to compare healthy individuals with cancer patients to identify potential drug targets. Only RNA data was available for the healthy patients, and therefore was used for this comparison. We identified the differentially expressed genes between cancer and healthy individuals. The same steps and parameters were used for this analysis, as for the differential expression analysis between the cancer subtypes.

4.3 Patient Stratification

The second line of analysis aims at identifying markers of patient survival. Patients' molecular profiles influence their response to treatment and disease progression. In the case of cancer, patient survival time is a reasonable measure of patient response. In a treatment context, markers associated with treatment response can stratify patients into groups of responsive and non-responsive patients. These markers will then be able to identify which group a new patient

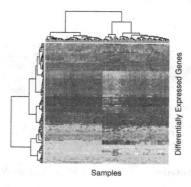

Fig. 3. Heirarchical clustering of expression for identified differentially expressed genes

belongs to and facilitate precision medicine through most effective treatment. Since gene expression is an intermediary between DNA and protein, it can be used to connect patient response with the molecular profile.

In this analysis, we integrate gene expression RNA level data with recurrence free survival information for the cancer patients, to answer the questions posed by the second line of analysis. We used the Cox regression to model survival time as a function of gene expression. The Cox regression model was used because of its ability to handle censored data [28]. Apart from the censored nature of survival data, another problem for the analysis is the high data dimensionality. Expression information is available for over 20,000 genes for the 87 samples with survival information. Therefore in order to identify high confidence genes as markers of patient survival, an appropriate dimensionality reduction technique needs to be applied. For this, we used the semi-supervised principle components based dimensionality reduction technique implemented in the R package SuperPC [6,7] to calculate the adjusted Cox regression coefficients. We used a training set constructed from a random set of 2/3rd of the samples to build the adjusted Cox regression model, and built a reduced model with the genes with the highest coefficients. We then tested the resulting model on the remaining 1/3rd samples (test set). This procedure was repeated 10 times, to obtain the best fitting model.

We used the genes from the final model to cluster all 93 lung cancer patients into 2 groups, with 78 and 9 patients each. While one of these groups showed a good survival probability (84 patients), the survival probabilities for the other group were very poor (Poor prognosis group: 9 patients). We then reapplied this analysis on the 78 patients who were part of the good survival probability group. This resulted in further subgrouping of the patients into two groups, both of which had better survival probabilities compared to the poor prognosis group. The survival probabilities for the resulting 3 groups of patients is shown in Fig. 4. These curves were generated using the R package ggplot2 [40]. Interestingly, all 9 patients in the poor prognosis group belong to the pure basaloid subtype. This indicates that these patients represent a particularly aggressive molecular profile seen in the pure basaloid patients.

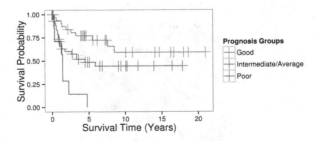

Fig. 4. Survival probability curves for identified molecular subgroups

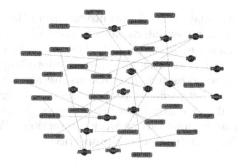

Fig. 5. Mapping of differentially expressed genes and SNPs. Genes are in blue/green and mutations are in pink. The sizes of gene nodes represent fold change, while the blue and green shades represent direction of change (Color figure online)

5   Multi-scale Integrative Analysis

The next stage of the analysis framework involves integration of the results from exploratory data analysis within a biologically meaningful context to improve our understanding of cancer and how the disease state develops. The type of multi-scale integration, and resulting inferences, depends on the available experimental datasets. With varied multi-scale datasets, the resulting disease model becomes richer, providing improved insights. For the lung cancer dataset, only DNA and RNA level molecular data are available, therefore we demonstrate the applicability of this step through DNA-RNA integration. From this analysis, we can identify the disease subtype associated DNA sequence mutations which lead to changes in RNA expression, thereby providing a mechanism for how these sequence changes are pathogenic.

We first annotated the 735 identified disease subtype associated DNA sequence alterations with genes based on their chromosomal location. The human genome build GrCH38 was used for the gene locations. This provided a list of 558 unique genes with disease associated mutations. We compared these to the differential gene expression analysis results between the basaloid and SCC subtypes, and identified genes which were also differentially expressed. This gene-mutation mapping, as visualized in Cytoscape (a tool for dynamic network visualization [1]), is shown in Fig. 5. Many of the genes discovered in this part of the analysis such as CLCA2, TIAM2 and BCL2 have been associated with progression and metastasis in various tumors [11,14,23].

6   Data Integration and Network Analysis

The final step of the analysis framework takes the results of the exploratory data analysis and multi-scale integration steps and combines them with existing biological knowledge-bases to finally answer the questions posed in the three analysis lines. We used network analysis to obtain insights from this stage of the analysis. This is because the complex interactions in the biological system are better understood when modeled as networks [22]. The networks provide information regarding the biological interactions and flow of information. When analyzing functional networks, key nodes and interactions are identified using centrality measures such as degree, betweenness, connectedness and eigenvector centrality. Node clustering is used to identify functional clusters. Node neighborhoods are analyzed for identifying interactions network interactions. We have used the R package igraph [13] for studying network properties.

6.1   Functional Characterization Databases

We used the information in the functional characterization databases for all the gene lists from the 3 types of exploratory data analysis, as well as the multi-scale integration analysis, for the first two lines of analysis. We used the R package GO.db [10] and 168 cancer and metabolic KEGG pathways [35] to annotate genes with their functional properties. Since these are non-random lists of genes, the functions they perform will be linked with the development of the disease state. In other words, these disease state associated functions will be over-represented for the gene list, than expected by chance. To identify these overrepresented gene functions, we used the Fisher's exact test, as implemented in XomPathways [38]. We modeled the results as a bipartite gene-function (pathway/GO) network, and the resulting gene-gene and function-function networks. The key functional properties and genes involved in the disease state were identified from the most central nodes in these networks. For the gene-biological processes functional annotation, the identified key processes were related to epithelial morphology, consistent with histology based subgrouping of the disease subtypes (Table 2).

6.2   Metabolic Network Reconstruction and Protein Interactions

The functional properties of genes provides a high level view of the contribution of genes to the disease state. At the core of these properties lies the metabolism.

Table 2. Biological process overrepresentation results. Top overrepresented biological processes for the genes expressed differentially between basaloid and SCC cancer subtypes. Degree and betweenness centrality measures for these genes in the process-process network are also given.

Biological process	Over-representation p-value	FDR adjusted q-value	Degree centrality	Betweenness centrality
Skin development	1.9E-9	7.1E-7	14	0.6
Epidermis development	3.8E-9	7.1E-7	14	0.6
Epithelial cell differentiation	1.1E-7	1.4E-5	6	5.1
Keratinocyte differentiation	1.6E-7	1.4E-5	10	0

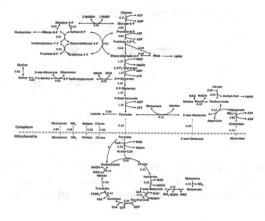

Fig. 6. Subset of human metabolic network. This image has been taken from [21]

Metabolism is centered around the processes of energy and biomass production, as these are the two core requirements for the cell. Some of the core metabolic reactions involved in energy production are depicted in Fig. 6. Diseases such as cancer develop due to metabolic changes brought about by protein changes. In order to identify potential drug targets for disease treatment, a mechanistic model is essential which considers the metabolite and protein interactions. Therefore, for our third line of analysis, we combined RNA based gene expression data, which is indicative of protein expression, with metabolic and protein interaction data, from reference databases.

Using the approach of the GIMME algorithm [8], we used expression data to identify reactions which were occurring in the disease and healthy states. For this we used an expression threshold such that about 25 % of the genes were assumed to be switched off. This information was used to initialize the metabolic model from RECON X. The metabolic models for both state were constructed using flux balance analysis, a type of constraint based modeling. Since the cancer cells show extensive growth and proliferation, the disease state network was optimized for maximum biomass production. The healthy lung cells are differentiated and primarily use energy for carrying out their functions. Therefore the healthy state network was optimized for maximizing energy production. Thermodynamically unfeasible cycles were removed from the models and the fluxes through all metabolic reactions were calculate. The R package sybil, sybilEFBA, sybilSBML and sybilcyclefreeflux were used for this analysis, along with glpkAPI [3,4,15,16].

We compared the fluxes through the reactions in both disease and healthy state metabolic models to identify the reactions with the most change in flux. From the information contained in Recon X, we identified the genes associated with these reactions. From a therapeutics point of view, these genes are potential targets for lung cancer. However, not all of them may be druggable. Additionally, targeting these genes may lead to high toxicity, or alteration in tumor properties

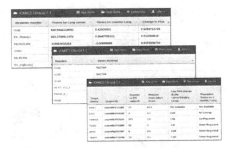

Fig. 7. Results from the analysis of cancer and healthy metabolic networks. The first step identifies altered reactions, the second step lists out the genes involved directly in the reactions. The final step identifies putative drug targets based on the protein interaction network.

rendering the drug ineffective. To solve these problems, we extended the identified gene list to include the other genes which directly interacted with these genes in the protein interaction network. These extra genes can indirectly modulate the metabolic reactions. The resulting gene list had 214 genes.

Out of these, the genes which interact with many other genes in the human protein interaction network (PIN) are likely to be inappropriate drug targets due to high toxicity. Therefore we calculated a degree score for each gene based on its degree centrality in the PIN. We also calculated a reaction score for each gene by summing its interactions with target reactions. Indirect interactions were weighted 0.5. Finally, we looked at whether the identified genes were differentially expressed between the healthy and tumor state, since this provided a mechanism by which the change in metabolic reactions was affected. Many well known cancer genes such as MYC, ERBB2, STAT3 and GSR, along with novel genes, were identified as therapeutic targets. Figure 7 gives the results from this analysis.

7   Conclusions

Here we described and illustrated the use of a big data multi-scale multi-omics framework for the identification of gene level biomarkers associated with lung cancer. Using this approach, we were able to identify diagnostic and prognostic biomarkers for the cancer subtypes, therapeutic targets for lung cancer, and even identified a hidden molecular subtype having dismal prognosis. We showed how different stages of the analysis framework come together to answer complex disease associated questions such as mechanism of disease development, processes influencing patient survival, and putative therapeutic targets. The results were all validated using bibliomic data (peer reviewed publications). While a basic meta-analysis framework for integrative analysis was described here, more comprehensive mathematical techniques can also be applied to get better results [33]. The identified target genes can be further validated as potential drug targets using an in-silico knockouts approach. This type of analysis uses iterative constraint based modeling on the metabolic network model, to study the effect of altering specific reactions on both the healthy and disease state [19]. We used the iOMICS platform in a semi-automated fashion for running the analysis. The input parameters and experimental data types were provided as input. User intervention was required for providing a biologically meaningful direction to the analyses, bringing them in line with the type of available data and hypotheses. This is an essential feature for the analysis of biological data.

While we have demonstrated the use of this analysis framework for cancer, it can be extended to other complex diseases such as neurological and heart diseases. It provides a general framework which can be used to combine multi-omics data to derive cross-scale inferences. For this purpose, the type of input experimental data decides the following analytics. Depending on the type of experiments conducted, the aspect of the disease state interactions unveiled by the analysis may vary. AlQuraishi et al. [2] looked at a complex disease such as cancer at the genomic scale, where they integrated biophysical data with genomic data to study tumor vs. normal state. On the other hand, an organ and system level view of drug interactions can provide useful insights regarding the efficacy and toxicity of drugs [29]. However, it does not depend on the specific type of experiment used to capture the same information. Although we have used data collected from genotyping and mRNA microarray experiments, the analytics approach can also be applied to cases with much larger quantities of data, collected from sequencing experiments, and can be integrated with data from knowledge-bases other than those used here.

References

1. Cytoscape. http://www.cytoscape.org/
2. AlQuraishi, M., Koytiger, G., Jenney, A., MacBeath, G., Sorger, P.K.: A multi-scale statistical mechanical framework integrates biophysical and genomic data to assemble cancer networks. Nat. Genet. **46**, 1363–1371 (2014)
3. Amer Desouki, A.: sybilcycleFreeFlux: cycle-Free Flux balance analysis: Efficient removal of thermodynamically infeasible cycles from metabolic flux distributions (2014). R package version 1.0.1
4. Amer Desouki, A.: sybilEFBA: Using Gene Expression Data to Improve Flux Balance Analysis Predictions (2015). R package version 1.0.2
5. Ashburner, M., Ball, C.A., Blake, J.A., Botstein, D., Butler, H., Cherry, J.M., Davis, A.P., Dolinski, K., Dwight, S.S., Eppig, J.T., et al.: Gene ontology: tool for the unification of biology. Nat. Genet. **25**(1), 25–29 (2000)
6. Bair, E., Hastie, T., Paul, D., Tibshirani, R.: Prediction by supervised principal components. J. Am. Stat. Assoc. **101**(473), 119–137 (2006)
7. Bair, E., Tibshirani, R.: Semi-supervised methods to predict patient survival from gene expression data. PLoS Biol. **2**(4), E108 (2004)
8. Becker, S.A., Palsson, B.O.: Context-specific metabolic networks are consistent with experiments. PLoS Comput. Biol. **4**(5), e1000082 (2008)
9. Brambilla, C., Laffaire, J., Lantuejoul, S., Moro-Sibilot, D., Mignotte, H., Arbib, F., Toffart, A.C., Petel, F., Hainaut, P., Rousseaux, S., et al.: Lung squamous cell carcinomas with basaloid histology represent a specific molecular entity. Clin. Cancer Res. **20**(22), 5777–5786 (2014)

10. Carlson, M.: GO.db: A set of annotation maps describing the entire Gene Ontology, R package version 3.1.2
11. Chen, J.S., Su, I.J., Leu, Y.W., Young, K.C., Sun, H.S.: Expression of t-cell lymphoma invasion and metastasis 2 (tiam2) promotes proliferation and invasion of liver cancer. Int. J. Cancer **130**(6), 1302–1313 (2012)
12. Collins, F.S., Varmus, H.: A new initiative on precision medicine. N. Engl. J. Med. **372**, 793–795 (2015)
13. Csardi, G., Nepusz, T.: The igraph software package for complex network research. Int. J. Complex Syst. **1695**(5), 1–9 (2006)
14. Del Bufalo, D., Biroccio, A., Leonetti, C., Zupi, G.: Bcl-2 overexpression enhances the metastatic potential of a human breast cancer line. The FASEB J. **11**(12), 947–953 (1997)
15. Gelius-Dietrich, G.: glpkAPI: R Interface to C API of GLPK (2015). R package version 1.3.0
16. Gelius-Dietrich, G., Desouki, A.A., Fritzemeier, C.J., Lercher, M.J.: sybil-efficient constraint-based modelling in R. BMC Syst. Biol. **7**(1), 125 (2013)
17. Hansen, J., Iyengar, R.: Computation as the mechanistic bridge between precision medicine and systems therapeutics. Clin. Pharmacol. Ther. **93**(1), 117–128 (2013)
18. Hucka, M., Finney, A., Sauro, H.M., Bolouri, H., Doyle, J.C., Kitano, H., Arkin, A.P., Bornstein, B.J., Bray, D., Cornish-Bowden, A., et al.: The systems biology markup language (sbml): a medium for representation and exchange of biochemical network models. Bioinformatics **19**(4), 524–531 (2003)
19. Jerby, L., Ruppin, E.: Predicting drug targets and biomarkers of cancer via genome-scale metabolic modeling. Clin. Cancer Res. **18**(20), 5572–5584 (2012)
20. Kanehisa, M., Goto, S.: Kegg: kyoto encyclopedia of genes and genomes. Nucleic Acids Res. **28**(1), 27–30 (2000)
21. Khazaei, T., McGuigan, A., Mahadevan, R.: Ensemble modeling of cancer metabolism. Front. Physiol. **3**, 135 (2012)
22. Kitano, H.: Systems biology: a brief overview. Science **295**(5560), 1662–1664 (2002)
23. Li, X., Cowell, J.K., Sossey-Alaoui, K.: CLCA2 tumour suppressor gene in 1p31 is epigenetically regulated in breast cancer. Oncogene **23**(7), 1474–1480 (2004)
24. Li, Y., Chen, L.: Big biological data: challenges and opportunities. Genomics, Proteomics Bioinform. **12**(5), 187–189 (2014)
25. Martın H, J.A., Bourdon, J.: Solving hard computational problems efficiently: asymptotic parametric complexity 3-coloring algorithm. PloS One **8**(1), e53437 (2013)
26. Mazocchi, F.: Complexity in biology. Exceeding the limits of reductionism and determinism using complexity theory. EMBO Rep. **9**, 10–14 (2008)
27. Mazocchi, F.: Complexity and the reductionism-holism debate in systems biology. Wiley Interdiscip. Rev. Syst. Biol. Med. **4**, 413–427 (2012)
28. Miller, R., Halpern, J.: Regression with censored data. Biometrika **69**(3), 521–531 (1982)
29. Moreno, J.D., Zhu, Z.I., Yang, P.C., Bankston, J.R., Jeng, M.T., Kang, C., Wang, L., Bayer, J.D., Christini, D.J., Trayanova, N.A., et al.: A computational model to predict the effects of class i anti-arrhythmic drugs on ventricular rhythms. Sci. Transl. Med. **3**(98), 98ra83 (2011)
30. Oosting, J., Eilers, P., Menezes, R.: quantsmooth: Quantile smoothing and genomic visualization of array data. R package version 1.35.0 (2014)

31. Orchard, S., Ammari, M., Aranda, B., Breuza, L., Briganti, L., Broackes-Carter, F., Campbell, N.H., Chavali, G., Chen, C., Del-Toro, N., et al.: The mintact projectintact as a common curation platform for 11 molecular interaction databases. Nucleic Acids Res. **42**, 358–363 (2013)

32. Purcell, S., Neale, B., Todd-Brown, K., Thomas, L., Ferreira, M.A., Bender, D., Maller, J., Sklar, P., De Bakker, P.I., Daly, M.J., et al.: Plink: a tool set for whole-genome association and population-based linkage analyses. Am. J. Hum. Genet. **81**(3), 559–575 (2007)

33. Ritchie, M.D., Holzinger, E.R., Li, R., Pendergrass, S.A., Kim, D.: Methods of integrating data to uncover genotype-phenotype interactions. Nat. Rev. Genet. **16**(2), 85–97 (2015)

34. Ritchie, M.E., Phipson, B., Wu, D., Hu, Y., Law, C.W., Shi, W., Smyth, G.K.: limma powers differential expression analyses for RNA-sequencing and microarray studies. Nucleic Acids Res. **43**, e47 (2015)

35. Segrè, A.V., Groop, L., Mootha, V.K., Daly, M.J., Altshuler, D., Consortium, D., Investigators, M., et al.: Common inherited variation in mitochondrial genes is not enriched for associations with type 2 diabetes or related glycemic traits. PLoS Genet. **6**(8), e1001058 (2010)

36. Sîrbu, A., Ruskin, H.J., Crane, M.: Cross-platform microarray data normalisation for regulatory network inference. PLoS One **5**(11), e13822 (2010)

37. Stephens, Z.D., Lee, S.Y., Faghri, F., Campbell, R.H., Zhai, C., Efron, M.J., Iyer, R., Schatz, M.C., Sinha, S., Robinson, G.E.: Big data: astronomical or genomical? PLoS Biol. **13**(7), e1002195 (2015)

38. Talukder, A.K., Ravishankar, S., Sasmal, K., Gandham, S., Prabhukumar, J., Achutharao, P.H., Barh, D., Blasi, F.: Xomannotate: analysis of heterogeneous and complex exome-a step towards translational medicine. PLoS ONE **10**, e0123569 (2015)

39. Thiele, I., Swainston, N., Fleming, R.M., Hoppe, A., Sahoo, S., Aurich, M.K., Haraldsdottir, H., Mo, M.L., Rolfsson, O., Stobbe, M.D., et al.: A community-driven global reconstruction of human metabolism. Nat. Biotechnol. **31**(5), 419–425 (2013)

40. Wickham, H.: ggplot2: Elegant Graphics for Data Analysis. Springer Science & Business Media, New York (2009)

Class Aware Exemplar Discovery
from Microarray Gene Expression Data

Shivani Sharma, Abhinna Agrawal, and Dhaval Patel[✉]

Department of Computer Science and Engineering,
Indian Institute of Technology-Roorkee, Roorkee, India
{pannicle, abhinnaagrawal}@gmail.com,
patelfec@iitr.ac.in

Abstract. Given a dataset, exemplars are subset of data points that can represent a set of data points without significance loss of information. Affinity propagation is an exemplar discovery technique that, unlike k–centres clustering, gives uniform preference to all data points. The data points iteratively exchange real–valued messages, until clusters with their representative exemplar become apparent.

In this paper, we propose a Class Aware Exemplar Discovery (CAED) algorithm, which assigns preference value to data points based on their ability to differentiate samples of one class from others. To aid this, CAED performs class wise ranking of data points, assigning preference value to each data point based on its class wise rank. While exchanging messages, data points with better representative ability are more favored for being chosen as exemplar over other data points.

The proposed method is evaluated over 18 gene expression datasets to check its efficacy for selection of relevant exemplars from large datasets. Experimental evaluation exhibits improvement in classification accuracy over affinity propagation and other state-of-art feature selection techniques. Class Aware Exemplar Discovery converges in lesser iterations as compared to affinity propagation thereby dropping the execution time significantly.

Keywords: Gene · Exemplar and clustering

1 Introduction

With the advent of microarray technology, simultaneous profiling of thousands of gene expression across multiple samples in a single experiment was made possible. The microarray technology generates huge amount of gene expression data whose competitive analysis is challenging. Moreover, it has been observed that gene expression datasets has large number of uninformative and redundant features which increases complexity of classification algorithms [1, 11–13].

To circumvent these problems many feature selection techniques are being proposed. The purpose of feature selection is extracting relevant features from the observed data which improves results of machine learning models. Compared with the dimensionality reduction techniques like Principal Component Analysis (PCA) and

© Springer International Publishing Switzerland 2015
N. Kumar and V. Bhatnagar (Eds.): BDA 2015, LNCS 9498, pp. 244–257, 2015.
DOI: 10.1007/978-3-319-27057-9_17

Linear Discriminate Analysis (LDA), feature selection algorithms only select the relevant subset of features instead of altering the original features. The selected relevant genes, also known as "biomarkers", find their application in medicine for discovery of new diseases, development of new pharmaceuticals [2, 12] etc. Existing work on feature subset selection from gene expression data can be categorized as (i) classification and (ii) clustering based approaches. The classification based approaches like ReliefF [3] and Correlation based Feature Selection [4], ranks features based on their intrinsic properties and select subset of top ranked features. The clustering based approaches like k-medoids [5] and affinity propagation [6] clusters the features based on their similarity with each other. The feature set is reduced to the representative of each cluster.

Affinity propagation proposed by Frey and Dueck in [6] for feature subset selection identifies subset of features which can represent the dataset. Such features are called exemplars. Affinity propagation takes similarity between features as input. Instead of specifying the number of clusters, a real number called preference value for all features is also passed as input to affinity propagation. The number of identified exemplars is influenced by the preference value. Larger the preference value more the clusters are formed. Features exchange real- valued messages until clusters with their representative exemplars emerge. Affinity propagation has found its application in the machine learning community, computational biology and computer vision. However, aforementioned approach gives uniform preference to all features and messages are exchanged iteratively between features irrespective of the capability of features to differentiate samples of one class from samples of other classes.

In this paper, we propose a Class Aware Exemplar Discovery (CAED) algorithm which calculates class wise ranking for all features and incorporates this information while assigning preference value to features. The features are clustered by exchanging two types of messages viz. responsibility and availability iteratively. The messages are exchanged in a way that the features ranked higher in class wise ranking are favored over the feature ranked lower which leads to better exemplar discovery.

We evaluated correctness of our approach by conducting experiments on 18 publicly available microarray gene expression datasets. We recorded classification accuracy as our performance metric. Improvement in classification accuracy over affinity propagation of three classifiers namely Support Vector Machine, Naive Bayes and C4.5 Decision Tree is achieved for 16, 17 and 13 datasets respectively.

2   Overview of Our Approach

The workflow of our approach is shown in Fig. 1. Gene expression matrix is transformed into similarity matrix using a distance measure. The diagonal values of similarity matrix also called preferences are updated using class aware ranking of features. The updated matrix is used for class aware clustering. The representative from each cluster called exemplar is extracted and the reduced set of features is evaluated over classifiers.

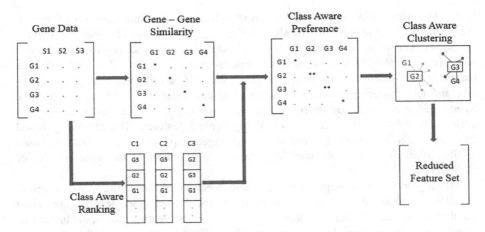

Fig. 1. Workflow of Class Aware Exemplar Discovery (CAED)

2.1   Gene Data

We selected 18 publicly available microarray datasets (available at http://faculty.iitr.ac. in/~patelfec/index.html) for experimental evaluation of Class Aware Exemplar Discovery algorithm. Microarray datasets are gene expression matrices, where expression value for each gene is measured over different samples. Generally total numbers of samples are very few compared to the features.

2.2   Gene-Gene Similarity

For a gene expression matrix $D_{n \times m}$, with n features and m samples, similarity between every two features is calculated and stored in similarity matrix $S_{n \times n}$. The similarity $s(i, k)$ indicates how well the feature with index k is suited to be the exemplar for feature i. The aim is to maximize the similarity, so we take negative of the distance between each feature. We used negative of Euclidean distance as the similarity measure for experimental evaluation.

2.3   Class Aware Preference

The affinity propagation algorithm takes similarity matrix and a real number called preference for each feature as input. For a similarity matrix $S_{n \times n}$, the value $s(i, i)$ where $i = \{1, 2, 3 \ldots, n\}$ is the preference value. These values are called preferences since the feature i with larger values $s(i, i)$ is more likely to be chosen as exemplar. The number of identified exemplars (number of clusters) is influenced by the values of input preference. Larger the value more the clusters are formed. The preference value can be uniform or non-uniform. If all features are equally suitable as exemplars, the preference value is set to a common value. The preference value can be set as any number in the range of $\min_{j s.t. j \neq i} s(i, j)$ to $\max_{j s.t. j \neq i} s(i, j) : i, j = \{1, 2, 3 \ldots, n\}$.

Samples = {S1, S2, ..., Sm}

Features = {G1, G2, ..., Gn}

Classes = {C1, C2, C3, C4, C5}

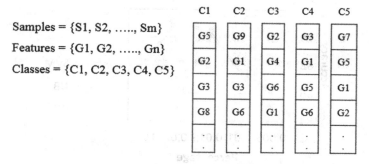

C1	C2	C3	C4	C5
G5	G9	G2	G3	G7
G2	G1	G4	G1	G5
G3	G3	G6	G5	G1
G8	G6	G1	G6	G2
.	.	.	.	.

Fig. 2. Depiction of class wise ranking of features

We propose assignment of preference value to a feature based on its ability to distinguish samples of one class from other classes. To aid this, we do class wise ranking of features using p-metric [1] by one versus all strategy. Top 0.015 % of features from each class is selected and are assigned preference value zero thereby increasing their probability of being chosen as exemplar.

Figure 2 depicts class wise ranking of features where each feature is assigned multiple ranks, one for each class. The high ranked features of each class are highlighted.

The other features are assigned uniform preference value i.e. $\underset{js.t.j\neq i}{median} s(i,j) : i.j = \{1,2,3...,n\}$. Figure 3 shows how accuracy of classifiers namely support vector machine (SVM), Naïve Bayes (NB) and C4.5 decision tree (DT) varied by changing the count of features which are assigned high value.

We observed that by selecting more than 0.015 % of features from each class no further improvement in classification accuracy of the classifiers was observed.

2.4   Class Aware Message Passing

The similarity matrix with class aware preference values is passed to affinity propagation for exemplar discovery. Affinity propagation is a message passing based clustering algorithm. Affinity propagation iteratively transmits real-valued messages among features until a good set of clusters with their representative exemplar emerge. The messages exchanged are of two kinds viz.

Responsibility message denoted as $r(i,k)$ is sent from feature i to candidate exemplar point k. It indicates the collected evidence for how appropriate feature k is to be chosen as exemplar for feature i.

Availability message denoted as $a(i,k)$ is sent from candidate exemplar point k to feature i.. It indicates the collected evidence of how appropriate it would be, for feature i to choose feature k as its exemplar.

We propose class aware message passing algorithm where strength of message exchanged between two features depends on their ability to discriminate samples among different classes.

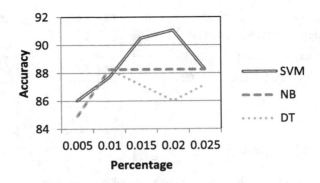

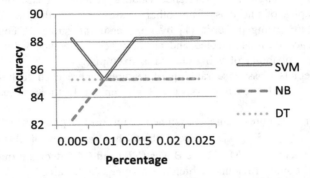

Fig. 3. Change in accuracy of classifiers by changing the percentage of high preference features on 2 datasets

Each iteration of affinity propagation has three steps:

Step 1. Calculating responsibilities r(i, k) given the availabilities
Step 2. Updating all availabilities a(i, k) given the responsibilities
Step 3. Combining the responsibilities and availabilities to generate clusters

Calculating Responsibilities $r(i,k)$ Given the Availabilities: For a dataset $D_{n \times m}$ with n features, m samples and p classes we calculate class wise rank for each feature using p–metric. Class wise rank of each feature i is denoted as $R_i = \{C_1, C_2, C_3. \ldots, C_p\}$ where $i = \{1, 2, 3..n\}$ and C_1 is rank of feature i for class 1. To calculate $r(i,k)$ we evaluate R_i and R_k. If rank of a feature i for class j is less than $\frac{n}{2}$ i.e. $C_j \leq \frac{n}{2}$, it lies in the upper half of the ranking and we denote it as H, else it lies in lower half and denoted as L. Hence, the ranking of feature i is changed to suppose $R_i = \{H, H, L, \ldots L\}$. Similarly ranking of feature k is changed to suppose $R_k = \{L, H, L \ldots, L\}$. The strength of responsibility message sent from i to k is governed by the occurrence of H in R_i and R_k.

Further calculation of responsibility $r(i, k)$ can be divided into two sections depending on the count of class labels of the dataset.

Two Class Label Dataset. For datasets with 2 classes, the class wise p-metric ranking of features is identical for both classes. The values in R_i and R_k can be of four kinds as listed below

$R_i = \{HH\} = R_k = (HH)$ – feature k should be assigned responsibility of serving as exemplar for feature i. Set $s(i, k) = \underset{vs.t.v \neq u}{max} s(u, v)$ where $u, v \in \{1, 2, 3 \dots n\}$

$R_i = (LL) R_k = (LL)$ – No change in $s(i, k)$

$R_i = (HH) R_k = (LL)$ - No change in $s(i, k)$

$R_i = (LL) R_k = (HH)$ – feature k should be assigned responsibility of serving as exemplar for feature i. Set $s(i, k) = \underset{vs.t.v \neq u}{max} s(u, v)$ where $u, v \in \{1, 2, 3 \dots n\}$.

Multi Class Label Dataset. Suppose $R_i = \{H, H, H, \dots L\}$ and $R_k = \{H, H, L, \dots L\}$ is class wise ranking for features i and k respectively. Count of occurrences of H in both sets is stored as H_i and H_k. If $H_k \geq H_i$ then, feature k should be assigned high responsibility of serving as exemplar for feature i. Set $s(i, k) = \underset{vs.t.v \neq u}{max} s(u, v)$ where $u, v \in \{1, 2, 3 \dots n\}$.

Then, the value of responsibilities is calculated using equation:

$$r(i, k) \leftarrow s(i, k) - \underset{k's.t.k' \neq k}{max}\{a(i, k') + s(i, k')\}$$

Setting $s(i, k)$ as maximum of all the similarities increases the strength of responsibility message sent from feature i to candidate exemplar point k.

Initially availabilities are set to zero. For the first iteration $r(i, k)$ is similarity between feature i and k as its exemplar, reduced by the maximum similarity between i and other features. Later, when features highly similar to i are assigned to some other exemplar, their availabilities as a candidate exemplar for i falls below zero. Such negative value will affect the similarity value $s(i, k')$ in the above equation.

Updating all availabilities $a(i, k)$ given the responsibilities. Availabilities are Calculated as:

$$a(i, k) \leftarrow min\{0, r(k, k) + \sum_{i's.t.i' \notin \{i,k\}} max\{0, r(i', k)\}\}$$

The value of availability can be zero or negative. Zero value indicates that k is available and k can be assigned as exemplar to i. If the value of $a(i, k)$ is negative, it indicates that k belongs to some other exemplar and it is not available to become exemplar for i.

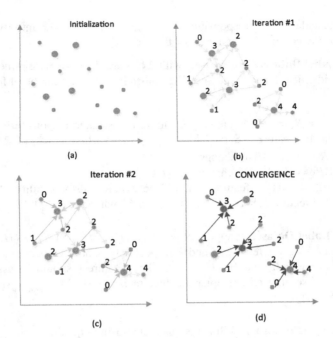

Fig. 4. (a) Two –dimensional features, sized according to their class aware preference value. (b) and (c) Messages are exchanged between features. The number associated with each feature corresponds to its count of occurrence in upper half of class wise ranking. The darkness of arrow directed from point i to point k corresponds to the strength of message that point i belongs to exemplar point k. (d) Clusters formed with their representative exemplar.

Combining the Responsibilities and Availabilities to Generate Clusters. For every iteration, the point j that maximizes $r(i,j) + a(i,j)$ is regarded as exemplar for point i. The algorithm terminate when changes in the message falls previously set threshold. Final result is list of all the exemplars which is an optimal subset of features. Figure 4 shows dynamics of Class Aware Exemplar Discovery algorithm when applied on 15 two-dimensional features with 4 class labels. Initially, features are sized according to their class aware preference. Each feature is numbered according to the count of classes in which it is high ranked. Class aware messages are exchanged between features. When convergence condition is satisfied, features are clustered with each cluster represented by red colored exemplar.

Algorithm 1 presents the steps followed by Class Aware Exemplar Discovery to select optimal set of features. The input to the algorithm is gene expression matrix with n specifying number of genes, m specifying number of samples and c classes. Three matrices namely responsibility, availability and similarity are initialized with zero. First we calculate negative of Euclidean distance between every pair of feature and store it in similarity matrix (Line 1). Next, we calculate class wise rank of all features (Line 2). We use N_c to denote ranked list of genes that is obtained for class c (Lines 3–11).

Class Aware Preference (Line 4) - We select top 0.015 % of features from N_c and assign them high preference value which is zero. To rest of the features median of similarities is assigned as preference value.

ALGORITHM 1. Class Aware Exemplar Discovery

Input: Gene Expression Matrix D_{nxm}
   C = set of class labels $\{c_1, c_2, c_3, \dots c_p\}$
   n = Number of genes
   m = Number of samples
Initialize: Similarity matrix $s[n][n]$
   Responsibility matrix $r[n][n]$
   Availability matrix $a[n][n]$
Output: ESet = List of exemplars

```
1.    Calculate S_nxm using D_nxm
2.    Let N_c, be ranked list of genes from D_nxm w.r.t
      class label c ∈ C;
3.    for each N_c
4.        Select 0.015% of top ranked genes; store in
          N_c';
5.    end for
6.    for each gene i ∈ N_c'
7.        set s(i, i) ←0;
8.    end for
9.    for each gene i ∉ N_c'
10.       set s(i, i) ← median       s(i, j);
                       js.t.j≠i
11.   end for
12.   for all i, j ∈ {1,2,3 …, n}
13.       set a[i][j] = 0;
14.   end for
15.   while the convergence conditions are not satisfied
16.       for each i, k
17.           Obtain class wise rank R_i and R_k of gene i
              and   kfor   p   classes   represented   as
              {C_1, C_2, C_3 ……, C_p};
18.           for each class wise rank C_j
19.               if C_j ≤ n/2
20.                   Set C_j = H;
21.                   else C_j = L;
22.               end if
23.               Let H_i and H_k be count of H in R_i and
                  R_k respectively;
24.               if c == 2 and R_k == HH
25.                   Set s(i, k) ←    max    s(u, v)
                                    vs.t.v≠u
                  where u, v ∈ {1,2,3 …, n};
26.               Else If c > 2 and H_k ≥ H_i
27.                   then,   Set   s(i, k) ←    max    s(u, v)   where
                                                 vs.t.v≠u
                  u, v ∈ {1,2,3 …, n};
28.           end for
29.           find   the   k' ≠ k   that   maximizes   a[i][k']
              +s[i][k']
30.               r(i, k) ← s(i, k) -  {a(i, k') + s(i, k')}.
31.           sum = 0;
32.           for each i' ∉ {i, k}
33.               if r[i'][k] > 0
34.                   do sum ← sum + r[i'][k];
35.               end if
36.           end for
37.           if i == k
38.               then a[i][k] ← sum;
39.               else if r[k][k] + sum < 0
40.                   then a[k][k] ← r[k][k] + sum;
41.                   else a[i][k] ← 0
42.               end if
43.       end for
44.       for each i
45.           Find the k that maximizes a[i][k] + r[i][k];
46.           Set k as the exemplar of i;
47.           Put point k in Eset;
48.       end for
49.   end while
50.   return Eset
```

Class Aware Message Passing (Lines 15–43). Then features are clustered by passing real valued class aware messages. The algorithm terminates when change in messages falls below previously set threshold. Exemplars are returned and can be used to accurately predict the class label of unlabeled samples.

3   Experimental Evaluation

We performed three set of experiments to evaluate the performance of our approach. In the first experiment we compared the performance of three different classifiers using features selected by CAED against the features selected by affinity propagation. In second experiment, we compared performance of CAED with CFS [4] for feature selection with greedy search strategy. WEKA [7] provided us with implementations of CFS. The third experiment compared the performance of classifiers using all the features versus features extracted by CAED. Details of all the three experiments are discussed in subsequent chapters. The experiments were carried out on 3.4 GHz Intel i7 CPU with 8 GB RAM machine running Windows-based operating system.

3.1   Description of Experimental Datasets

We performed experimental evaluation of Class Aware Exemplar Discovery over 18 publicly available microarray gene expression datasets [8–11]. Table 1 describes the

Table 1. Description of datasets

S.no.	Data set name	Attributes	Samples	Classes
1	chowdary-2006_database1	183	104	2
2	alizadeh-2000-v1	1096	42	2
3	nutt-2003-v3_database1	1153	22	2
4	pomeroy-2002-v1_database1	858	34	2
5	nutt-2003-v2_database1	1071	28	2
6	west-2001_database1	1199	49	2
7	meduloblastomiGSE468	1466	23	2
8	chen-2002	86	179	2
9	breast_A	1214	98	3
10	DLBCL_B	662	180	3
11	golub-1999-v2_database1	1869	72	3
12	liang-2005	1412	37	3
13	dyrskjot-2003_database1	1204	40	3
14	DLBCL_A	662	141	3
15	bredel-2005	1740	50	3
16	risinger-2003	1772	42	4
17	tomlins-2006-v2	1289	92	4
18	Breast_B	1214	49	4

datasets used for experimental study. The datasets used for experimental evaluation are picked from various cancer related research work.

3.2 Comparison of Class Aware Exemplar Discovery with Affinity Propagation

We evaluated the classification accuracy of three state-of- art classifiers namely support vector machine (SVM), Naïve Bayes (NB) and C4.5 decision tree (DT) using the exemplars generated by Affinity Propagation (AP) and the exemplars generated by Class Aware Exemplar Discovery. The classification accuracy is calculated using 10 fold cross validation approach.

To visualize the results we performed "Win-Loss Experiment". If the classification accuracy of CAED is better than baseline approach the result is declared as win, if the classification accuracy has degraded the result is declared as loss otherwise declared as draw. Figure 5 shows results of "Win-Loss Experiment", obtained when classification accuracy of three classifiers using exemplars generated by affinity propagation is compared against Class Aware Exemplar Discovery.

We observed that Class Aware exemplar discovery generates less exemplar in comparison to Affinity propagation. Figure 6 shows drop in count of clusters (i.e., number of examples) from affinity propagation to CAED.

We also observed that Class Aware Exemplar Discovery converges in lesser message passing iteration in comparison to affinity propagation. This reduces the execution time tremendously. Figure 7 shows drop in execution time, Y axis is measured in seconds.

3.3 Comparison of Class Aware Exemplar Discovery with Standard Feature Subset Selection Techniques

We compare the effectiveness of CAED with features generated using CFS (Correlation based Feature Selection). The maximum achievable 10 fold cross validation classification accuracy is recorded as performance metric. Figure 8 shows results of "Win-Loss Experiment", obtained when classification accuracy of three classifiers using feature subset generated by CFS is compared against exemplars generated by Class Aware Exemplar Discovery.

3.4 Comparison of Class Aware Exemplar Discovery with All Features

We evaluated the performance of three classifiers support vector machine (SVM), Naïve Bayes (NB) and C4.5 decision tree (DT) using all features of the 18 datasets. We compared these results with the classification accuracy obtained using features produced by Class Aware Exemplar Discovery.

Figure 9 shows results of "Win-Loss Experiment" obtained when classification accuracy of three classifiers using all features is compared against Class Aware Exemplar Discovery.

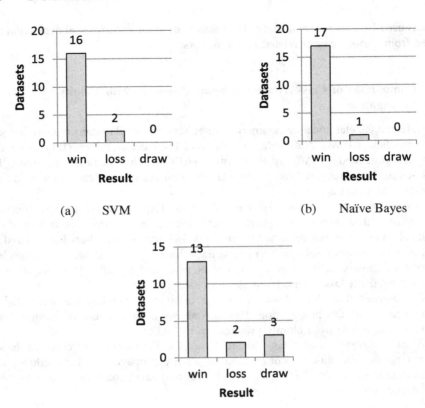

(a)   SVM

(b)   Naïve Bayes

(c) Decision Tree

Fig. 5. Win – loss depiction of CAED versus affinity propagation carried over classifiers (a) support vector machine (b) Naïve Bayes (c) C4.5 decision tree

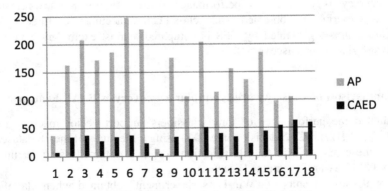

Fig. 6. Drop in count of clusters in 18 dataset

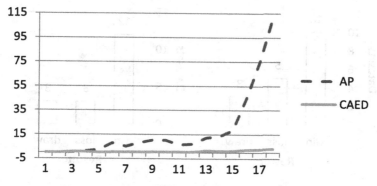

Fig. 7. Drop in execution time

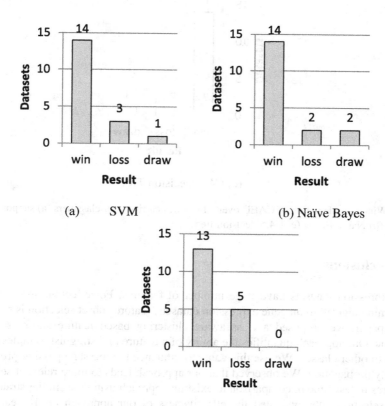

(a)   SVM

(b) Naïve Bayes

(c) C4.5 Decision Tree

Fig. 8. Win – loss depiction of CAED over CFS carried over classifiers (a) support vector machine (b) Naïve Bayes (c) C4.5 decision tree

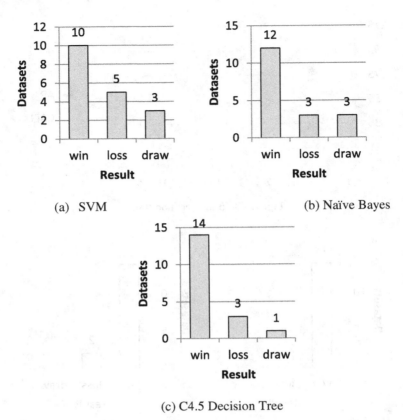

(a) SVM

(b) Naïve Bayes

(c) C4.5 Decision Tree

Fig. 9. Win- Loss depiction of CAED over all features carried over classifiers (a) support vector machine (b) Naïve Bayes (c) C4.5 decision tree

4 Conclusions

Gene expression datasets have large number of features. For effective application of any learning algorithm on gene expression datasets, feature subset selection is required. In this paper, we proposed a class aware clustering based feature subset selection technique. Our approach quantifies the ability of a feature to distinguish samples of one class from other classes. We use this value to influence the message passing procedure of affinity propagation. We observed that our approach leads to more relevant selection of features in less time in comparison to existing approach using the similar strategy for feature selection. We evaluated the effectiveness of our approach on 18 real world cancer datasets.

We evaluated Class Aware Exemplar Discovery against affinity propagation. Experiments have shown have shown that our technique outruns Affinity propagation in terms of classification accuracy. In comparison to affinity propagation, CAED converges in less number of iteration leading to huge drop in execution time.

We also evaluated the feature set generated by CAED against state-of-art feature selection technique. Experimental results have shown CAED gives better classification accuracy for all the classifiers used. Motivated by recent growth in parallel computing [13] and NVIDIA CUDA Research Center Support, we are developing a GPU based parallel algorithm for CAED. We are also working on improving the readability of mathematical symbol in the printed version of the submitted paper.

References

1. Inza, I., Larrañaga, P., Blanco, R., Cerrolaza, A.J.: Filter versus wrapper gene selection approaches in DNA microarray domains. Artif. Intell. Med. **31**(2), 91–103 (2004)
2. De Abreu, F.B., Wells, W.A., Tsongalis, G.J.: The emerging role of the molecular diagnostics laboratory in breast cancer personalized medicine. Am. J. Pathol. **183**(4), 1075–1083 (2013)
3. Kononenko, I., Šimec, E., Robnik-Šikonja, M.: Overcoming the myopia of inductive learning algorithms with RELIEFF. Appl. Intell. **7**(1), 39–55 (1997)
4. Hall, M.A.: Correlation-based feature selection for machine learning. Doctoral dissertation, The University of Waikato (1999)
5. Kashef, R., Kamel, M.S.: Efficient bisecting *k*-medoids and its application in gene expression analysis. In: Campilho, A., Kamel, M. (eds.) ICIAR 2008. LNCS, vol. 5112, pp. 423–434. Springer, Heidelberg (2008)
6. Frey, B.J., Dueck, D.: Clustering by passing messages between data points. Science **315** (5814), 972–976 (2007)
7. Hall, M., Frank, E., Holmes, G., Pfahringer, B., Reutemann, P., Witten, I.H.: The WEKA data mining software: an update. ACM SIGKDD Explor. Newsl. **11**(1), 10–18 (2009)
8. De Souto, M.C., Costa, I.G., de Araujo, D.S., Ludermir, T.B., Schliep, A.: Clustering cancer gene expression data: a comparative study. BMC Bioinf. **9**(1), 497 (2008)
9. Foithong, S., Pinngern, O., Attachoo, B.: Feature subset selection wrapper based on mutual information and rough sets. Expert Syst. Appl. **39**(1), 574–584 (2012)
10. Mramor, M., Leban, G., Demšar, J., Zupan, B.: Visualization-based cancer microarray data classification analysis. Bioinformatics **23**(16), 2147–2154 (2007)
11. Blum, A., Langley, P.: Selection of relevant features and examples in machine learning. Artif. Intell. **97**(1/2), 245–271 (1997)
12. Chandrashekar, G., Sahin, F.: A survey on feature selection methods. Comput. Electr. Eng. **40**, 16–28 (2014)
13. Soufan, O., Kleftogiannis, D., Kalnis, P., Kalnis, B.: Bajic DWFS: a wrapper feature selection tool based on a parallel genetic algorithm. PLoS ONE **10**, e0117988 (2015). doi:10.1371/journal.pone.0117988

Multistage Classification for Cardiovascular Disease Risk Prediction

Durga Toshniwal, Bharat Goel[✉], and Hina Sharma

Department of Computer Science and Engineering,
Indian Institute of Technology, Roorkee, Roorkee, Uttarakhand, India
{durgatoshniwal,bharat.goel10,hs250193}@gmail.com

Abstract. Cardiovascular diseases are the prominent causes of death each year. Data mining is an emerging area which has numerous applications specifically in healthcare. Our work suggests a system for predicting the risk of a cardiovascular disease using data mining techniques and is based on the ECG tests. It further recommends nearby relevant hospitals based on the prediction. We propose a multistage classification algorithm in which the first stage is used to classify normal and abnormal ECG beats and the next stage is used to refine the prediction done by the first stage by reducing the number of false negatives. In this work experiments have been conducted on the MIT-BIH Arrhythmia dataset which is a benchmark dataset. The results of the experiments show that the proposed technique is very promising.

Keywords: ECG · Classification · MIT-BIH · Random Forest

1 Introduction

Cardiovascular diseases are the number one cause of deaths globally, as claimed by WHO [1]. Early detection of unusual heart activity can avoid sudden cardiac death. To detect the abnormality of the heart activity, a continuous ECG signal monitoring is required. The Electrocardiogram (ECG or EKG) signals are the bioelectric signals that indicate the electrical activity of the heart that are recorded by placing electrodes on patient's body. During the various cardiovascular diseases, such as myocardial infarction, arrhythmia, myocarditis, bundle branch block etc., there is a deviation in the electrical activity of the cardiovascular system and hence in the ECG signals. ECG has various features some of which get distorted from the normal features and similar cardiovascular disease have a similar change in the ECG features [2, 3]. If an unknown ECG has features similar to that of an ECG signal with arrhythmia, it could be deduced that this unknown signal has the similar arrhythmia. Thus, using the ECG signal, it is easy to predict the disease of the patient. In real life, ECG recordings are often corrupted by noise.

2 Related Work

Various works [4–10] have been done for arrhythmia classification using different statistical method, machine learning models, neural networks and reasonable accuracies have been achieved.

© Springer International Publishing Switzerland 2015
N. Kumar and V. Bhatnagar (Eds.): BDA 2015, LNCS 9498, pp. 258–266, 2015.
DOI: 10.1007/978-3-319-27057-9_18

Various statistical methods have been used such as in [4] a time-frequency spectral method was developed to process atrial activities which produced an accuracy of 88 % using a Bayesian based method to analyze ECG signals.

Artificial neural networks also has been used for this purpose like a multi-layer perceptron (MLP) model with back-propagation was used to classify ECG arrhythmias [5] which produced an accuracy of 99 %. A novel ECG arrhythmia classification model with a modular mixture of experts and negatively correlated learning neural network was proposed [6] and produced an accuracy of 96.02 % using MIT-BIH repository. A probabilistic ANN classifier was used to discriminate eight types of arrhythmia from ECG beats using MIT-BIH data sets [7] with accuracy rates of 99.71 %.

Data samples from machine resistance and patients' heart rates were first collected from participants performing exercise on a cyclo-ergometer [8]. A non-linear autoregressive exogenous (NARX) neural network was used to obtain the optimal training configuration [8].

Some works have used other techniques for example, based on ECGs from patients with heart failures, Chi-square based decision trees were produced to differentiate patients with varying levels of risk [9]. A classification tree based on condition combination competition was proposed for ischemia detection of spatiotemporal ECGs, and an accuracy rate of 98 % was achieved [10]. An ensemble classifier based on extremely randomized decision trees was used for classification of ECG signals in [11].

Support vector machines have been used in [9, 12–15]. Data sets from MIT-BIH and BIDMC Congestive Heart Failure Database (CHFD) were widely used with different support vector machine (SVM) models, as reviewed in this section. The SVM model was used for ECG arrhythmia analysis in [12]. Feature extraction was accomplished using six different methods for comparison purposes. Using the MIT-BIH data sets, the highest accuracy rate achieved was 92.2 %. To enhance the accuracy rate of ECG signals classification, a statistical method for segmenting heartbeats from ECG signals was used [13]. Based on the MIT-BIH data sets the highest accuracy rate acquired by the SVM classifier was 99.45 %.

A wavelet filter was used for feature extraction. Based on the MIT-BIH data sets, the highest recorded accuracy rate was 96.19 % [14]. ECG beats were classified using the SVM model in [9]. The QRS complexes were segmented after pre-processing the ECG signals obtained from the MIT-BIH repository. Accuracy rates from 97.2 % to 98.8 % were reported [9]. Based on the MIT-BIH data sets, a combination of thirteen metrics was tested, and the best combination was selected for further evaluation [15]. The SVM model was used for classifying the data samples, which led to an accuracy rate of 99.34 % [15].

Although different types of classifiers have been employed for prediction of arrhythmia very few focus on time efficiency for classification. Also very few focus on reducing the false negatives during the classification stage. But the possibility of using ensemble methods has not been used. Further the existing method do not focus on time efficiency of the classification but in the real world, time efficiency may be of importance when we are treating patients therefore there is a need to improve the time efficiency of the classifier model.

3 Proposed Work

The aim of the proposed work is to predict cardiovascular disease risk based on ensemble methods while reducing the false positives. Further it also provides a prototype for the recommendation for the nearest hospital based on the prediction. Figure 1 summarizes the flow of the proposed work, the shaded blocks indicate the work on which research was focused.

In the present work a Multi-stage classifier has been used for prediction of cardiovascular disease. The first stage aims to segregate the normal vs. abnormal records. Further in the second stage the aim is to improve the accuracy by reducing the false negatives. Here the false negatives are more in focus because that is of more importance clinically because a diseased patient should not be classified as normal. However reasonable rate of false positives is still acceptable in medical domain.

As per the proposed framework in Fig. 1 first of all signals were pre-processed using Butterworth filter to remove noise. Then the features were extracted from the annotated database using R-peak locations. Since this gave a large feature set, these features are reduced using wavelet transform with Daubechies of order 8. After this Fast ICA algorithm was used to computationally disintegrate the multivariate signal into additive subcomponents. These features were then collectively reduced using PCA (Principal Component Analysis). Finally 4 more features were then appended to the feature set [12]. Further correlation feature selection was employed to select relevant features. For the classification various classifiers were used such as SVM, Naïve Bayes, AdaBoost1, Random Forest, etc., from which Random Forest gave the best accuracy with 120 trees and hence we used Random Forest with 120 trees for our classification.

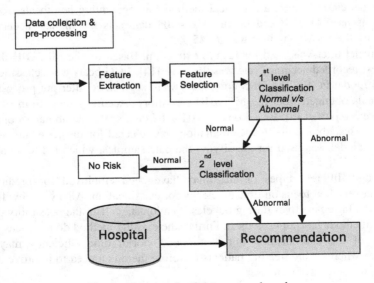

Fig. 1. Framework of the proposed work

Further work is going on for recommendation. After classification all the diseased patients can be recommended their nearby hospitals using the hospital database.

3.1   Data Set

We have used MIT-BIH Arrhythmia Dataset [16] for the experiments that contain half hour two lead ambulatory ECG recordings from 47 real patients. The recordings are digitized at 360 samples per second per channel (2 channels). Each record is annotated by cardiologists. According to AAMI (Association for the Advancement of Medical Instrumentation) recommendations, only 44 recordings from the MIT-BIH Arrhythmia Dataset should be used for evaluation of cardiac arrhythmia signal classification methods, excluding the four recordings that contain paced beats (records 102, 104, 107, and 217).

Table 1 shows the summary of the number of instances in each class. DS1 refers to the dataset 1 and DS2 is the smaller dataset (dataset 2) obtained by random sampling from DS1.

Table 1. Summary of the datasets DS1 and DS2

Heart beat type	Annotation	DS1 instances	DS2 instances
Normal	N	38083	19054
Left bundle branch block	L	3948	2003
Right bundle branch block	R	3781	1829
Nodal escape beat	j	16	10
Premature ventricular contraction	V	3683	1837
Ventricular escape beat	E	105	55
Nodal premature beat	J	32	14
Atrial escape beat	e	16	5
Supraventricular premature beat	S	2	1
Atrial premature beat	A	809	433
Fusion of ventricular and normal beat	F	415	203
Aberrated atrial premature beat	a	100	49
Total		50990	25494

4   Experiments and Results

4.1   Pre-processing

The raw ECG signals were first preprocessed to remove the noise using Butterworth filter to reduce the signal to noise ratio (Fig. 2).

The baseline wandering is also removed by subtracting the mean of the signal. The preprocessed signal was used for the subsequent processing. MATLAB was used for signal preprocessing and feature extraction.

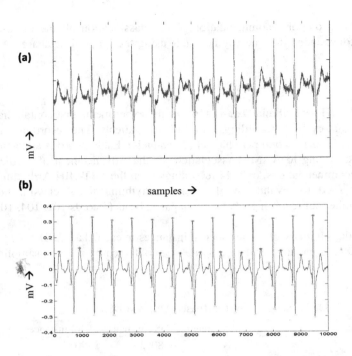

Fig. 2. (a) Original signal (b) signal after noise and baseline wandering removal with fiducial points

4.2 Feature Extraction

One beat in the ECG signal consists of P wave, QRS complex and a T wave as shown in Fig. 3.

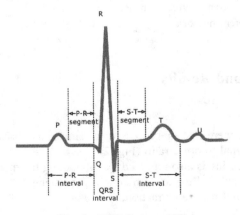

Fig. 3. ECG features [17]

The R-peaks locations annotated from the database were used to segment the heartbeats. The records have a sampling rate of 360 Hz thus, each heartbeat segment contains 100 samples before the R-peak that will include the P and Q waves, and 200 samples after the R-peak that will include the S and T waves. This method eliminates the error involved in marking fiducial points and also it takes into account, the shapes of the waveforms. The limitation of this method is that when heart beats faster than normal, heartbeat segments of 300 samples can contain information from neighboring heartbeats.

Biomedical signals usually exhibit characteristics that change over time or position. Wavelet Transform extracts information in both temporal and frequency domains. Therefore, in this paper, we have used WT with Daubechies of order 8 as the mother wavelet. The feature set includes the detail coefficients of level 3(D3) and level 4(D4) and approximation coefficients of level 4 (A4).

Apart from WT, we have also used the Independent Component Analysis of signals using the Fast ICA algorithm. 14 ICAs were derived for each heartbeat that yielded the best results among the varying values from 10 to 30. One hundred and fourteen wavelet features and 18 ICA features were concatenated and then reduced using PCA to obtain 52 features. Besides the above structural features, 4 RR interval features such as previous RR, post RR, local RR and average RR are also used [12]. Previous RR is the interval between previous and current R peaks. Similarly, post RR is the distance between current and following R peaks. Local RR interval is computed by calculating the mean of all RR intervals in a window of 10 s. Average RR interval is obtained as the average of RR intervals in the past 5 min. All the features together are again reduced using supervised correlation feature selection.

4.3   Classification

In this particular work a two stage classifier has been used. There are various classifiers we tried multiple of them, some of those which gave the best results have been listed out here in Table 2 such as AdaBoost1, Naïve Bayes, SVM, and Random Forest. Out of all these Random Forest gave the highest accuracy. Therefore we choose to use Random Forest for further classification in all stages. In case of Random Forest different numbers of trees were iterated upon and the best results were obtained with 120 trees. However the results of that have not been included in due to space constraints.

Classification is done using features from one lead at a time. Our experiments concluded that the only one lead (MLII) is enough to predict, as it gives higher accuracy than V5 lead. This can be useful for a user as he needs to store only one lead

Table 2. Comparison of different classifiers.

Classifiers	Accuracy
Random Forest (120 trees)	98.49 %
AdaBoost1	98.42 %
SVM	98.41 %
Naïve Bayes	88.44 %

data to predict the disease. The first stage classifies the ECG signal into one of the 12 classes. A second stage is introduced to further classify the normal subclass in order to reduce the false negatives improving the abnormal class accuracies and hence the overall accuracy.

The relevant features from Normal subclass are selected again using correlation feature selection for the second stage classification performed to reduce the false negatives.

Figures 4 and 5 show the confusion matrix of the classification for the 1st and 2nd stages respectively.

Table 3 shows the result of improvement in the accuracy as a result of the introduction of 2nd stage.

Predicted Class →

s	e	J	E	f	j	F	a	V	A	R	L	N	
0	0	0	0	0	0	0	0	0	0	0	0	2	S
0	0	0	0	0	0	0	0	0	1	0	0	15	e
0	0	6	0	0	0	0	0	0	0	18	0	8	J
0	0	0	98	0	0	0	0	0	0	0	0	7	E
0	0	0	0	0	0	0	0	0	0	0	0	0	f
0	0	0	0	0	2	0	0	0	0	4	0	10	j
0	0	0	0	0	0	288	0	33	0	0	0	94	F
0	0	0	0	0	0	0	60	10	0	0	0	29	a
0	0	0	0	0	9	0	0	3543	0	1	7	123	V
0	0	0	0	0	0	4	0	4	591	4	1	205	A
0	0	0	0	0	0	0	6	0	0	3731	0	44	R
0	0	0	0	0	0	0	15	0	0	0	3899	36	L
0	0	0	0	0	0	0	0	47	15	0	3	38018	N

Fig. 4. Confusion matrix for 1st stage

Predicted Class →

S	e	J	E	f	j	F	a	V	A	R	L	N	
0	0	0	0	0	0	0	0	0	0	0	0	2	S
0	5	0	0	0	0	0	0	0	0	0	0	10	e
0	0	2	0	0	0	0	0	0	0	0	0	6	J
0	0	0	0	0	0	0	0	0	0	0	0	7	E
0	0	0	0	0	0	0	0	0	0	0	0	0	f
0	0	0	0	0	2	0	0	0	0	1	0	7	j
0	0	0	0	0	0	19	0	0	0	0	0	75	F
0	0	0	0	0	0	0	3	0	0	0	0	26	a
0	0	0	0	0	0	0	0	1	0	0	0	122	V
0	0	0	0	0	0	0	0	0	6	0	0	199	A
0	0	0	0	0	0	0	0	0	0	0	0	44	R
0	0	0	0	0	0	0	0	0	0	0	0	36	L
0	0	0	0	0	0	0	0	0	0	1	0	38017	N

Fig. 5. Confusion matrix for 2nd Stage

Table 3. Comparison of accuracies

Super class	Accuracy after 1st stage	Accuracy after 2nd stage
Normal	99.82 %	99.82 %
Abnormal	94.55 %	94.85 %
Overall	98.49 %	98.57 %

Experiments suggest that a third stage or any more stages does not further improve the classification accuracy because after the second stage the number of misclassified records are very few therefore there is no substantial gain in accuracy by increasing the number of levels.

The work can be summarized as follows- we assume that the user has the MLII lead ECG data, the system detects the R peaks and predict the disease of the user where Abnormality and Normality of the ECG is more important than the individual classification of the signal. The system then recommends nearby hospitals if the user has a risk of any cardiovascular disease.

5 Conclusion

Cardiovascular diseases are risk to life therefore it is very important to be able to predict them at an early stage. There have been different methods that have been proposed in this regard. However most of the existing methods make use of single stage classification. The aim of the present work is to use a multistage classification for the purpose of improving accuracy and reducing the false negatives. For the experiment MIT-BIH Arrhythmia Dataset which is a real life and benchmark dataset has been used. The performances of different kinds of classifiers have been studied and it was concluded that Random Forest (ensemble method) gave the best result. Thus for our work we choose Random Forest with 120 trees. Firstly we pre-processed the signals using Butterworth filter and then features were extracted using R-peaks of the annotated dataset. Then various techniques were applied to reduce the feature set such as wavelet transform with Daubechies, Fast ICA algorithm, PCA and others. After the feature selection classification was done for first level. Further the Normal class results of first level classification were again classified into normal and abnormal in the second level. Since the work is related to medical domain the very minute improvement in accuracy is of great importance. The accuracy attained by the proposed work is 98.57 % which is better than most of the existing accuracies.

We can explore the possibility of using it in real time and the database for recommendation system for hospitals can be enlarged and some application can be developed that integrates this prediction along with recommendation.

Acknowledgement. We are thankful to Dr. Ajay Bhargava (a cardiologist) for his guidance regarding the ECG features for disease prediction.

References

1. World Health Organisation. http://www.who.int/mediacentre/factsheets/fs317/en/
2. Qian, B., Wang, X., Cao, N., Li, H., Jian, Y.: A relative similarity based method for interactive patient risk prediction. Data Min. Knowl. Disc. **29**(4), 1070–1093 (2015). Online first: (2014)
3. Vafaie, M.H., Ataei, M., Koofigar, H.R.: Heart diseases prediction based on ECG signals' classification using a genetic-fuzzy system and dynamical model of ECG signals. Biomed. Signal Process. Control **14**, 291–296 (2014)
4. Lee, J., McManus, D.D., Bourrell, P., Sörnmo, L., Chon, K.H.: Atrial flutter and atrial tachycardia detection using Bayesian approach with high resolution time–frequency spectrum from ECG recordings. Biomed. Signal Process. Control **8**, 992–999 (2013)
5. Özbay, Y., Ceylan, R., Karlik, B.: Integration of type-2 fuzzy clustering and wavelet transform in a neural network based ECG classifier. Expert Syst. Appl. **38**(1), 1004–1010 (2011)
6. Javadi, M., et al.: Classification of ECG arrhythmia by a modular neural network based on mixture of experts and negatively correlated learning. Biomed. Signal Process. Control **8**(3), 289–296 (2013)
7. Wang, J.S., Chiang, W.C., Hsu, Y.L., Yang, Y.T.C.: ECG arrhythmia classification using a probabilistic neural network with a feature reduction method. Neurocomputing **116**, 38–45 (2013)
8. Irigoyen, E., Miñano, G.: A NARX neural network model for enhancing cardiovascular rehabilitation therapies. Neurocomputing **109**, 9–15 (2013)
9. Zidelmal, Z., Amirou, A., Ould-Abdeslam, D., Merckle, J.: ECG beat classification using a cost sensitive classifier. Comput. Methods Programs Biomed. **111**(3), 570–577 (2013)
10. Fayn, J.: A classification tree approach for cardiac ischemia detection using spatiotemporal information from three standard ECG leads. IEEE Trans. Biomed. Eng. **58**(1), 95–102 (2011)
11. Scalzo, F., Hamilton, R., Asgari, S., Kim, S., Hu, X.: Intracranial hypertension prediction using extremely randomized decision trees. Med. Eng. Phys. **34**(8), 1058–1065 (2012)
12. Luz, E.J.D.S., Nunes, T.M., De Albuquerque, V.H.C., Papa, J.P., Menotti, D.: ECG arrhythmia classification based on optimum-path forest. Expert Syst. Appl. **40**(9), 3561–3573 (2013)
13. Wu, Y., Zhang, L.: ECG classification using ICA features and support vector machines. In: Lu, B.-L., Zhang, L., Kwok, J. (eds.) ICONIP 2011, Part I. LNCS, vol. 7062, pp. 146–154. Springer, Heidelberg (2011)
14. Daamouche, A., Hamami, L., Alajlan, N., Melgani, F.: A wavelet optimization approach for ECG signal classification. Biomed. Signal Process. Control **7**, 342–349 (2012)
15. Li, Q., Rajagopalan, C., Clifford, G.D.: A machine learning approach to multi-level ECG signal quality classification. Comput. Methods Programs Biomed. **117**(3), 435–447 (2014)
16. Goldberger, A.L., Amaral, L.A.N., Glass, L., Hausdorff, J.M., Ivanov, P.C., Mark, R.G., Mietus, J.E., Moody, G.B., Pang, C.-K., Stanley, H.E.: PhysioBank, physiotoolkit, and physionet: components of a new research resource for complex physiologic signals. Circulation **101**(23), e215–e220 (2000). (Circulation Electronic Pages; http://circ.ahajournals.org/cgi/content/full/101/23/e215)
17. Pantech Solutions. https://www.pantechsolutions.net/blog/what-is-biosignal/ecg-signal/

Author Index

Printed in the United States
By Bookmasters